Liver Metastases

Jean-Nicolas Vauthey · Paulo M. G. Hoff ·
Riccardo A. Audisio · Graeme J. Poston
Editors

Liver Metastases

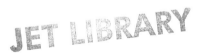

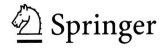 Springer

Editors

Jean-Nicolas Vauthey, MD, FACS
Department of Surgical Oncology
The University of Texas M.D. Anderson
 Cancer Center
Houston, TX, USA

Paulo M. G. Hoff, MD, FACP
Centro de Oncologia
Hospital Sirio Libanes
Sao Paulo, Brazil

Riccardo A. Audisio, MD, FRCS
Department of General Surgery
Whiston Hospital
University of Liverpool
Prescot, Merseyside, UK

Graeme J. Poston, MB MS FRCS
Digestive Diseases, Critical Care and Anaesthesia
Centre for Digestive Diseases
University Hospital Aintree
Liverpool, UK

ISBN 978-1-84628-946-0   e-ISBN 978-1-84628-947-7
DOI 10.1007/978-1-84628-947-7

British Library Cataloguing in Publication Data
A catalogue record for this book is available from the British Library

Library of Congress Control Number: 2008936486

Printed on acid-free paper

Springer Science+Business Media
springer.com

Preface

The concept for *Liver Metastases* arose from the need for an authoritative treaty in this important subject. Contrasting with the usual paradigm, in which the treatment of liver metastases is just a chapter in a broader surgical or medical oncology textbook, our work extensively addresses the contemporary multidisciplinary management of liver metastases. Throughout the text, experiences from the paradigms of colorectal cancer metastases treatment strategies are used to point to the new directions in the management of liver metastases. The goal is to present the information in a logical and informative way, including the natural history, diagnosis, staging, prognosis, and treatment of liver metastases, with emphasis in the collaborative, multidisciplinary approach.

The treatment of liver metastases is one of the most exciting areas in medicine in the early twenty-first century thanks to the diligent work of innovative investigators. Over the last few decades, the imaging techniques have been refined, surgical indications and techniques have been perfected, and a large number of effective systemic treatments have been developed. Patients who were deemed incurable just a few years ago can now be offered the hope for a normal life. One of the prime examples is in the treatment of colorectal cancer metastatic to the liver, where institutions are now reporting 5-year survival rates approaching 60% in resectable disease.

We have gathered contributions from some of the most important investigators in the field, and believe that we have achieved our goal. Our aim is to produce a textbook that is easy to read and that can be used as a reference by all healthcare providers involved in the treatment of patients with liver metastases. We hope you agree with us.

Texas, USA — Jean-Nicolas Vauthey
Sao Paulo, Brazil — Paulo M. G. Hoff
Prescot, UK — Riccardo A. Audisio
Liverpool, UK — Graeme J. Poston

Contents

1 Radiological Imaging of Liver Metastases 1
   Carlos Valls, Laura Martínez, Sandra Ruiz, and Esther Alba

2 Biology of Colorectal Cancer Liver Metastases 15
   Curtis J. Wray, Ami N. Shah, Russell S. Berman, and Syed A. Ahmad

3 Surgery for Colorectal Metastases 25
   Dario Ribero, Yun Shin Chun, and Jean-Nicolas Vauthey

4 Destructive Therapies for Colorectal Cancer Metastases 39
   Dan G. Blazer III, Daniel A. Anaya, and Eddie K. Abdalla

5 Systemic Therapy for Non-operable Colorectal Cancer Metastases 51
   Paulo M. G. Hoff and Scott Kopetz

6 Locoregional Chemotherapy for Hepatic Metastasis
   of Colorectal Cancer 59
   Simon H. Telian, Byron E. Wright, and Anton J. Bilchik

7 Oncosurgical Strategies for Unresectable Liver Metastases 69
   Robbert J. de Haas, Dennis A. Wicherts, and René Adam

8 Adjuvant Chemotherapy 83
   Christophe Penna and Bernard Nordlinger

9 Biologicals for Colorectal Cancer Metastases 91
   Gunnar Folprecht

10 Internal Radiation for the Treatment of Liver Metastases 99
   Douglas M. Coldwell and Andrew S. Kennedy

11 Surgical Treatment of Colorectal Liver Metastases in Elderly Patients 111
   *Barbara L. van Leeuwen, N. de Liguori Carino, G.J. Poston,
   and R.A. Audisio*

12 Health-Related Quality of Life and Palliative Care in Colorectal
    Liver Metastases   117
    Clare Byrne and Mari Lloyd-Williams

13 Carcinoid Liver Metastases: The Carcinoid Syndrome   129
    John Bendelow, Louise Jones, and Graeme J. Poston

14 Gastrointestinal Stromal Tumors   137
    Dan Byrd and Charles Blanke

15 Surgery for Breast Cancer Liver Metastases   149
    Georges Vlastos and Daria Zorzi

16 Liver-Directed Therapy for Metastatic Melanoma to the Liver   155
    Debashish Bose and Timothy M. Pawlik

17 Non-colorectal Gastrointestinal Liver Metastases   169
    Thomas A. Aloia

Index   179

Contributors

Eddie K. Abdalla, MD, Associate Professor Department of Surgical Oncology, The University of Texas M.D. Anderson Cancer Center, Houston, TX, USA

René Adam, MD, PhD, Professor Centre Hépato-Biliaire, AP-HP Hôpital Paul Brousse, Villejuif, France

Syed A. Ahmad, MD, Assistant Professor of Surgery Department of Surgery, University of Cincinnati, Cincinnati, OH, USA

Esther Alba, Department of Radiology, Bellvitge University Hospital, Barcelona, Spain

Thomas A. Aloia, MD, Assistant Professor of Surgery Department of Surgery, Weill-Cornell Medical College, The Methodist Hospital, Houston, TX, USA

Daniel A. Anaya, MD, Fellow Department of Surgical Oncology, The University of Texas M.D. Anderson Cancer Center, Houston, TX, USA

Riccardo A. Audisio, MD, FRCS Department of General Surgery, Whiston Hospital, University of Liverpool, Prescot, Merseyside, UK

John Bendelow, MB, ChB, Resident in Surgery Centre for Digestive Diseases, University Hospital Aintree, Liverpool, UK

Russell S. Berman, MD, Assistant Professor Department of Surgical Oncology, New York University School of Medicine, New York, NY, USA

Anton J. Bilchik, MD, PhD, FACS, Professor of Clinical Medicine and Medical Director California Oncology Research Institute, University of California Los Angeles, Santa Monica, CA, USA

Charles Blanke, MD, FACP, Professor of Medicine Department of Medicine, Division of Medical Oncology, University of British Columbia and the British Columbia Cancer Agency, Vancouver, BC, Canada

Dan G. Blazer III, MD, Fellow Department of Surgical Oncology, The University of Texas M.D. Anderson Cancer Center, Houston, TX, USA

Debashish Bose, MD, PhD, Fellow Department of Surgical Oncology, The University of Texas M.D. Anderson Cancer Center, Houston, TX, USA

Dan Byrd, MD Department of Medicine, OHSU Cancer Institute, Vancouver, BC, Canada

Clare Byrne, MSC RN, Advanced Nurse Practitioner Liverpool Supra-Regional Hepatobiliary Unit, University Hospital Aintree, Liverpool, UK

Nicola de Liguori Carino, MD Supra-Regional Hepatobiliary Unit, University Hospital Aintree, Liverpool, UK

Yun Shin Chun, MD, Fellow Department of Surgical Oncology, The University of Texas M.D. Anderson Cancer Center, Houston, TX, USA

Douglas M. Coldwell, PhD, MD Interventional Radiologist, Department of Radiology, Jane Phillips Medical Center, Bartlesville, OK, USA

Robbert J. de Haas, MD Centre Hépato-Biliaire, AP-HP Hôpital Paul Brousse, Villejuif, France

Gunnar Folprecht, MD, Professor Medical Department I, University Hospital Carl Gustav Carus, Dresden, Germany

Paulo M. G. Hoff, MD, FACP, Executive Director Centro de Oncologia, Hospital Sirio Libanes, Sao Paulo, Brazil

Louise Jones, MSc, Advanced Nurse Practitioner Centre for Digestive Diseases, University Hospital Aintree, Liverpool, UK

Andrew S. Kennedy, MD, FACRO, Co-Medical Director Wake Radiology Oncology, Cary, NC, USA

Scott Kopetz, MD, Assistant Professor Department of Gastrointestinal Medical Oncology, The University of Texas M.D. Anderson Cancer Center, Houston, TX, USA

Mari Lloyd-Williams, MD, FRCGP, FRCP, MMedSci, Professor Academic Palliative and Supportive Care Studies Group, School of Population, Community and Behavioural Sciences, University of Liverpool, Liverpool, UK

Laura Martínez, Department of Radiology, Bellvitge University Hospital, Barcelona, Spain

Bernard Nordlinger, MD, Professor Hôpital Ambroise Paré, Boulogne, France

Timothy M. Pawlik, MD, MPH, Assistant Professor of Surgery Department of Surgery, Division of Surgical Oncology, Johns Hopkins Hospital, Johns Hopkins University School of Medicine, Baltimore, MD, USA

Christophe Penna, MD, Professor of Surgery Department of Digestive Surgery and Oncology, Ambroise Pare Hospital, Boulogne, France

Graeme J. Poston, MB, BS, MS, FRCS(Eng), FRCS(Ed), Director Division of Surgery, Digestive Diseases, Critical Care and Anaesthesia, Centre for Digestive Diseases, University Hospital Aintree, Liverpool, UK

Dario Ribero, MD Department of Hepato-Biliary-Pancreatic and Digestive Surgery, Mauriziano Hospital Umberto I, Torino, Italy

Sandra Ruiz, Department of Radiology, Bellvitge University Hospital, Barcelona, Spain

Ami N. Shah, MD, Resident Department of Surgery, University of Illinois at Chicago, Chicago, IL, USA

Simon H. Telian, MD, Surgical Oncology Fellow John Wayne Cancer Institute, Santa Monica, CA, USA

Carlos Valls, MD, PhD Department of Radiology, Bellvitge University Hospital, Barcelona, Spain

Barbara L. van Leeuwen, MD, PhD Department of Surgery, University Medical Center Groningen, Gronigen, The Netherlands

Jean-Nicolas Vauthey, MD, Professor of Surgery Department of Surgical Oncology, The University of Texas M.D. Anderson Cancer Center, Houston, TX, USA

Georges Vlastos, MD, Associate Attending Department of Gynecology and Obstetrics, Division of Gynecology, Senology and Surgical Gynecologic Oncology Unit, Geneva University Hospitals, Geneva, Switzerland

Dennis A. Wicherts, MD Centre Hépato-Biliaire, AP-HP Hôpital Paul Brousse, Villejuif, France

Curtis J. Wray, MD, Fellow Department of Surgical Oncology, The University of Texas M.D. Anderson Cancer Center, Houston, TX, USA

Byron E. Wright, MD, FACS Senior Surgical Oncology Fellow, Department of Surgical Oncology, John Wayne Cancer Institute, Santa Monica, CA, USA

Daria Zorzi, MD, Fellow Department of Surgical Oncology, The University of Texas M.D. Anderson Cancer Center, Houston, TX, USA

Radiological Imaging of Liver Metastases

Carlos Valls, Laura Martínez, Sandra Ruiz, and Esther Alba

Introduction

Liver metastases are frequently incurable events in disseminated cancers. Barely 30 years ago, such metastases were near-universally regarded as incurable. However, significant progress in both medical and surgical oncology now means that long-term survival is often achievable; for an ever-increasing number of patients, timely radical surgery now offers the real possibility of cure. Much of this progress has been achieved in the field of colorectal cancer, so this chapter will concentrate on imaging liver metastases using our experience in this disease as a paradigm on which to base future strategies for the management of other malignant diseases that spread to the liver.

The liver is the commonest distant site for metastatic spread in patients with colorectal carcinoma (CRC) [1, 2, 3] and in a significant proportion of patients who die from metastatic disease, metastases are located exclusively in the liver [3, 4]. Although the prognosis for non-treated liver metastases remains dismal, some patients with limited hepatic disease can benefit from hepatic resection. Recent experience has shown that hepatic surgery for CRC metastasis provides an effective therapeutic approach in a substantial proportion of patients. Recent surgical series report 5-year survival rates of up to 20%–40% [5, 6, 7]. Consequently, as perioperative mortality and morbidity rates became acceptable, hepatic resection has become the only curative option for isolated hepatic metastasis.

Earlier reports suggested that only a small proportion (<10%) of patients with colorectal metastases are candidates for resection with curative intent [3]. Furthermore, tumor recurrence is rreported in up to 60% of the patients who underwent resection or ablation [5, 7, 8, 9, 10].

Diagnosis and Staging of Liver Metastasis

The natural progression of colorectal cancer is determined by the biology of its pathways of spread. Sites of distant metastases are influenced by the venous drainage of the primary tumor. The portal vein is the main route of delivery of metastatic colorectal cancer cells to the liver. The venous drainage of the colon and upper rectum is via the portal venous system, which provides 80% of the blood flow to the liver. Therefore the liver is the most frequent site of metastases from colorectal cancer and acts as a filter for these malignant cells. On the other hand, lower rectal tumors can disseminate via veins draining into the internal iliac veins, which may explain the apparent relative increase in lung metastases seen with lower rectal cancers when compared to other CRCs. Modern imaging techniques may detect liver metastasis with high accuracy and therefore are critically important when planning treatment. However, benign lesions (which are found in up to 10% of the population and so will exist in 10% of patients diagnosed with cancer) are not infrequently confused with liver metastasis. Therefore accurate radiologic diagnosis and staging is essential in order to get effective treatment to potentially curable patients [11, 12].

Once the liver is involved, metastases may spread beyond the lungs, bones endocrine system, and the brain. In the lower rectum, the dissemination further occurs through the hemorrhoidal plexus without the involvement of the portal system. The superior hemorrhoidal veins drain into the inferior mesenteric vein and then into the portal vein to the liver. The middle and inferior hemorrhoidal veins, however, drain into the pelvic veins and then directly into the inferior vena cava. In the absence of hepatic metastases, the incidence of pulmonary metastases in CRC is lower than 5% while the incidence of bone and brain metastases is less than 1%.

C. Valls (✉)
Department of Radiology, Bellvitge University Hospital,
Barcelona, Spain

J.-N. Vauthey et al. (eds.), *Liver Metastases*, DOI 10.1007/978-1-84628-947-7_1,
© Springer-Verlag London Limited 2009

Radiologic–Pathologic Correlation

Hepatic colorectal cancer metastases are generally hypovascular lesions when compared to the hepatic parenchyma and often appear as hypodense lesions, which are best visualized during the portal venous phase of liver enhancement. This radiologic behavior is due to a combination of factors: vascularization that is mainly arterial rather than portal, a relative lack of glycogen in tumor tissue, and a relative increase in the amount of water in the extracellular spaces or tumor matrices [13]. During the portal venous phase, normal liver parenchyma usually enhances intensely, while liver metastases (with their dominant arterial supply) appear as relatively hypovascular nodules. However, the enhancement pattern of liver metastasis can be extremely variable depending on the extent of vascularization and the type of contrast injection protocol. In general, colorectal liver metastases appear as hypovascular lesions with rim peripheral enhancement (Fig. 1.1). This pattern of enhancement is best seen in portal phase imaging, when the maximum

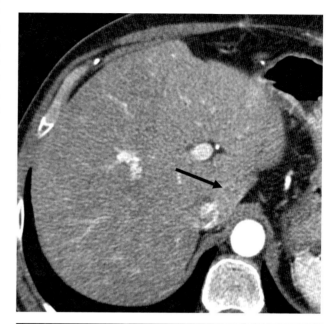

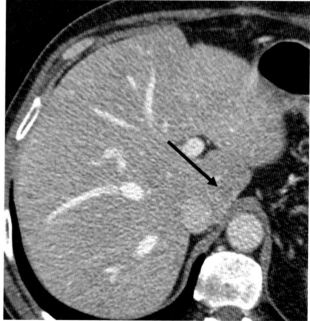

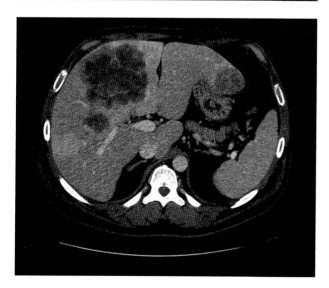

Fig. 1.1 Large hepatic metastases. Contrast-enhanced CT shows multiple low attenuation hepatic metastases and bilateral tumor infiltration

Fig. 1.2 Tiny liver metastases from colon carcinoma. **A.** Contrast-enhanced arterial dominant phase shows the metastasis as an area of intense ring enhancement (*arrow*). **B.** Contrast-enhanced portal venous phase showing the tumor as an ill-defined area of low density (*arrow*). Axial T2-weighted fast spin-echo (FSE) image. **C.** The metastases that have moderately high signal intensity compared with the liver

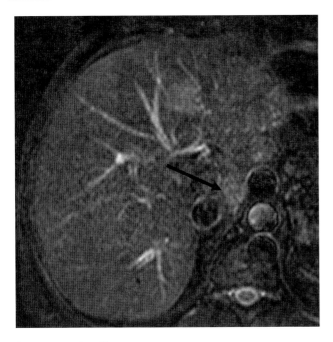

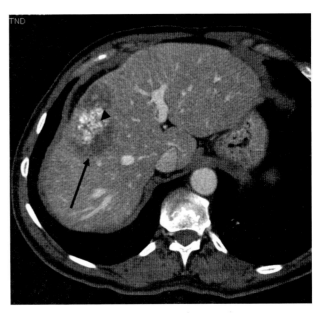

Fig. 1.3 (continued)

Fig. 1.2 (continued)

difference in attenuation between the liver and hypovascular lesions is achieved. In small-size liver metastasis, arterial dominant-phase imaging may be useful to detect faint peripheral rim enhancement of metastatic nodules (Fig. 1.2). Liver metastases from colorectal cancer may show cystic or calcified degeneration. Calcified metastases are usually large nodules with amorphous central or peripheral calcification and heterogeneous contrast

enhancement (Fig. 1.3). Calcification is seen more frequently in mucinous tumors and after chemotherapy. Metastases from other tumors may appear as hypervascular lesions (e.g., carcinoid and other neuroendocrine tumors); these lesions are then best visualized during the arterial phase of liver imaging.

Imaging Modalities for the Detection of Hepatic Metastases

Recent advances in imaging techniques, such as computed tomography (CT), magnetic resonance imaging (MRI), ultrasound (US), positron emission tomography (PET), and integrated PET–CT imaging, have increased our ability to detect and characterize focal liver lesions [14]. There is no consensus in the literature on which is the best imaging method for the detection of hepatic metastases in patients with colorectal cancer. The non invasive nature of US and its low cost make this imaging technique a useful tool in the diagnosis of liver metastasis. However, since US is operator dependent, in some patients certain parts of the liver may not be clearly visualized. In routine daily practice, US may be useful as an initial searching technique in symptomatic patients, but it does not play an important role in screening for CRC hepatic metastases. Helical CT (HCT) is the technique of choice for tumor staging at the abdominal and thoracic level. In patients with contraindications to iodinated contrast or known severe hepatic steatosis, gadolinium-enhanced MRI offers the best diagnostic

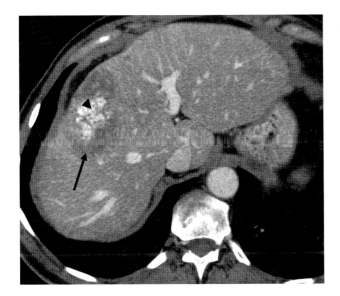

Fig. 1.3 Calcified liver metastases of colon carcinoma. Contrast-enhanced portal phase (**A**) and delayed phase (**B**) exhibit a hypodense mass (*arrow*) with internal calcium deposits (*arrowhead*)

alternative. PET with 18-Fluorodeoxyglucos (FDG) is another technique now used widely in staging. However, its sensitivity in detecting liver metastasis is not superior to that of HCT. Its use is better suited for the detection and staging of extrahepatic metastatic lesions, even though its sensitivity appears to be lower than initially thought [15].

The reported sensitivities of imaging methods range from 57% to 100% for US, from 36% to 94% for CT, from 86% to 96% for MRI, and from 86% to 99% for PET in a meta-analysis published in the nuclear medicine literature in 2000 [16]. In a more recent meta-analysis published by Bipat et al. [13], the authors report sensitivity, on a per-patient basis, for HCT (64.7%), MRI (75.8%), and FDG PET (94.6%). On a per-lesion basis, sensitivity estimates were as follows: HCT (68.2%), MRI (78.2%), and FDG PET (75.9%). FDG PET had significantly higher sensitivity on a per-patient but not on a per-lesion basis.

Ultrasound

Real-time US evaluation offers a rapid, non-invasive method for screening patients with suspected liver metastases. However, it is not widely used in comparison to other imaging modalities, especially for the primary diagnosis of liver lesions. US has relative disadvantages, is significantly more operator dependent than the other imaging methods, and fails to show parts of the liver in certain patients. However, US is highly efficient in distinguishing patients with diffuse hepatic metastases that involve all the liver.

We use 3.5 MHz–5 MHz curved-array transducers to detect liver metastases using percutaneous transabdominal US evaluation. Findings suggestive of metastases include multiple solid lesions and the presence of a hypoechoic halo surrounding a liver mass. US evaluation has a low sensitivity with a false negative ratio above 50% and low specificity [17]. The advances in US, such as power Doppler and second-harmonic imaging with contrast agents, have improved detection and characterization of liver metastases. Still the success of sonographic evaluation depends not only on these technical innovations but also on the experience of the examiner.

Computed Tomography

The introduction of multidetector CT (MDCT) has provided unique capabilities that are especially valuable for hepatic volume acquisition, combining short scan times, narrow collimation, and the ability to obtain multiphase data. These features result in improved lesion detection and characterization [18].

Short acquisition time MDCT provides the opportunity to capture peak enhancement in visceral organs by optimizing contrast injection and scan protocols. Technical protocols are extremely varied, depending on the available technology. However, the minimum technical requirements for an assessment of CRC hepatic metastases should include helical techniques, a slice thickness less than 5 mm, extension to include both the pelvis and thorax, and adequate contrast enhancement using (2 ml/kg) non-ionic contrast media injected intravenously at a rate of 3–5 ml/s.

There is no consensus in the literature regarding the optimal phases for imaging liver metastasis using CT. Double- or triple-phase HCT of the liver has been shown to be useful in the detection of hypervascular hepatic tumors. However, no definitive superiority has been established for the detection of hypovascular metastases. Hypovascular lesions such as CRC metastases are best detected during the portal venous phase of liver enhancement; the delay time recommended to detect these lesions is around 60–70 s after contrast injection [19]. Although the arterial-dominant phase does not help to depict additional hepatic metastases not visible on portal-dominant phase images, the authors believe that studies of liver metastases should include a dual-phase evaluation with image acquisition during hepatic arterial and portal venous phases. This will accurately detect segmental localization of hepatic tumors as well as hepatic and portal venous anatomy, which is important for surgical planning. Occasionally, arterial phase imaging may help to detect peripheral enhancement in small liver metastasis without definite enhancement on portal phase imaging (Fig. 1.2). Arterial phase imaging can also be useful to detect and characterize benign hypervascular nodules such as focal nodular hyperplasia (FNH) or small angiomas that can be mistaken for metastases.

Delayed CT images of the liver should be obtained 4–5 min after the initiation of contrast injection. These delays are helpful in cases of hepatic masses that are believed to possibly represent cavernous hemangioma, where progressive enhancement of the hemangioma is one of its characteristic features, or cystic lesions. Multiplanar Volume Rendering (VR) and Maximum Intensity Projection (MIP) techniques allow for the evaluation of feeding vessels and vascular variants. Vascular delineation also results in accurate segmental localization that is essential before hepatic resection.

Magnetic Resonance Imaging

In most comparative studies, MRI is not superior to CT in the evaluation of the liver metastases. In our experience, MRI is a complementary method for the study of CRC hepatic metastases. Although MRI allows an adequate study of hepatic parenchyma, its sensitivity for detection of extrahepatic extension is smaller than CT [20]. In general MRI is considered the technique of choice in patients with contraindications to iodinated contrast, in patients with fatty infiltration of the liver, and in detection and characterization of small liver metastases, especially in distinguishing small metastases from small cysts (Fig. 1.4).

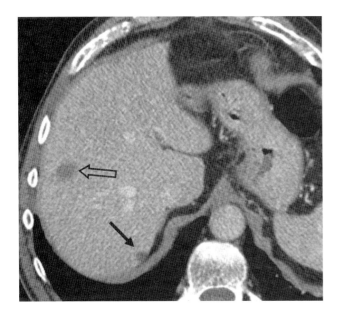

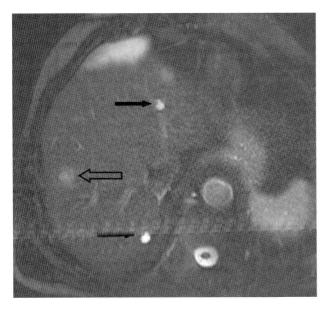

Fig. 1.4 Colorectal metastases with coincidental multiple liver cyst. (**A**) Axial CT in portal phase in a patient who has colon carcinoma shows a hypodense metastasis in segment VIII (*open arrow*) and a second lesion (*arrow*) "too small to characterize." (**B**) Axial T2-weighted fast spin-echo shows a metastasis (*open arrow*) that has moderately high signal intensity compared with the liver and much lower signal intensity than the bright fluid-like signal intensity of the cysts (*arrows*)

MRI for the study of hepatic metastases is usually performed with 1.5 T units, with high-amplitude gradients and phased-array coils. Technical parameters include chemical shift imaging with T1-weighted in-phase and out-phase imaging to rule out fatty change, T2-weighted with or without fat-saturation to characterize fluid lesions such as cysts and hemangiomas, and dynamic multiphasic gadolinium-enhanced imaging T1-weighted 2-D or 3-D sequences to detect focal solid lesions.

The majority of colorectal liver metastases show several typical findings. The lesions appear as low signal intensity on T1-weighted images and as moderately high signal intensity lesions on T2-weighted images with fat suppression. Metastases with intratumoral hemorrhage, coagulative necrosis, or mucin production may exhibit mixed signal intensity on T1-weighted images, and those with a desmoplastic reaction may exhibit low signal intensity on T2-weighted images.

Contrast injection is routinely performed for the evaluation of liver metastases. Gadolinium is distributed in blood vessels and extracellular space rapidly after intravenous bolus injection. After administration of gadolinium, most colorectal metastases are hypointense during the portal phase.

In addition to the extracellular contrast agent, contrast agents specific to the liver, such as superparamagnetic iron oxide (SPIO) and manganese-based MR contrast, have been introduced to improve the detection of hepatic metastases.

Ferumoxides are a liver-specific SPIO-MR contrast agent taken up predominantly by the Kupfer cells of the macrophage–monocytic phagocytic system. During this processes, SPIO causes T2-shortening effects, leading to a marked reduction in signal intensity of liver parenchyma. Because hepatic metastases do not have the reticuloendothelial cells of normal parenchyma, there is no SPIO uptake and so they remain high in signal intensity. A review of the current literature shows that an SPIO-enhanced MRI has a better diagnostic performance than CT [20, 21], whereas gadolinium-enhanced MRI has a better diagnostic performance than SPIO-enhanced MRI for focal liver lesions [22, 23]. A study by Marsini and collaborators [24] reported sensitivities for liver metastases by gadolinium and SPIO-enhanced MRI of 63% versus 43%.

Mangafodipir trisodium (Mn DPDP, Teslascan) is another T1-shortening MR contrast agent which also has potential as a hepatobiliary agent. Comparison of gadolinium-DTPA and Mn DPDP as MRI agents showed no observable differences in terms of both detection and characterization of liver metastases [25].

Presently, gadolinium is used more often as a non-liver-specific contrast agent for liver imaging. When compared to liver-specific contrast agents, the results appear to be slightly less superior [26]. According to some authors, MRI performed with specific contrasts could have a higher sensitivity than CT scans or gadolinium MRI. However, at present there is no scientific evidence to support its use in CRC patients with hepatic metastases.

Differential Diagnosis

CT scan has demonstrated great accuracy in the diagnosis of hepatic metastases; however, possible differential diagnoses have to take into account the following three clinical conditions.

Hemangioma

This is the most frequent benign solid hepatic tumor, with a prevalence close to 8% within the general population. Given this prevalence, it is often seen in cancer patients. In 85% of cases, tri-phase HCT (arterial, portal, and equilibrium phases) will demonstrate characteristic radiological features that allow a definitive diagnosis. The presence of complete arterial hyper-enhancement in all phases or globular, peripheral, and discontinuous enhancement in the portal phase has a positive predictive value (PPV) of 100% for hemangioma [11]. MRI should be done in any uncertain situations.

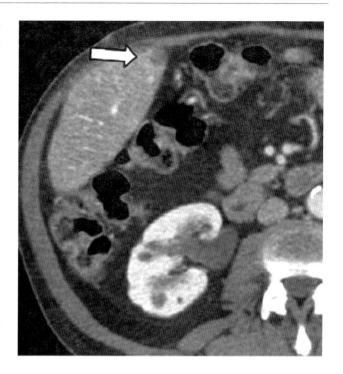

Focal Steatosis

This condition presents with hepatic parenchyma showing hypodense lesions due to fatty infiltration. Focal fatty change is usually localized in specific areas such as segments III–IV, anterior to the portal vein, around the gallbladder or lying sub-capsularly. In other instances, it can show a nodular appearance, which cannot be differentiated from the metastatic lesions. In these cases, it is necessary to perform MRI with chemical shift imaging (in-phase and out-phase) to confirm the presence of steatosis. In- and out-phase chemical shift MRI sequences are very useful in the setting of fatty liver, as they allow splitting of the signal between protons from the water and those of the fat due to the difference in the resonance frequency. Areas with fatty change will show a marked drop of signal in opposed phase imaging, so allowing confident differentiation from solid metastatic lesions (Fig. 1.5)

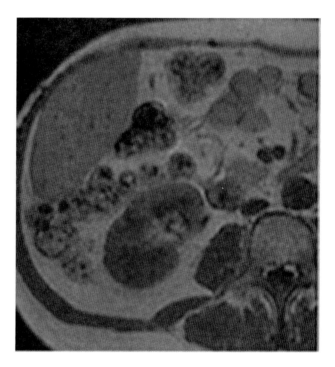

Sub-Centimeter Focal Lesions

Sub-centimeter lesions continue to be difficult to characterize by radiological techniques. Eighty per cent of these lesions will turn out to be benign. Given that these lesions

Fig. 1.5 Focal hepatic steatosis in a patient with liver metastases from colorectal cancer. (**A**) Axial CT image shows diffuse fatty infiltration of liver and hypodense lesion (*arrow*) suspicious for metastasis in segment V. Axial in-phase (**B**) and out-phase (**C**) images show greater signal drop of lesion in **D** (*arrow*), consistent with hypersteatosis (more fatty) compared with diffusely fatty infiltrated liver

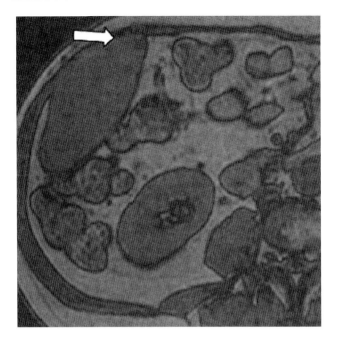

Fig. 1.5 (continued)

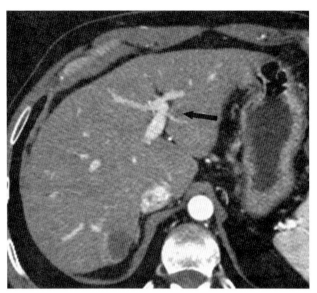

Fig. 1.6 Atypical angiomas. CT shows large hypodense lesion in segment VII consistent with metastasis. In addition another small hypodense lesion (*arrow*) is seen in segment IV which was considered metastasis. Histological examination demonstrated atypical hemangioma

cannot be characterized by any technique, it is necessary to perform follow-up every 3–6 months to confirm their continuing stability [12].

Staging of Hepatic Metastases in Potentially Resectable Patients

Accurate and careful preoperative selection of patients with colorectal metastases who are most likely to benefit from surgery is critical to avoid unnecessary surgery. Preoperative imaging with radiological techniques is therefore crucial for these patients. This radiological assessment of potentially resectable liver metastases should address the following five critical issues.

Evaluation of Possible Liver Metastases

Are all visible lesions metastases, or are there any benign lesions such as hemangioma or FNH (Fig. 1.6)? Radiological examination has to determine the number, size, and location of the tumor(s) according to Couinaud's segments, as well as vascular invasion of critical portal or hepatic vein structures. In addition, the final radiological report should alert the surgeon to any anatomic variant that may change the surgical approach, such as portal trifurcation, vestigial left lateral segment, or variations in hepatic venous drainage (Fig. 1.7)

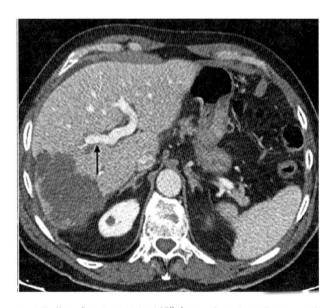

Fig. 1.7 Portal variant. Helical CT shows a large hypodense mass in segment VI consistent with a metastasis. Note right anterior portal vein originating from the left portal vein (*arrow*)

Possible Hilar Lymph Node Involvement

Nodal involvement at the porta hepatis carries a poor prognosis, because involvement of these lymph nodes represents metastases from the established hepatic metastasis. Overall survival rate in these patients after surgical resection ranges between 3% and 12% [27] and in many institutions such a finding may represent a

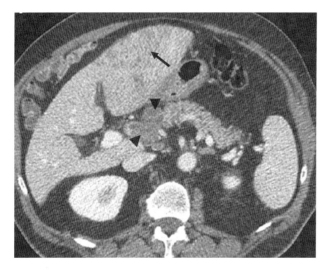

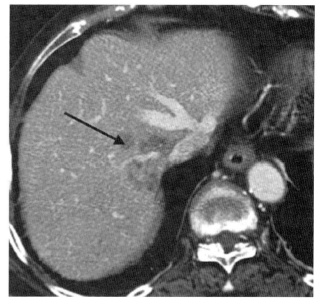

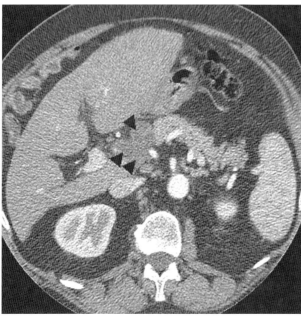

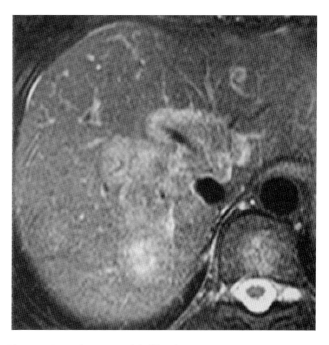

Fig. 1.8 Enlarged lymph nodes in a patient with colorectal carcinoma. Contrast-enhanced portal venous phase (**A**), and arterial phase (**B**), showing multiple metastases (*arrows*) and lymph-node metastases in the hepatic hilar region (*arrowhead*)

Fig. 1.9 Vascular tumoral infiltration. **A**. CT at the level of the hepatic dome shows liver metastasis in segments VII and VIII infiltrating the right hepatic vein (*arrow*). **B**. MRI in another patient shows extensive tumoral infiltration of the three hepatic veins

contraindication to liver surgery. Hilar lymph nodes can be suspected preoperatively if the nodes are large enough (Fig. 1.8), but in most cases their small size precludes an adequate preoperative diagnosis.

Vascular Invasion

Assessment of vascular invasion is critical when deciding the appropriate surgical strategy in patients with liver metastasis. Tumoral infiltration of both right and left

portal pedicles or all three hepatic veins close to the vena cava (Fig. 1.9) is often considered contraindications to surgical resection, and these patients should undergo chemotherapy and re-evaluation with further imaging to assess response to this chemotherapy [28]. Vascular infiltration of portal or hepatic vascular structures of one lobe is not a contraindication to surgery, although carrying a poorer prognosis.

Liver Volumetry

Radiologic studies of liver metastases in potentially resectable patients must also include volumetric data to determine the volume of future remnant liver when considering extended (beyond a hemi-liver) resections. In most institutions insufficient residual volume of liver parenchyma (<20%–25%) is a contraindication to surgical resection. Preoperative portal vein embolization to create hypertrophy of the uninvolved portions of the liver may be used in case of presumed insufficient residual liver volume.

Presence of Extrahepatic Disease

Extrahepatic disease in the lung, other solid viscera (adrenal, spleen, para- and pre-aortic lymph nodes), or retroperitoneum is usually readily detected with preoperative imaging (Figs. 1.10 and 1.11). However, in patients coming to laparotomy for possible resection of hepatic metastasis, one of the commonest causes of unresectability is previously unsuspected peritoneal or extrahepatic spread. Peritoneal carcinomatosis often presents as small and superficial peritoneal nodules which are extremely difficult to detect preoperatively (Fig. 1.12). When peritoneal disease is more extensive, omental tumoral infiltration is easily detected as mass--like tumoral enhancement of the greater omentum ("omental cake") associated with large peritoneal nodules and loculated peritoneal fluid, with occasional thickening of the peritoneum (Fig. 1.13).

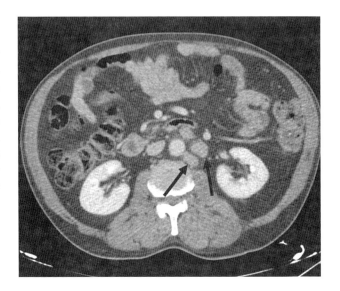

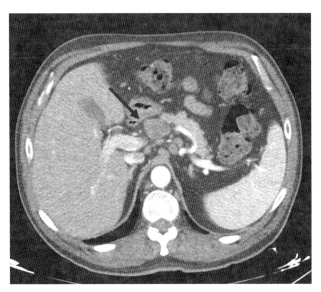

Fig. 1.11 Enlarged lymph nodes in a patient with metastatic colon cancer. Contrast-enhanced CT scan shows enlarged portocaval, aorto-caval; and porta hepatis nodes

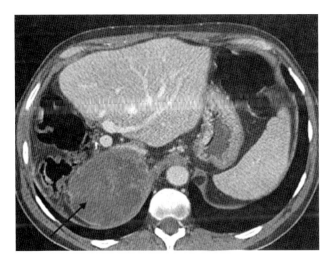

Fig. 1.10 Adrenal metastasis (*arrow*) in a patient following liver resection for colorectal metastases

We are routinely using PET–CT for the detection of extrahepatic metastatic disease. However, although the sensitivity of PET–CT is higher than CT (Fig. 1.14) in that setting, the PPV of PET–CT is relatively low (Fig. 1.15). Over the last 3 years, we have prospectively studied 63 patients with metachronous liver metastases, using abdominal HCT and FDG-PET–CT scan as part of the preoperative staging work-out before surgical resection. HCT correctly detected 98 of 136 (72%) hepatic metastases from colorectal cancer, while FDG-PET–CT detected 83 of 136 (61%), with a false positive ratio of 8.1% and 6%, respectively. With specific regard to extrahepatic disease, the sensitivity and PPV were 25% and

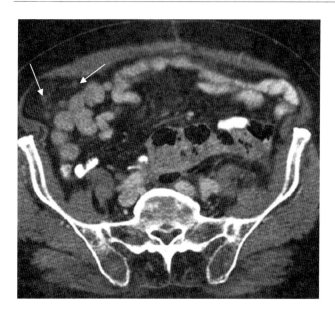

Fig. 1.12 Peritoneal carcinomatosis. CT shows small hypodense nodules in the greater omentum (*arrow*) consistent with peritoneal carcinomatosis

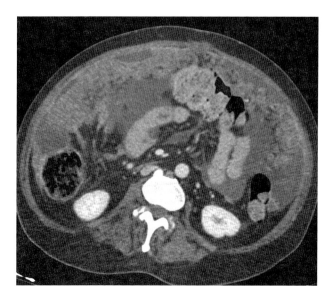

Fig. 1.13 Massive peritoneal carcinomatosis. Contrast-enhanced CT scan reveals large tumoral omental implants giving typical "omental cake" appearance

50% for CT and 80% and 30.7% for FDG-PET–CT. The results for CT were better than PET–CT in detecting liver metastases, while for extrahepatic disease the sensitivity of PET–CT was better than CT. However, in our experience the PPV of PET–CT for extrahepatic disease is much lower than previously reported (30.7%) and therefore no patient should be denied surgery on the basis of PET–CT findings alone. PET–CT findings suggesting non-resectability should be confirmed histologically.

Follow-Up for Recurrent Metastatic Disease

At present, there are no published data reviewing or meta-analyzing follow-up protocols on patients who have undergone resection or thermal ablation of liver metastases. The usual practice in most institutions for patients with colorectal cancer consists of periodic determinations of carcinoembryonic antigen (CEA) levels, with a sensitivity of 59% and specificity of 84% [29], complemented with imaging techniques when the CEA rises. On the other hand, the results of detecting recurrent colorectal cancer by periodic CEA determinations in patients following resection of CRC liver metastases are lower than those seen using image-driven protocols. In a report by Freeny et al. [29], only 50% of those patients with liver metastases (5/10) had elevated CEA levels. CT is usually accepted as the conventional imaging modality to demonstrate recurrent liver metastases; however, it fails to detect hepatic lesions in up to 7% of these patients [30].

Follow-Up of Patients After Surgical Resection of CRC Hepatic Metastases

Although there is no consensus in the literature and no study has demonstrated benefits in statistical terms, in our center we recommend testing serum CEA and performing abdominal, pelvic, and chest CT scans every 6 months during the first 2 years and annually for the next 3 years.

The detection of tumor recurrence after hepatectomy remains difficult. US scan remains a good technique to study the liver; however, it is operator dependent, and the results can be influenced by artifacts such as post-surgical changes, obesity, and steatosis. HCT is a more sensitive technique, but invasive, as it requires high doses of contrast (150–170 ml) at a high injection rate. Not every hospital CT scan unit (including helical) is able to produce high-quality diagnostic images or carry out follow-up to an agreed protocol. Each center has to adapt to the available technology and equipment.

Imaging and Follow-Up After Radiofrequency Ablation

Radiofrequency ablation (RFA) has become an increasingly utilized technique for the treatment of unresectable liver tumors [31, 32]. Multiphasic contrast-enhanced CT

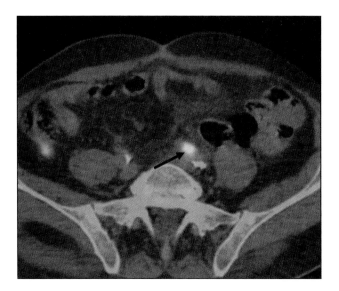
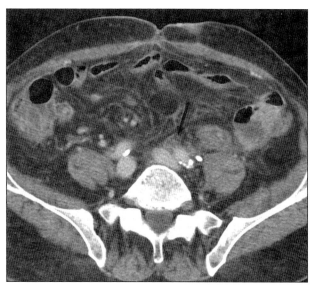

Fig. 1.14 False positive finding of PET–CT. Post-surgical fibrosis in a patient with colorectal carcinoma resection. **A.** Transverse FDG-PET–CT images show avid focus (*arrow*) with FDG uptake in the retroperitoneal space that was considered metastatic. **B.**

Activity seen on PET–CT coincides with fibrous changes after surgery on CT without evidence of metastasis foci. At histopathological examination the lesion was benign (granulomatous reaction)

and dynamic MRI demonstrate a similar capability to detect early tumor recurrences after RFA. Dromain et al. [33] reported a higher sensitivity for the early detection of local recurrence using MRI when compared to CT, but these differences were not significant ($p = 0.12$). Following RFA, follow-up should be performed every 3 months for 1 year, and every 6 months thereafter. On enhanced CT, the ablation area is expected to be non-enhancing (Fig. 1.16). Although occasional rim enhancement may be seen in the arterial phase related to hyperemia following the thermal injury, no focal enhancement should be present within the ablation area, which if present, is suspicious for residual or recurrent tumor.

Differentiation of reactive hyperemia from residual tumor may be difficult, and in equivocal cases early follow-up is necessary. The MRI signals of coagulation

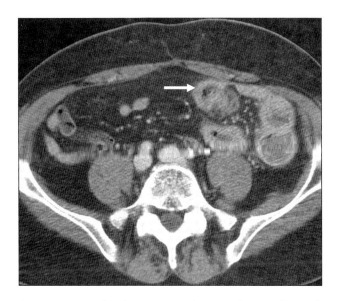
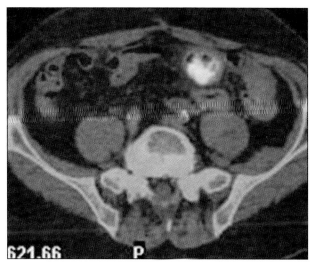

Fig. 1.15 Locoregional recurrence after resection. **A.** CT at the level of the iliac crests shows post-surgical changes after right colectomy without evidence of tumor recurrence. **B.** PET–CT

shows highly metabolic area adjacent to ileocolic anastomosis (*arrow*) consistent with tumor recurrence

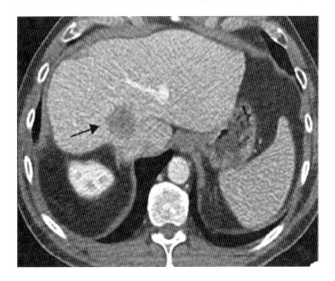

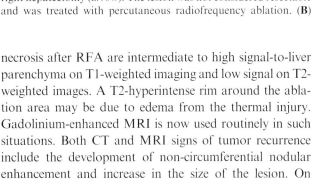

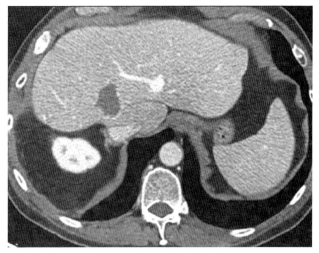

Fig. 1.16 (**A**) CT shows tumoral recurrence in segment IV after right hepatectomy (*arrow*). The lesion was not considered resectable and was treated with percutaneous radiofrequency ablation. (**B**)

Follow-up CT 6 months later shows hypodense lesion without contrast enhancement consistent with necrosis of the lesion without evidence of tumor recurrence

necrosis after RFA are intermediate to high signal-to-liver parenchyma on T1-weighted imaging and low signal on T2-weighted images. A T2-hyperintense rim around the ablation area may be due to edema from the thermal injury. Gadolinium-enhanced MRI is now used routinely in such situations. Both CT and MRI signs of tumor recurrence include the development of non-circumferential nodular enhancement and increase in the size of the lesion. On MRI, T1-hypointense and T2-hyperintense signal areas should raise the possibility of recurrent or residual tumor.

References

1. Parker SL, Tong T, Bolden S, et al. Cancer Statistics. CA Cancer J Clin. 1996; 65: 5–27.
2. Baker ME, Pelley R. Hepatic metastases: Basic principles and implications for radiologists. Radiology. 1995; 197: 329–337.
3. Weiss L, Grundmann E, Torhorst J, et al. Haematogenous metastatic patterns in colonic carcinoma: An analysis of 1541 necropsies. J Pathol. 1986; 150: 195–203.
4. Gilbert HA, Kagan AR. Metastases: Incidence, detection, and evaluation without histologic confirmation. In: Weiss L, ed. Fundamental Aspects of Metastasis. Amsterdam: North-Holland Pub. Co.; 1976:385–405.
5. Scheele J, Stang R, Altendorf-Hofmann A, et al. Resection of colorectal liver metastases. World J Surg. 1995; 19: 59–71.
6. Sugarbaker PH. Surgical decision making for large bowel cancer metastatic to the liver. Radiology. 1990; 174: 621–626.
7. Fong Y, Cohen AM, Fortner JG, et al. Liver resection for colorectal metastases. J Clin Oncol. 1997; 15: 938–946.
8. Ohlson B, Stenram U, Tranberg KG. Resection of colorectal liver metastases: 25-year experience. World J Surg. 1998; 22: 268–277.
9. Jemal A, Tiwari RC, Murray T. Cancer statistics 2007. Cancer J Clin. 2004; 57: 43–66.
10. Yoon SS, Tanabe TK. Surgical treatment and other regional treatments for colorectal cancer liver metastases. Oncologist. 1999; 4: 197–208.
11. Van Leeuwen MS, Noordzij J, Feldberg MA, et al. Focal liver lesions: Characterization with triphasic spiral CT. Radiology. 1996; 201: 327.
12. Schwartz LH, Gandras EJ, Colangelo SM, et al. Prevalence and importance of small hepatic lesions found at CT in patients with cancer. Radiology. 1999; 210: 71–74.
13. Bipat S, Glas A, Slors F. Rectal cancer: local staging and assessment of lymph node involvement with endoluminal US, TC, and MR imaging, a meta-analysis. Radiology. 2004; 232: 733–783.
14. Choi J. Imaging of hepatic metastases. Cancer Control. 2006; 13(1) 6–12.
15. Truant S, Huglo D, Hebbar M, et al. Prospective evaluation of the impact of [18F]fluoro-2-deoxy-D-glucose positron emission tomography of resectable colorectal liver metastases. Br J Surg. 2005; 92(3) 362–9.
16. Huebner RH, Parker KC, Shepherd JE, et al. A meta-analysis of the literature for whole-body FDG PET detection of recurrent colorectal cancer. J Nucl Med. 2000; 41: 1177–1189.
17. Hagspiel KD, Neidi KF, Eichenberger AC, et al. Detection of liver metastases: Comparison of supermagnetic iron oxide-enhanced and unenhanced MR imaging at 1.5T with dynamic CT, intraoperative US, and percutaneous US. Radiology. 1995; 196: 471–478.
18. Foley WD, Mallisee TA, Hohenwalter MD, et al. Multiphase hepatic CT with a multirow detector CT scanner: AJR Am J Roentgenol. 2000; 175: 679–85.
19. Kanematsu M, Goshima S, Kondo H, et al. Optimizing scan delays of fixed duration contrast injection in contrast-enhanced biphasic multidetector-row CT for the liver and the detection of hypervascular hepatocellular carcinoma. J Comput Assist Tomogr. 2005; 29: 195–201.
20. Schmidt J, Strotzer M, Fraunhofer S, et al. Intraoperative ultrasonography versus helical computed tomography and computed tomography with arterioportography in diagnosing colorectal liver metastases: Lesion-by-lesion analysis. World J Surg. 2000; 24: 43–8.

21. Ward J, Naik KS, Guthrie IA, et al. Hepatic lesion detection: Comparison of MR imaging after the administration of super-paramagnetic iron oxide with dual-phase CT by using alternative-free response receiver operating characteristic analysis. Radiology. 1999; 210(2) 459–66.

22. Kim T, Federle MP, Baron RL, et al. Discrimination of small hepatic hemangiomas from hypervascular malignant tumors smaller than 3 cm with three-phase helical CT. Radiology. 2001; 219: 699–706.

23. Reimer P, Jahnke N, Fiebich M, et al. Hepatic lesion detection and characterization: Value of nonenhanced MR imaging, supermagnetic iron oxide-enhanced MR imaging, and spiral CT-ROC analysis. Radiology. 2000; 217(1) 152–8.

24. Matsuo M, Kanematsu M, Itoh K, et al. Detection of malignant hepatic tumors: Comparison of gadolinium- and ferum-oxide-enhanced MR imaging. Am J Roentgenol. 2001; 177: 637–43.

25. Kettritz U, Schlund JF, Wilbur K, et al. Comparison of gadolinium chelates with manganese-DPDP for liver lesion detection and characterization: Preliminary results. Magn Reson Imaging. 1996; 14(10) 1185–90.

26. Delbke D, Martin WH. PET-CT for evaluation of colorectal carcinoma. Semin Nucl Med. 2004; 34(3) 209–23.

27. Simmonds P, Colquitt J, Primrose JN, et al. Surgical resection of hepatic metastases from colorectal cancer: A systematic review of published series. Br J Cancer. 2006; 94: 982–99.

28. Poston GJ, Adam R, Alberts S, et al. OncoSurge: a strategy for increasing resectability with curative intent in liver metastases from colorectal cancer. J Clin Oncol. 2005; 23: 7125–34.

29. Rymer R. Detection of hypovascular hepatic metastases at triple-phase helical CT: sensitivity of phases and comparison with surgical and histopathologic findings. Radiology. 2004; 231(2) 413–20.

30. Freeny PC, Marks WM, Ryan JA, Bolen JW. Colorectal carcinoma evaluation with CT: preoperative staging and detection of postoperative recurrence. Radiology. 1986; 158: 347–353.

31. Lencioni R, Cioni D, Bartolozzi C. Percutaneous radiofrequency thermal ablation of liver malignancies: Techniques, indications, imaging findings, and clinical results. Abdom Imaging. 2001; 26: 345–360.

32. Goldberg SN, Gazelle GS, Mueller PR. Thermal ablation therapy for focal malignancy: A unified approach to underlying principles, techniques, and diagnostic imaging guidance. Am J Radiol. 2000; 174: 323–331.

33. Dromain C, de Baere T, Elias D, et al. Hepatic tumors treated with percutaneous radio-frequency ablation: CT and MR imaging follow-up. Radiology. 2002; 223: 255–262.

Biology of Colorectal Cancer Liver Metastases

2

Curtis J. Wray, Ami N. Shah, Russell S. Berman, and Syed A. Ahmad

Colorectal Hepatic Metastases Formation

Progression to metastatic disease is an inefficient sequence of events. Primary tumors shed enormous quantities of cells into the vasculature; yet, only 0.001% of these cells form tumor foci [1]. The evolution of colorectal cancer (CRC) is recognized to be a complex, multistage progression in which the transformation from normal epithelial colonocytes to metastatic CRC cells involves numerous epigenetic changes that lead to numerous phenotypic alterations. This hypothesis describes an accumulation of genetic events and somatic mutations, each conferring a distinct growth advantage of the colonocyte, which eventually results in uncontrolled cell proliferation, clonal tumor development, and progression from adenoma to invasive carcinoma. The characteristics and capabilities of cells following malignant transformation include the following: (1) autocrine growth signaling; autocrine loop of growth factors; (2) resistance to inhibitory factors; (3) resistance to apoptosis (avoidance of destruction by immune mechanisms); (4) unlimited replication potential; (5) sustained angiogenesis (recruitment of nutritional supply to the tumor mass); (6) tissue invasion and metastasis. In this review, we will focus on the latter events of this sequence.

Alteration of Cell–Cell and Cell–Matrix Interactions

Epithelial to Mesenchymal Transition

Recently, adhesion molecules have taken center stage in the context of metastatic CRC. At the "invasive" or

leading front of CRC, tumor cells have been shown to undergo a change to a more dedifferentiated cell type. These changes are accompanied with a more metastatic and invasive program, termed epithelial to mesenchymal transition (EMT) [2]. EMT was initially described in embryonic development in which cells lose epithelial characteristics and gain mesenchymal properties; allowing them to migrate in an extracellular environment in processes such as gastrulation and neural crest formation. EMT plays a role in more than embryonic processes. It has shown to be important in gastric cancer, head and neck tumors, breast cancers, pancreatic cancers, melanoma, bladder, and most recently CRC [3, 4, 5]. In CRC, tumor cells undergoing EMT are able to escape from the constraints of epithelial cells bound together by adhesion molecules and are able to become more fibroblastic, and become an invasive, metastatic CRC (Fig. 2.1). The key changes noted in cells that undergo EMT are as follows: (1) the loss of E-cadherin causing disruption of adherens junctions and loss of cell polarity, (2) the nuclear translocation of β (beta)-catenin leading to a more metastatic and invasive transcriptional program, (3) gain of vimentin, a mesenchymal marker, and (4) the upregulation of the Snail family of transcription factors. Evidence for the importance of EMT in CRC comes from several sources. Spaderna et al. demonstrated an increase in EMT markers in CRC tissue specimens, and this correlated with increased metastasis and poorer patient survival [6]. In addition, many of the molecules central to EMT have been shown to be critical in the formation of metastatic CRC disease.

Loss of E-cadherin expression is one of the most heavily involved processes in EMT and in metastatic CRC (Fig. 2.2). E-cadherin is a type I cadherin that mediates homophilic interactions by forming bonds between immunoglobulin domains in their extracellular region and actin filaments via the (α, β, γ) (alpha, beta, gamma) catenin family in the cytoplasm [7]. Loss of E-cadherin in vitro confers invasive properties to noninvasive cells and conversely, introduction

S.A. Ahmad (✉)
Assistant Professor of Surgery, University of Cincinnati, Cincinnati, OH, USA

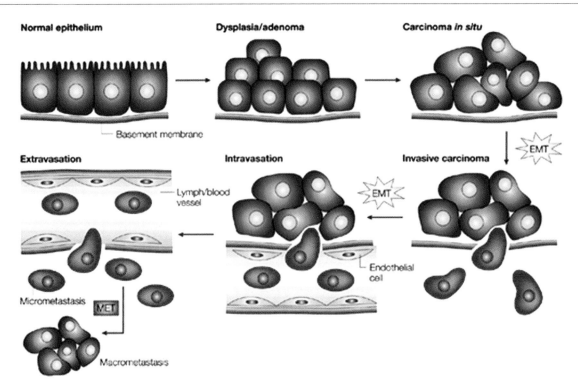

Fig. 2.1 Sites of EMT in the emergence and progression of carcinoma. Epithelial cells lined by the basement membrane can proliferate locally to give rise to an adenoma. Further transformation by epigenetic changes and genetic alterations leads to a carcinoma in situ, still outlined by an intact basement membrane. Continued alterations induce local dissemination of carcinoma cells, possibly through an epithelial—mesenchymal transition (EMT), and the basement membrane becomes fragmented. The cells can intravasate into lymph or blood vessels, allowing their passive transport to distant organs

of E-cadherin into invasive epithelial cell lines blocks invasive properties. Therefore, E-cadherin is considered a suppressor of invasion and metastasis, and its functional inactivation represents a critical step in the acquisition of this capability [8].

The importance of E-cadherin downregulation in CRC is evident in several studies which demonstrated that decreased expression is an independent adverse prognostic factor for a higher T stage, higher N stage, vascular invasion and worse survival [9]. Abnormal expression of E-cadherin at invasive front of CRC, demonstrating cytoplasmic, rather than membranous expression, has been correlated with higher risk of disease recurrence [10]. Reduction and complete absence of E-cadherin expression were observed more often in patients with CRC liver metastases than in patients without metastases [11]. Gene expression demonstrates that decreased E-cadherin mRNA was greatest in patients with CRC liver metastases [12]. While multiple mechanisms are known to cause abnormal or reduced E-cadherin expression, including mutations or deletions of the E-cadherin gene, mutations in the β (beta)-catenin gene, and transcriptional repression of the E-cadherin gene by promoter hypermethylation or chromatin rearrangements; it is not yet clear which of these is relevant in CRC.

Another crucial factor in the progression of EMT to metastatic CRC is β (beta)-catenin. Increased expression and over activity of β (beta)-catenin directly leads to loss of epithelial cell differentiation [13]. Over 80% of sporadic CRCs demonstrate a mutation in the Adenomatous Polyposis Coli (APC) tumor suppressor gene. The APC protein is known to interact with β-catenin, negatively regulating downstream β (beta)-catenin interactions. With the mutation in the APC gene, Wnt signaling pathway activation leads to β (beta)-catenin accumulation in the nucleus leading to transcriptional activation of the T cell factor/lymphocyte enhancer factor (TCF/LEF) family. Several genes including cyclin D1 and c-Myc, which control cell growth and proliferation, contain multiple TCF responsive elements in their promoters and are upregulated by nuclear translocated β (beta)-catenin. Also, when E-cadherin is downregulated from the plasma membrane it is no longer able to bind to cytoplasmic β (beta)-catenin, allowing for the cytoplasmic accumulation of β (beta)-catenin, overwhelming tightly controlled degradation mechanisms, allowing for nuclear translocation and activity of β (beta)-catenin [2].

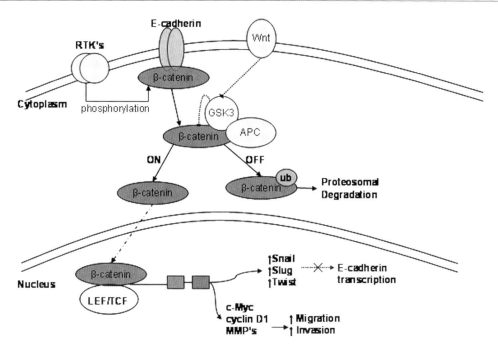

Fig. 2.2 Molecular mechanisms of EMT in colon cancer metastasis. Any number of receptor tyrosine kinases (RTK) can activate the EMT pathway. One proposed pathway is the phosphorylation of β (beta)-catenin by receptor tyrosine kinases releasing it from E-cadherin. Another mechanism of activation is the Wnt pathway, activating a transmembrane domain that inhibits GSK3β (beta). GSK3β (beta) is responsible for the ubiquitination and proteosomal degradation of β (beta)-catenin. However, GSK3β (beta) needs APC to form the complex that allows for the degradation of β (beta)-catenin. If β (beta)-catenin is not targeted for degradation or the amount of cytoplasmic β (beta)-catenin translocation is greater than what can be degraded, β (beta)-catenin can then be translocated to the nucleus. Once translocated to the nucleus it can bind to TCF/LEF and become transcriptionally active. β (beta)-catenin also binds to several other molecules not shown here. β (beta)-catenin can then upregulate Snail, Slug, and Twist that block the transcription of E-cadherin. β (beta)-catenin also can upregulate c-Myc, cyclin D1, and the productions of MMPs that increase migration and invasion

The absolute level of nuclear β (beta)-catenin appears to increase from early adenomas to later stage adenocarcinomas [14]. In invasive CRC, nuclear β (beta)-catenin is accumulated at the invasive front that has undergone EMT [15]. Wong et al. demonstrated that in 100% of metastatic CRC specimens there was nuclear expression of β (beta)-catenin and that high immunohistochemical staining correlated with lymph node metastases [16]. In addition, several investigators have found a significant correlation between decreased survival and increased nuclear β (beta)-catenin expression [16, 17]. Further support for the importance of β (beta)-catenin comes from a recent study by Lugli et al. which included over 1,420 CRC specimens that demonstrated increased nuclear β (beta)-catenin staining is an adverse prognostic factor [18]. The nuclear staining of β (beta)-catenin at the invasive front is suggestive of a higher likelihood of aggressive and metastatic disease leading to a poorer prognosis.

Vimentin, an intermediate filament that is an important part of the cytoskeletal structure of cells, is often overexpressed in cells that have undergone EMT [19]. In breast cancer, invasive, aggressive cells were shown to differentially express vimentin over cells that were non-invasive and in both breast and prostate cancer, tumor cell overexpression of vimentin was associated with a more malignant phenotype [20, 21, 22]. Interestingly, proteomic studies identified vimentin as a gene expressed in CRC but not in normal colonic tissue [23]. Recently, vimentin overexpression in the tumor stroma of CRC has been shown to be associated with a shorter survival and was a more sensitive prognostic marker for recurrence for patients with stage II and stage III rather than lymph node status [24]. This may suggest that overexpression of vimentin at the tumor–stroma interface is a marker for more aggressive and metastatic disease; however, this is still an area under investigation.

The Snail family of nuclear transcription factors which includes Snail, Slug, and Twist has been shown to be an important part of the EMT process. In vitro studies with carcinoma cell lines that lack E-cadherin produce significant amounts of Snail, and the transfection of E-cadherin-positive lines with Snail results in the induction of EMT [25]. The nuclear translocation of β (beta)-catenin can upregulate the activity of the Snail family of transcription factors that can then bind to an inhibitory promoter of E-cadherin and directly repress E-cadherin transcription, furthering the EMT phenotype [26]. In CRC, Slug expression is an independent prognostic factor for a worse prognosis and associated with distant metastatic disease [27]. The Snail family of transcription factors is under intense scrutiny and may lead to novel therapeutic targets in CRC.

Invasion and Metastasis

For a CRC cell to metastasize to a distant organ, it must be able to invade and traverse the basement membrane (BM) and the extracellular matrix (ECM). Numerous mechanisms of tumor cell invasion of the BM have been described [28]. Anomalous survival and resistance to apoptosis are hallmarks of CRC invasion and progression to metastatic disease [29]. While the molecular mechanisms underlying EMT are currently being elucidated, little notice has been given to the possibility that aberrant cell survival mechanisms are a crucial element. Nonetheless, following EMT, CRC cells migrate and survive despite the lack of cell–cell contact, implying that the phenotypic alteration results in an escape from the constraints of adhesion-dependent survival.

CRC cells generate a wide variety of proteolytic enzymes. The family of proteases that has received the most interest has been the matrix metalloproteinases (MMPs). MMPs play an essential role in normal homeostatic physiology because the ECM and BM is a dynamic template of structural proteins, growth factors and enzymes, which is constantly being remodeled. The range of physiologic activities is impressive: MMPs can mediate cell death, cell proliferation, cell differentiation, tumor-associated angiogenesis, and malignant conversion [30]. MMPs are collectively able to degrade practically all ECM components, i.e., collagens, laminins, fibronectin, vibronectin, enactin, and proteoglycans [31]. There are at least 24 MMPs that have been historically divided into four subfamilies according to ECM substrate specificity and homology to other MMPs. Examination of MMP expression in human tumor tissue sections revealed that MMPs are largely produced by reactive stromal cells recruited to the neoplastic environment. The protease expression directly correlates to an invasive phenotype and tumor progression. Additional MMPs are essential to CRC liver metastases formation. Several investigators have shown that MMP-7 overexpression is associated with CRC metastases development and progression [32, 33].

Src in CRC Metastasis

Src, a nonreceptor tyrosine kinase, has been identified as playing a central role in tumor invasion and motility through changes in focal adhesion kinases and changes in adherens junctions. In CRC Src has been shown to be elevated in premalignant colon polyps, higher in primary CRC and highest in CRC liver metastasis [34]. c-Src is also activated in other sites of colon cancer metastasis [35]. Src may cooperate with tyrosine kinase receptors such as epidermal growth factor (EGF) and hepatocyte growth factor (HGF) to induce migration and invasion [36]. While the mechanisms of Src activation are still unclear, many cell lines have demonstrated that the increased levels of Src activation are due to an increase in the total protein level [37]. In experimental studies, elevated Src correlated with the ability to metastasize to the liver after intrasplenic injections, but did not affect cell growth rates [38]. c-SRC overexpression may also lead to an increase in angiogenesis and the reduction in Src activity has shown to be associated with a decrease in vascular endothelial growth factor (VEGF) [39]. Currently, several Src inhibitors, including Dasatinib (Bristol–Myers Squibb, Princeton, NJ, has been approved for CML) are in clinical trials. While Src inhibitors have not been shown to affect cell proliferation and growth in vitro, they may affect the rate of metastases.

Migration and Motility

Cell migration is necessary for tumor cells to gain access to the microvasculature. Cell migration is dependent upon the interaction of the tumor cells' cytoskeleton, forming membrane ruffles, filopodia and pseudopodia, and the ECM. This complicated interaction is stimulated by cytokines such as HGF and transforming growth factor β (beta) (TGF-β [beta]). HGF is a protein secreted by mesodermal cells and its receptor, c-met, is a transmembrane tyrosine kinase receptor that is expressed mainly in epithelial tissues [40]. In vitro experiments have shown that treatment of CRC cell lines with HGF leads to c-met activation and induces human CRC cell motility [41]. Activation of HGF/c-met leads to increased survival and growth in anchorage-independent conditions, as well as increased in vitro migration [42]. In human pathology specimens, concentrations of c-met mRNA have been demonstrated to be higher in hepatic metastases than in primary CRC tumors [43]. Approximately 50% of primary CRCs overexpress c-met, whereas up to 70% of liver metastases overexpress c-met compared with the primary colorectal tumor [44].

These studies imply that overexpression of the c-met protein and HGF may be essential to promoting the development of CRC metastases.

Growth factors and Tumor Angiogenesis

Once a tumor cell becomes fixed into the hepatic parenchyma, it must be able to interact appropriately with the microenvironment. Proliferation, which is a decisive step in the growth of clinically significant metastases, may occur secondary to constitutively activated oncogenes or other microenvironmental stimuli, such as growth factors [45]. Growth factors function by binding to specific tyrosine kinase receptors, thereby transducing an extracellular signal. It is the activation of these receptors that leads to the transcription of genes that regulate metastatic tumor growth [46]. Growth factor ligands thought to be involved in the growth of colorectal liver metastases include EGF, insulin-like growth factor (IGF) and HGF [47].

The EGF axis comprises the EGF receptor (EGFR) and its ligands, EGF and transforming growth factor-α (alpha) [48]. These ligands mediate growth, proliferation, and metastases of CRC cells [49]. In vitro cell migration assay experiments have shown that treatment of CRC cells with EGF induces a chemomigratory response [50]. EGFR expression in primary cultures of established human CRC cell lines is significantly higher in cell lines from patients with American Joint Committee on Cancer (AJCC) stage III tumors than in lines established from earlier stage lesions. In addition, in vivo work has shown that increased EGFR expression correlates directly with the ability to produce liver metastases [51].

Parker et al. have shown that increased EGFR gene expression and functional protein levels correlate with metastatic potential of human CRC cells in athymic nude mice [52]. In this experiment, monoclonal antibodies specific for phosphorylated EGFR demonstrated increased immunoreactivity in metastatic liver lesions when compared to primary cecal or subcutaneous tumors. This implies that CRC liver metastases growth is dependent upon response to distant organ-derived growth factors and activation of cell-surface tyrosine kinase receptors.

Once a tumor ascertains an invasive phenotype in the organ of metastasis, it must establish its own neovascular blood supply. Amplified vascularity may allow not only an increase in tumor growth but also a better chance of hematogenous tumor embolization [53]. Preliminary work in the field of angiogenesis was based on a simple model in which a tumor cell would secrete a soluble factor that would bind to an endothelial cell receptor and induce proliferation. Current models suggest that angiogenesis is dependent upon the balance among stimulatory and inhibitory molecules (see Table 2.1).

Vascular Endothelial Growth Factor

Vascular endothelial growth factor (VEGF) is probably the most studied and best-characterized angiogenic effector molecule. VEGF is known to be upregulated in CRC, and the relationship of VEGF level with the metastatic potential of colon cancers and overall patient survival has been well described [54]. VEGF, VEGF-receptors, and vessel counts have been shown to be present in higher amounts in metastatic rather than nonmetastatic tumors, and directly correlated with the degree of neovascularization and proliferation [55].

In a following paper, VEGF and vessels counts were evaluated for their ability to serve as prognostic markers in node-negative CRC patients [56]. These study patients

Table 2.1 Endogenous stimulatory and inhibitory angiogenic factors

Stimulatory	Inhibitory
Acidic fibroblast growth factor (FGF)	Angiostatin
Basic FGF	Endostatin
Angiogenin	Vasculostatin
HGF	Interferon α, β, γ (alpha, beta, gamma)
IL-8	IP-10
MMP	Platelet factor 4
Placenta growth factor	Prolactin fragment
Platelet derived growth factor (PDGF)	Thrombospondin-1,2
Transforming growth factor-α, β (TGF)-α, β (alpha, beta)	TIMP 1–4
Tumor necrosis factor-α (alpha)	Others
VEGF/vascular permeability factor	
Others	

were not given adjuvant chemotherapy and were observed for a minimum of 5 years. Low vessel counts correlated with a favorable prognosis and higher vessels counts were associated with disease recurrence. Patients whose tumors had low VEGF expression had improved outcomes and survival rates than patients with elevated VEGF expression.

VEGF has also been identified as a candidate survival factor whose expression is increased in response to EMT [57]. Concomitant upregulation of Flt-1, a tyrosine kinase VEGF receptor, accompanied the increase in VEGF production. Importantly, we characterized this VEGF/Flt-1 autocrine interaction as necessary for survival of the CRC cells, since disruption of Flt-1 function causes significant apoptosis in cells that underwent EMT. Significantly, this finding defined the acquisition of the self-regulated survival pathway as an essential component of the EMT process itself.

Liver Metastases and Apoptosis

Another means by which CRC liver metastases survive and proliferate in the new microenvironment is by avoiding the intrinsic process of apoptosis [58, 59]. Apoptosis was initially described as a physiologic process of cellular suicide or "programmed cell death" [60]. Apoptosis is vital for normal homeostasis and the apoptotic machinery is present in virtually all eukaryotes. Cellular stress leading to the activation of death-inducing factors or the withdrawal of surviving factors can trigger apoptosis. A complex balance between pro- and anti-apoptotic proteins regulates this process. Colorectal metastases can exploit these factors to bypass the normal pathways that would normally trigger apoptosis. The upregulation of anti-apoptotic genes (Bcl-2, Bcl-X_L, and Mcl-1) and the downregulation of pro-apoptotic genes are mechanisms to avoid apoptosis (Bax, Bak, Bad, Bim, Noxa, and Puma) [61]. Altered expression and function in these Bcl-2 family of proteins, a major apoptosis-regulatory protein family, often occurs in cancers.

During the adenoma to carcinoma sequence, decreased expression of p53 has demonstrated a loss of regulatory apoptosis and cell cycle arrest. Numerous groups have studied the expression of Bcl-2 (B cell lymphoma 2) family members during colon tumorigenesis [62]. Bcl-X_L overexpression has been observed in colon adenocarcinoma and in some adenomas, implying that upregulation of the anti-apoptotic Bcl-X_L is a relatively early event in adenoma to carcinoma transition [63]. Decreased expression of the pro-apoptotic genes Bak and Bax may also be associated with tumor progression and escape from

apoptotic control. Development of novel agents that (1) inhibit upregulated pro-survival mechanisms and (2) function as pro-apoptotic mimetics remains an active area of interest.

Anti-Angiogenic Treatment of Liver Metastases

Anti-VEGF Therapy

It is well understood that angiogenesis is essential for both tumor growth and metastases formation. This fact has led to a monumental research effort in an effort to discover novel anti-angiogenic compounds. However, angiogenesis is not only a pathologic process, but is also crucial for homeostasis. Normal physiologic angiogenesis is essential for reproduction, wound healing, menses, as well as a compensatory response to ischemia in both coronary artery and peripheral vascular disease [64]. Therefore, therapeutic efficacy of anti-angiogenic therapy requires equilibrium where angiogenesis in tumors is inhibited without interrupting physiologic angiogenesis.

The fact that VEGF signaling is an autocrine loop that appears to be a consequence of EMT is consistent with the notion that autocrine signaling of survival is manifested during the later stages of carcinoma progression [65]. Obviously, the acquisition of an inherent ability to inhibit apoptosis, in an autocrine manner, could play a chief role in CRC tumorigenesis. These findings are substantiated by other reports of both VEGF and Flt-1 gene expression as being upregulated during neoplastic progression of the colonic epithelia mucosa, as well as the increased Flt-1 mRNA in hepatic CRC metastases [66]. The identification of VEGF/Flt-1-mediated survival may have therapeutic implications for CRC, substantiating the clinical utility of EMT. In several mouse models, transfection of Flt-1, which acts in a dominant-negative manner to the endogenously expressed receptor, has been effective for a variety of cancer types, including colon, ovarian, pancreatic, and lung [67, 68, 69]. These studies concluded that the suppression of primary tumor growth and prolonged animal survival were based on the ability of the soluble receptor to block angiogenesis. Thus, anti-angiogenic gene therapy using soluble Flt-1 is considered to be a potential avenue for therapeutic exploitation. In this regard, it is interesting to note that VEGF inhibitors represent a new class of novel therapeutic agents for the treatment of CRC [70]. Warren et al. first reported the inhibitory effects of a VEGF monoclonal antibody (mAb) on the growth of CRC hepatic metastases [71]. These mAbs significantly decreased the growth of human CRC cell lines in the livers of nude mice, when compared to isotopic control antibody mice. Another anti-angiogenic strategy utilizes anti-VEGF receptor antibodies. DC101 (Imclone, Brooklyn, NY, USA), a mAb directed against VEGFR-2 (KDR), has been shown to be anti-angiogenic, inhibiting both EC survival and VEGF-mediated ascites formation in a murine model of colon cancer carcinomatosis [72].

Another mAb that has revolutionized anti-angiogenic or targeted therapy is bevacizumab (Genentech, San Francisco, CA, USA). It has been involved in several clinical trials with results that have demonstrated improved survival when compared to previous regimens for advanced CRC. This humanized antibody binds to VEGF-A and neutralizes its function by steric hindrance; thus its effects in vivo have been interpreted as acting via an inherent ability to inhibit angiogenesis. However, since clinical trials are often limited to patients who have metastatic disease it is possible that bevacizumab may also be affecting VEGF-mediated survival pathways that are elaborated as a consequence of EMT.

Kabbinavar et al. reported promising results from a phase II trial comparing bevacizumab plus 5-FU/leucovorin vs. 5-FU/leucovorin alone in the treatment of metastatic CRC [73]. Compared with the control patients, those treated with bevacizumab plus 5-FU/leucovorin resulted in higher response rates, longer progression-free survival (PFS), and longer median survival. In a landmark phase III trial, bevacizumab plus irinotecan/5-FU/ leucovorin (IFL) was demonstrated to be more effective than a standard IFL chemotherapy regimen [74]. In this report, Hurwitz et al. demonstrated a median survival of 20.3 months in the patients given bevacizumab/IFL compared to only 15.6 months in the control group. In the experimental group, the median PFS was longer (10.6 months vs. 6.2 months, P value<0.00001). Those patients receiving bevacizumab/IFL demonstrated higher response rates (44.9%) than IFL chemotherapy alone (34.7%) (see Table 2.2).

In another important clinical trial, Giantonio et al. presented results of ECOG 3200 a 3-arm phase III study of 822 patients with progressive metastatic CRC after 5-FU and irinotecan who had not received prior oxaliplatin or Avastin [75]. Patients were randomized to receive FOLFOX, Avastin (10 mg/kg), or the combination.

Patients treated with FOLFOX + Avastin had an approximately 2-month improvement in PFS and overall survival (OS) and improved response rate compared to FOLFOX monotherapy. Response rates were improved by approximately 10% with the addition of bevacizumab. Avastin monotherapy was inferior to both other arms. It is important to note that ECOG 3200 excluded patients who had previously received bevacizumab. Therefore, it does not address the second-line use of Avastin after failure of an Avastin-containing regimen. Instead, the study serves to validate Avastin's contribution of additional benefit to FOLFOX.

Inhibitors of Epidermal Growth factor

Antibodies directed against EGFR have received considerable interest for the treatment of CRC [76]. Clinical trials using anti-EGFR strategies have also shown effective results in stage IV CRC [77]. Saltz et al. have reported on the use of cetuximab (Erbitux®, Imclone Systems Inc. New York, NY, USA), a chimeric monoclonal antibody that binds selectively to EGFR with high affinity, competes for ligand binding, and downregulates receptor expression on the cell surface [78]. In this study, cetuximab was used in combination with irinotecan (Pfizer Oncology, New York, NY, USA) in patients with refractory and advanced CRC. Twenty-one patients (17%) achieved a partial response, and an additional 37 patients (31%) had stable disease or minor responses. Cetuximab associated toxicities are minor, yet an interesting toxicity is the development of a cutaneous rash. There is a significant association between rash severity and cetuximab clinical response [79].

In another important trial, Cunningham et al. compared the efficacy of cetuximab in combination with irinotecan with that of cetuximab alone in metastatic CRC that was refractory to treatment with irinotecan [80]. The investigators randomly assigned 329 patients whose disease had progressed during or within 3 months after treatment with an irinotecan based regimen to receive either cetuximab and irinotecan or cetuximab monotherapy. The patients were evaluated for tumor response and also for the time to tumor progression, survival, and side

Table 2.2 Summary of bevacizumab plus IFL compared to IFL chemotherapy only

Survival and response rates	IFL/placebo ($n=412$)	IFL/BV ($n=403$)	P value
Median survival (months)	15.6	20.3	0.00003
Progression-free survival	6.24	10.6	<0.00001
Objective response	35%	45%	0.0029
Duration of response (months)	7.1	10.4	0.0014

effects of treatment. Response rates in the combination-therapy group were significantly higher than that in the monotherapy group (22.9% vs. 10.8%, $P = 0.007$). The median time to progression was significantly greater in the combination-therapy group (4.1 vs. 1.5 months, $P < 0.001$). The median survival time was 8.6 months in the combination-therapy group and 6.9 months in the monotherapy group ($P = 0.48$). The authors conclude that cetuximab has clinically significant activity when given alone or in combination with irinotecan in patients with irinotecan-refractory CRC.

To date, there has not been a published clinical trial comparing bevacizumab to cetuximab; however, an ongoing CALGB/SWOG trial CTSU/C80405 is designed to address this issue [81]. This is a phase III study in which irinotecan/5-FU/leucovorin or oxaliplatin/5-FU/leucovorin with bevacizumab, cetuximab (C225), or with the combination of bevacizumab and cetuximab therapies are being used in patients with untreated metastatic CRC. Current clinical trial data support the use of bevacizumab as first-line treatment of metastatic CRC [82]. Outside of a clinical trial or off-protocol use of cetuximab is likely to be used in patients who cannot take bevacizumab or have failed bevacizumab therapy.

Summary

The study of tumor interaction with the surrounding microenvironment has increased our understanding of the biologic mechanisms regulating metastatic development. The capacity to develop effective biologic or targeted therapies will depend on understanding of the underlying complex mechanisms between endothelial and tumor cells. Biologic therapies must be directed at both the primary site and metastatic focus. By the time of metastatic formation, the majority of steps in the cascade have been accomplished. Specific therapy to down-regulate or interrupt the final stages of metastases, proliferation, angiogenesis, and other tumor pro-survival mechanisms appear to be the most promising areas of clinical research.

References

1. Butler TP, Gullino PM. Quantitation of cell shedding into efferent blood of mammary adenocarcinoma. Cancer Res. 1975; 35 (3) 512–6.
2. Thiery JP. Epithelial-mesenchymal transitions in tumour progression. Nat Rev Cancer. 2002; 2 (6) 442–54.
3. Katoh M. Epithelial-mesenchymal transition in gastric cancer (Review). Int J Oncol. 2005; 27 (6) 1677–83.
4. Horikawa T, Yang J, Kondo S, et al. Twist and epithelial-mesenchymal transition are induced by the EBV oncoprotein latent membrane protein 1 and are associated with metastatic nasopharyngeal carcinoma. Cancer Res. 2007; 67 (5) 1970–8.
5. Vasko V, Espinosa AV, Scouten W, et al. Gene expression and functional evidence of epithelial-to-mesenchymal transition in papillary thyroid carcinoma invasion. Proc Natl Acad Sci USA. 2007; 104 (8) 2803–8.
6. Spaderna S, Schmalhofer O, Hlubek F, et al. A transient, EMT-linked loss of basement membranes indicates metastasis and poor survival in colorectal cancer. Gastroenterology. 2006; 131 (3) 830–40.
7. Kemler R. From cadherins to catenins: Cytoplasmic protein interactions and regulation of cell adhesion. Trends Genet. 1993; 9 (9) 317–21.
8. More H, Humar B, Weber W, et al. Identification of seven novel germline mutations in the human E-cadherin (CDH1) gene. Hum Mutat. 2007; 28 (2) 203.
9. Hugh TJ, Dillon SA, Taylor BA, et al. Cadherin-catenin expression in primary colorectal cancer: A survival analysis. Br J Cancer. 1999; 80 (7) 1046–51.
10. Elzagheid A, Algars A, Bendardaf R, et al. E-cadherin expression pattern in primary colorectal carcinomas and their metastases reflects disease outcome. World J Gastroenterol. 2006; 12 (27) 4304–9.
11. Delektorskaya VV, Perevoshchikov AG, Golovkov DA, Kushlinskii NE. Expression of E-cadherin, beta-catenin, and CD-44v6 cell adhesion molecules in primary tumors and metastases of colorectal adenocarcinoma. Bull Exp Biol Med. 2005; 139 (6) 706–10.
12. Kim JC, Roh SA, Kim HC, et al. Coexpression of carcinoembryonic antigen and E-cadherin in colorectal adenocarcinoma with liver metastasis. J Gastrointest Surg. 2003; 7 (7) 931–8.
13. Mariadason JM, Bordonaro M, Aslam F, et al. Down-regulation of beta-catenin TCF signaling is linked to colonic epithelial cell differentiation. Cancer Res. 2001; 61 (8) 3465–71.
14. Brabletz T, Jung A, Kirchner T. Beta-catenin and the morphogenesis of colorectal cancer. Virchows Arch. 2002; 441 (1) 1–11.
15. Brabletz T, Jung A, Spaderna S, et al. Opinion: migrating cancer stem cells—an integrated concept of malignant tumour progression. Nat Rev Cancer. 2005; 5 (9) 744–9.
16. Wong SC, Lo ES, Lee KC, et al. Prognostic and diagnostic significance of beta-catenin nuclear immunostaining in colorectal cancer. Clin Cancer Res. 2004; 10 (4) 1401–8.
17. Cheah PY, Choo PH, Yao J, et al. A survival-stratification model of human colorectal carcinomas with beta-catenin and p27kip1. Cancer. 2002; 95 (12) 2479–86.
18. Lugli A, Zlobec I, Minoo P, et al. Prognostic significance of the wnt signalling pathway molecules APC, beta-catenin and E-cadherin in colorectal cancer: A tissue microarray-based analysis. Histopathology. 2007; 50 (4) 453–64.
19. Lee JM, Dedhar S, Kalluri R, Thompson EW. The epithelial-mesenchymal transition: New insights in signaling, development, and disease. J Cell Biol. 2006; 172 (7) 973–81.
20. Nagaraja GM, Othman M, Fox BP, et al. Gene expression signatures and biomarkers of noninvasive and invasive breast cancer cells: Comprehensive profiles by representational difference analysis, microarrays and proteomics. Oncogene. 2006; 25 (16) 2328–38.
21. Zajchowski DA, Bartholdi MF, Gong Y, et al. Identification of gene expression profiles that predict the aggressive behavior of breast cancer cells. Cancer Res. 2001; 61 (13) 5168–78.
22. Lang SH, Hyde C, Reid IN, et al. Enhanced expression of vimentin in motile prostate cell lines and in poorly differentiated and metastatic prostate carcinoma. Prostate. 2002; 52 (4) 253–63.

23. Alfonso P, Nunez A, Madoz-Gurpide J, et al. Proteomic expression analysis of colorectal cancer by two-dimensional differential gel electrophoresis. Proteomics. 2005; 5 (10) 2602–11.
24. Ngan CY, Yamamoto H, Seshimo I, et al. Quantitative evaluation of vimentin expression in tumour stroma of colorectal cancer. Br J Cancer. 2007; 96 (6) 986–92.
25. Cano A, Perez-Moreno MA, Rodrigo I, et al. The transcription factor snail controls epithelial-mesenchymal transitions by repressing E-cadherin expression. Nat Cell Biol. 2000; 2 (2) 76–83.
26. Conacci-Sorrell M, Simcha I, Ben-Yedidia T, et al. Autoregulation of E-cadherin expression by cadherin-cadherin interactions: The roles of beta-catenin signaling, Slug, and MAPK. J Cell Biol. 2003; 163 (4) 847–57.
27. Shioiri M, Shida T, Koda K, et al. Slug expression is an independent prognostic parameter for poor survival in colorectal carcinoma patients. Br J Cancer. 2006; 94 (12) 1816–22.
28. Gutman M, Fidler IJ. Biology of human colon cancer metastasis. World J Surg. 1995; 19 (2) 226–34.
29. Jaattela M. Escaping cell death: Survival proteins in cancer. Exp Cell Res. 1999; 248 (1) 30–43.
30. Coussens LM, Fingleton B, Matrisian LM. Matrix metalloproteinase inhibitors and cancer: Trials and tribulations. Science. 2002; 295 (5564): 2387–92.
31. McCawley LJ, Matrisian LM. Matrix metalloproteinases: They're not just for matrix anymore! Curr Opin Cell Biol. 2001; 13 (5) 534–40.
32. Masaki T, Matsuoka H, Sugiyama M, et al. Matrilysin (MMP-7) as a significant determinant of malignant potential of early invasive colorectal carcinomas. Br J Cancer. 2001; 84 (10) 1317–21.
33. Wilson CL, Heppner KJ, Labosky PA, et al. Intestinal tumorigenesis is suppressed in mice lacking the metalloproteinase matrilysin. Proc Natl Acad Sci USA. 1997; 94 (4) 1402–7.
34. Termuhlen PM, Curley SA, Talamonti MS, et al. Site-specific differences in pp60c-src activity in human colorectal metastases. J Surg Res. 1993; 54 (4) 293–8.
35. Talamonti MS, Roh MS, Curley SA, Gallick GE. Increase in activity and level of pp60c-src in progressive stages of human colorectal cancer. J Clin Invest. 1993; 91 (1) 53–60.
36. Leu TH, Maa MC. Functional implication of the interaction between EGF receptor and c-Src. Front Biosci. 2003; 8: s28–38.
37. Mao W, Irby R, Coppola D, et al. Activation of c-Src by receptor tyrosine kinases in human colon cancer cells with high metastatic potential. Oncogene. 1997; 15 (25) 3083–90.
38. Jones RJ, Avizienyte E, Wyke AW, et al. Elevated c-Src is linked to altered cell-matrix adhesion rather than proliferation in KM12C human colorectal cancer cells. Br J Cancer. 2002; 87 (10) 1128–35.
39. Ellis LM, Staley CA, Liu W, et al. Down regulation of vascular endothelial growth factor in a human colon carcinoma cell line transfected with an antisense expression vector specific for c-src. J Biol Chem. 1998; 273 (2) 1052–7.
40. Harvey P, Clark IM, Jaurand MC, et al. Hepatocyte growth factor/scatter factor enhances the invasion of mesothelioma cell lines and the expression of matrix metalloproteinases. Br J Cancer. 2000; 83 (9) 1147–53.
41. Li HW, Shan JX. Effects of hepatocyte growth factor/scatter factor on the invasion of colorectal cancer cells in vitro. World J Gastroenterol. 2005; 11 (25) 3877–81.
42. Herynk MH, Tsan R, Radinsky R, Gallick GE. Activation of c-Met in colorectal carcinoma cells leads to constitutive association of tyrosine-phosphorylated beta-catenin. Clin Exp Metastasis. 2003; 20 (4) 291–300.
43. Fujita S, Sugano K. Expression of c-met proto-oncogene in primary colorectal cancer and liver metastases. Jpn J Clin Oncol. 1997; 27 (6) 378–83.
44. Di Renzo MF, Olivero M, Giacomini A, et al. Overexpression and amplification of the met/HGF receptor gene during the progression of colorectal cancer. Clin Cancer Res. 1995; 1 (2) 147–54.
45. Pawlik TM, Choti MA. Shifting from clinical to biologic indicators of prognosis after resection of hepatic colorectal metastases. Curr Oncol Rep. 2007; 9 (3) 193–201.
46. Cruz J, Ocana A, Del Barco E, Pandiella A. Targeting receptor tyrosine kinases and their signal transduction routes in head and neck cancer. Ann Oncol. 2007; 18 (3) 421–30.
47. Itoh Y, Joh T, Tanida S, et al. IL-8 promotes cell proliferation and migration through metalloproteinase-cleavage proHB-EGF in human colon carcinoma cells. Cytokine. 2005; 29 (6) 275–82.
48. Malecka-Panas E, Kordek R, Biernat W, et al. Differential activation of total and EGF receptor (EGF-R) tyrosine kinase (tyr-k) in the rectal mucosa in patients with adenomatous polyps, ulcerative colitis and colon cancer. Hepatogastroenterology. 1997; 44 (14) 435–40.
49. Markowitz SD, Molkentin K, Gerbic C, et al. Growth stimulation by coexpression of transforming growth factor-alpha and epidermal growth factor-receptor in normal and adenomatous human colon epithelium. J Clin Invest. 1990; 86 (1) 356–62.
50. Suzuki E, Ota T, Tsukuda K, et al. nm23-H1 reduces in vitro cell migration and the liver metastatic potential of colon cancer cells by regulating myosin light chain phosphorylation. Int J Cancer. 2004; 108 (2) 207–11.
51. Buchanan FG, Gorden DL, Matta P, et al. Role of beta-arrestin 1 in the metastatic progression of colorectal cancer. Proc Natl Acad Sci USA. 2006; 103 (5) 1492–7.
52. Parker C, Roseman BJ, Bucana CD, et al. Preferential activation of the epidermal growth factor receptor in human colon carcinoma liver metastases in nude mice. J Histochem Cytochem. 1998; 46 (5) 595–602.
53. Rmali KA, Puntis MC, Jiang WG. Tumour-associated angiogenesis in human colorectal cancer. Colorectal Dis. 2007; 9 (1) 3–14.
54. Tonra JR, Hicklin DJ. Targeting the vascular endothelial growth factor pathway in the treatment of human malignancy. Immunol Invest. 2007; 36 (1) 3–23.
55. Reinmuth N, Parikh AA, Ahmad SA, et al. Biology of angiogenesis in tumors of the gastrointestinal tract. Microsc Res Tech. 2003; 60 (2) 199–207.
56. Takahashi Y, Tucker SL, Kitadai Y, et al. Vessel counts and expression of vascular endothelial growth factor as prognostic factors in node-negative colon cancer. Arch Surg. 1997; 132 (5) 541–6.
57. Bates RC, Goldsmith JD, Bachelder RE, et al. Flt-1-dependent survival characterizes the epithelial-mesenchymal transition of colonic organoids. Curr Biol. 2003; 13 (19) 1721–7.
58. Bernet A, Mehlen P. Dependence receptors: When apoptosis controls tumor progression. Bull Cancer. 2007; 94 (4) E12–7.
59. Blank M, Shiloh Y. Programs for cell death: Apoptosis is only one way to go. Cell Cycle. 2007; 6 (6) 686–95.
60. Kerr JF, Wyllie AH, Currie AR. Apoptosis: A basic biological phenomenon with wide-ranging implications in tissue kinetics. Br J Cancer. 1972; 26 (4) 239–57.
61. Willis SN, Adams JM. Life in the balance: How BH3-only proteins induce apoptosis. Curr Opin Cell Biol. 2005; 17 (6) 617–25.
62. Backus HH, Van Groeningen CJ, Vos W, et al. Differential expression of cell cycle and apoptosis related proteins in

colorectal mucosa, primary colon tumours, and liver metastases. J Clin Pathol. 2002; 55 (3) 206–11.

63. Rupnarain C, Dlamini Z, Naicker S, Bhoola K. Colon cancer: genomics and apoptotic events. Biol Chem. 2004; 385 (6) 449–64.

64. Pang RW, Poon RT. Clinical implications of angiogenesis in cancers. Vasc Health Risk Manag. 2006; 2 (2) 97–108.

65. Mercurio AM, Bachelder RE, Bates RC, Chung J. Autocrine signaling in carcinoma: VEGF and the alpha6beta4 integrin. Semin Cancer Biol. 2004; 14 (2) 115–22.

66. Andre T, Kotelevets L, Vaillant JC, et al. VEGF, VEGF-B, VEGF-C and their receptors KDR, FLT-1 and FLT-4 during the neoplastic progression of human colonic mucosa. Int J Cancer. 2000; 86 (2) 174–81.

67. Kuo CJ, Farnebo F, Yu EY, et al. Comparative evaluation of the antitumor activity of antiangiogenic proteins delivered by gene transfer. Proc Natl Acad Sci USA. 2001; 98 (8) 4605–10.

68. Takayama K, Ueno H, Nakanishi Y, et al. Suppression of tumor angiogenesis and growth by gene transfer of a soluble form of vascular endothelial growth factor receptor into a remote organ. Cancer Res. 2000; 60 (8) 2169–77.

69. Hasumi Y, Mizukami H, Urabe M, et al. Soluble FLT-1 expression suppresses carcinomatous ascites in nude mice bearing ovarian cancer. Cancer Res. 2002; 62 (7) 2019–23.

70. Diaz-Rubio E. New chemotherapeutic advances in pancreatic, colorectal, and gastric cancers. Oncologist. 2004; 9 (3) 282–94.

71. Warren RS, Yuan H, Matli MR, et al. Regulation by vascular endothelial growth factor of human colon cancer tumorigenesis in a mouse model of experimental liver metastasis. J Clin Invest. 1995; 95 (4) 1789–97.

72. Shaheen RM, Tseng WW, Vellagas R, et al. Effects of an antibody to vascular endothelial growth factor receptor-2 on survival, tumor vascularity, and apoptosis in a murine model of colon carcinomatosis. Int J Oncol. 2001; 18 (2) 221–6.

73. Kabbinavar F, Hurwitz HI, Fehrenbacher L, et al. Phase II, randomized trial comparing bevacizumab plus fluorouracil (FU)/leucovorin (LV) with FU/LV alone in patients with metastatic colorectal cancer. J Clin Oncol. 2003; 21 (1) 60–5.

74. Hurwitz H, Fehrenbacher L, Novotny W, et al. Bevacizumab plus irinotecan, fluorouracil, and leucovorin for metastatic colorectal cancer. N Engl J Med. 2004; 350 (23) 2335–42.

75. Giantonio B, Catalano P, Meropol N. High-dose bevacizumab improves survival when combined with FOLFOX4 in previously treated advanced colorectal cancer: Results from the Eastern Cooperative Oncology Group E3200. In: Proceedings of American Society of Clinical Oncology, Orlando FL, 2005, Abstract #2.

76. Chu E. Targeted therapy. Clin Colorectal Cancer. 2007; 6 (5) 336.

77. Chung KY, Saltz LB. Antibody-based therapies for colorectal cancer. Oncologist. 2005; 10 (9) 701–9.

78. Saltz LB, Meropol NJ, Loehrer PJ Sr, et al. Phase II trial of cetuximab in patients with refractory colorectal cancer that expresses the epidermal growth factor receptor. J Clin Oncol. 2004; 22 (7) 1201–8.

79. Perez-Soler R, Saltz L. Cutaneous adverse effects with HER1/EGFR-targeted agents: Is there a silver lining? J Clin Oncol. 2005; 23 (22) 5235–46.

80. Cunningham D, Humblet Y, Siena S, et al. Cetuximab monotherapy and cetuximab plus irinotecan in irinotecan-refractory metastatic colorectal cancer. N Engl J Med. 2004; 351 (4) 337–45.

81. Southwest Oncology Group. A Phase III trial of irinotecan/5-FU/leucovorin or oxaliplatin/5-FU/leucovorin with bevacizumab, or cetuximab (C225), or with the combination of bevacizumab and cetuximab for patients with untreated metastatic adenocarcinoma of the colon or rectum. http://www.swog.org/Visitors/ViewProtocolDetails.asp?ProtocolID = 1999 Accessed May 23, 2007.

82. de Gramont A, Tournigand C, Andre T, et al. Adjuvant therapy for stage II and III colorectal cancer. Semin Oncol. 2007; 34 (2 Suppl 1): S37–40.

Dario Ribero, Yun Shin Chun, and Jean-Nicolas Vauthey

Introduction

Colorectal adenocarcinoma is the most common gastro-intestinal malignancy and the second leading cause of cancer-related death in the United States. In the year 2007, over 150,000 new patients are expected to be diagnosed with colorectal cancer, and over 50,000 patients will die of the disease [1]. The liver is the most common site of distant metastases from colorectal cancer with approximately 25% of patients diagnosed with synchronous colorectal liver metastases (CLM) at presentation. A further 30% of patients develop metachronous CLM, usually within the first 2 years following primary tumor resection [2]. Without treatment, the median survival of patients with CLM is measured in months, and 5-year survival is almost nil. Although the development of new chemotherapeutic and biologic agents has led to increased response rates, the median survival for patients treated with the best available systemic therapy alone remains 20 months [3, 4]. Complete hepatic resection is the only potentially curative therapy for patients with CLM, resulting in 5-year overall survival rates of up to 58% [5]. The objectives of this chapter are to describe selection criteria of patients for hepatic resection, the current definition of resectability, strategies to increase resectability, anesthetic and operative considerations, and surgery in the era of multimodality treatment for CLM.

Selection of Patients for Hepatic Resection

The identification of patients who are appropriate candidates for hepatic resection depends upon patients' medical fitness, tumor resectability, and anticipated extent of resection. The goal of a curative hepatic resection is to resect all tumors with microscopically negative margins while ensuring that sufficient functional liver parenchyma remains.

Patients' General Medical Fitness

Despite advances in perioperative care and surgical technique, morbidity rates after liver resection are significant, ranging between 22% and 45% [6, 7, 8]. In addition to ensuring adequate hepatic reserve, as outlined later in this chapter, preoperative considerations include patients' cardiopulmonary condition, comorbidities, and performance status. Most studies suggest that in the absence of major comorbidities, advanced age is not an independent predictor of increased perioperative morbidity [9, 10].

Assessment of Tumor Resectability and Anticipated Extent of Resection

The objectives of preoperative imaging studies are to anatomically define tumors and their relationship to vascular and biliary structures, identify the presence of extrahepatic disease, and plan the extent of resection. Helical, triple-phase computed tomography (CT) of the thorax, abdomen, and pelvis is the preferred preoperative imaging modality, with the portal venous phase providing the greatest discrimination for CLM. Recent studies of multi-detector helical CT show that sensitivity for detection of CLM ranges between 70% and 95% [11, 12]. In patients with fatty livers, magnetic resonance imaging (MRI) is more sensitive than CT.

Some authors have advocated the use of 18F-fluoro-deoxyglucose-positron emission tomography (FDG-PET) as the most accurate imaging tool for CLM,

J.-N. Vauthey (✉)
Professor of Surgery, Department of Surgical Oncology,
The University of Texas M.D. Anderson Cancer Center, Houston,
TX, USA

J.-N. Vauthey et al. (eds.), *Liver Metastases*, DOI 10.1007/978-1-84628-947-7_3,
© Springer-Verlag London Limited 2009

detecting CT-occult disease in approximately 25% of patients [13]. However, FDG-PET, based on increased glucose uptake by malignancies, is not tumor specific, and false-positive results can arise in benign conditions, including inflammation and infection [14]. Moreover, in patients who have recently received chemotherapy, glucose uptake by tumors is diminished, resulting in reduced sensitivity of FDG-PET [15]. In addition, the spatial resolution of FDG-PET remains inferior to that of CT or MRI, failing to provide the anatomic detail necessary for surgical planning. Thus, while some groups routinely use FDG-PET in the preoperative evaluation of patients with CLM, the risk of false-positive findings and increased costs should be considered.

Diagnostic laparoscopy has been used to identify patients with occult peritoneal or extrahepatic nodal disease missed on preoperative imaging. However, most studies show a relatively low yield of laparoscopy, preventing unnecessary laparotomy in only 5–10% of patients, at the expense of increased operative time and costs [16, 17].

Definition of Resectability—A Changing Paradigm

Previously, assessment of the resectability of CLM focused on morphologic characteristics of tumors. Current criteria of resectability focus on the liver that remains after resection rather than what is removed. Table 3.1 outlines changes in criteria of irresectability. In a recent expert consensus statement, resectability of CLM was defined as the ability to achieve a margin-negative resection while preserving two contiguous hepatic segments with adequate vascular inflow and outflow as well as biliary drainage, while ensuring that sufficient functional liver remains (more than 20% of the total estimated liver volume) [18].

Table 3.1 Changing paradigm in criteria of irresectability in patients with CLM

Traditional criteria	Contemporary criteria
Four or more metastases	Inability to perform R0 resection
Size >5 cm	
Bilateral disease	
Surgical margin <1 cm	Histologically positive margin
Extrahepatic metastases	Inability to resect all detectable disease
Clinicopathologic prognostic scoring systems, predating modern chemotherapy	Disease progression on modern chemotherapy

Multinodular and/or Bilateral Disease

In the past, liver resection was contraindicated in patients with multiple, bilateral CLM because of poor survival [19, 20]. However, in a contemporary study of 159 patients who received preoperative chemotherapy before resection of 4 or more metastases, a 5-year survival of 51% was achieved [21]. Similarly, Kokudo and coworkers found that survival of patients with four or more metastases was similar to that observed in patients with fewer metastases [22]. Thus, with modern chemotherapy and improvements in surgical technique, the presence of multiple bilateral disease should not preclude potentially curative hepatectomy [21].

Size >5 cm

Historically, patients who underwent resection of metastases with diameter greater than 4 or 5 cm were reported to have poorer survival rates. Recently, Minagawa and associates showed that in 235 patients undergoing resection of CLM, maximum tumor diameter did not affect patient survival [23]. Similarly, Hamady's group found that patients who underwent resection of metastases with diameter 8 cm or larger had comparable survival rates as patients with smaller metastases [24]. Thus, tumor diameter > 5 cm is not a contraindication to hepatectomy in CLM.

Surgical Margin

Older studies advocated 1 cm as the minimum surgical margin necessary for hepatectomy in CLM to achieve better disease-free survival [20, 25]. In 2006, a multicenter series of 557 patients was published, which demonstrated that the width of surgical margin does not affect recurrence or survival rates, provided the margin is histologically negative (Fig. 3.1). Similarly, in a study by Adam and colleagues of 138 patients with initially unresectable CLM who responded to chemotherapy and underwent secondary hepatectomy, 5-year overall survival was 33%, despite two-thirds of patients having a 0 mm margin [26]. Thus, an anticipated margin of less than 1 cm is not a contraindication for resection.

Hepatic and Pulmonary Metastases

Several reports have shown that surgical resection of isolated hepatic and pulmonary metastases from colorectal

Fig. 3.1 Survival after hepatic resection for CLM, stratified by margin status. There was no significant difference in survival among patients with a negative surgical margin, regardless of the width of the margin. Reprinted with permission from Pawlik et al. [91]

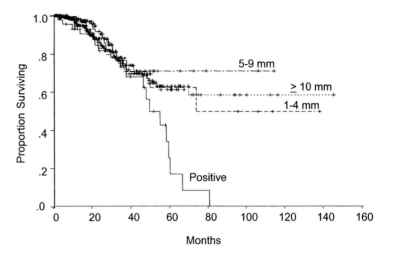

cancer is safe and associated with extended survival in selected patients, with 5-year overall survival rates ranging between 30% and 45% [27, 28, 29]. Factors shown to be associated with poorer survival are short disease-free interval between metastases (<1 year), multiple hepatic lesions, thoracic lymph node metastases, and elevated serum level of carcinoembryonic antigen (CEA) (>5 ng/mL) [27, 28].

Other Sites of Extrahepatic Disease

The classic contraindication to hepatic resection in CLM was the presence of extrahepatic disease, including peritoneal implants, extrahepatic nodal disease, and ovarian metastases. However, emerging data indicate that as a result of more effective chemotherapy, preoperative imaging, and surgical technique, selected patients with extrahepatic disease can undergo resection of all sites of metastases and have prolonged survival. Such patients with liver and extrahepatic diseases may be designated as borderline resectable [30]. In 2002, Jaeck and associates reported on the outcome of complete hilar lymphadenectomy for patients with CLM [31]. Although there were few 5-year survivors, 12% of patients survived 3 years, despite the presence of metastases in the periportal lymph nodes. In 2004, Elias and coworkers reported a 28% 5-year overall survival rate after simultaneous R0 resection of CLM and extrahepatic disease [32]. In a subsequent study, Elias' group found that the total number of resected metastases was a better predictor of survival than the number and location of anatomic sites, provided complete resection of all detectable disease was achieved [33]. Thus, even patients with multiple extrahepatic sites of disease may be selected for metastatectomy and achieve prolonged survival.

Prognostic Factors

Conventional clinicopathologic factors associated with poor outcome after hepatic resection for CLM include node-positive primary, disease-free interval of <12 months from primary to metastases, multiple hepatic tumors, size >5 cm, and CEA >200 ng/ml [34]. Using these criteria, Fong and colleagues at the Memorial Sloan-Kettering Cancer Center (MSKCC) devised a scoring system that was predictive of outcome. Notably, these prognostic factors were determined before the advent of effective systemic chemotherapy, and their utility as prognostic indicators in the era of modern chemotherapy is unknown. In a study from the Mayo Clinic, 662 patients were reviewed for risk factors on outcome after hepatic resection [35]. Perioperative blood transfusions and positive hepatoduodenal nodes were the major determinants of survival and recurrence. When applying three scoring systems from MSKCC [34], University of Pittsburgh [36], and a multicenter French study [37], the authors found that none of the scoring systems were predictive of survival or recurrence. They concluded that since no preoperative scoring system can predict which patients will have prolonged survival, hepatectomy should be performed if all gross disease can be resected.

In contrast to the limitations of traditional clinico-pathologic scoring systems, response to chemotherapy is emerging as a powerful prognostic tool and surrogate marker of tumor biology. Rubbia-Brandt and coworkers examined pathologic specimens in patients undergoing hepatectomy after preoperative chemotherapy and graded tumor regression [38]. They found that higher tumor regression grade was associated with improved overall and disease-free survival. This finding is in agreement with other studies showing that response to preoperative chemotherapy is predictive of improved survival after hepatic resection [26, 30].

Ensuring Sufficient Functional Hepatic Reserve and Strategies to Increase Resectability

By traditional criteria, only 10–15% of all patients with CLM are eligible for curative hepatectomy. Novel methods have been employed to allow more patients with CLM to be candidates for hepatic resection. These strategies include portal vein embolization (PVE), two-stage hepatectomy, and repeat hepatectomy. In patients who undergo aggressive treatment with such strategies, careful assessment of the remnant liver function is imperative to avoid postoperative hepatic failure.

Measuring the Future Liver Remnant (FLR)

When selecting patients for extended hepatectomy or hemihepatectomy with anticipated small remnant liver, a key determinant to ensuring adequate functional parenchyma remains is preoperative measurement of the future liver remnant (FLR) volume. The FLR volume is predictive of remnant liver function and has been shown to be predictive of postoperative clinical course [39, 40, 41, 42, 43]. The FLR volume is measured directly with three-dimensional CT and standardized to the total estimated liver volume (TELV), which is calculated using a formula based on the association between total liver volume and body surface area (BSA): TELV (cm^3) = $-794.41 + 1267.28 \times$ BSA (m^2). The ratio of the CT-measured FLR volume to the TELV is termed the "standardized FLR volume (sFLR)". Abdalla and colleagues showed that in patients without chronic liver disease undergoing extended hepatectomy, with or without PVE, patients with sFLR of $\leq 20\%$ had a complication rate of 50%, contrasted with a 13% complication rate in patients with sFLR $> 20\%$ [44]. Calculating the sFLR provides a standardized measurement of the functional remnant liver, allowing a uniform comparison of FLR volume, with or without PVE.

The minimum sFLR necessary for successful hepatic resection depends on multiple factors including the complexity of the anticipated resection, simultaneous procedures, patients' comorbidities, and underlying liver disease. Most patients with CLM have normal underlying liver, although more Western patients are presenting with liver disease associated with the metabolic syndrome, as well as chemotherapy-induced liver injury. In general, an sFLR of 20% is considered the minimum safe volume needed in patients with normal underlying liver, while an sFLR of 40% is required in patients with cirrhosis or

hepatitis. In patients who receive extensive chemotherapy before hepatic resection, an sFLR volume limit for safe resection of 30% has been proposed [45].

Portal Vein Embolization (PVE)

In patients who are otherwise candidates for major hepatectomy, an inadequate sFLR may be the only obstacle to curative resection. In such patients, preoperative PVE is a safe, minimally invasive procedure that redistributes intrahepatic portal flow to induce hypertrophy of the anticipated FLR [46]. PVE is usually performed through a percutaneous transhepatic ipsilateral approach, which uses ultrasound-guided puncture of a portal branch followed by portography and embolization of the entire portal territory to be resected with microparticles and microcoils [47]. In patients with inadequate sFLR, PVE has been demonstrated to result in significant increase in FLR volume, allowing safe and potentially curative major resection in patients who would otherwise not be candidates for resection based on inadequate remnant liver [44, 48].

Hypertrophy of the remnant liver follows a nonlinear kinetic profile during the first 2 months after PVE (Fig. 3.2). The greatest increase in liver volume (75%) occurs within 3 weeks after PVE, after which a plateau phase of minimal regeneration is reached [49]. Thus, the optimum interval time to assess response to PVE is 4 weeks. At this time, repeat CT volumetry is performed to determine whether a sufficient liver volume has been reached and to assess the degree of hypertrophy, defined as the difference in sFLR before and after PVE. Ribero and associates demonstrated that patients with slow liver growth during the first 3 weeks, specifically degree of hypertrophy of $\leq 5\%$, had a significantly worse clinical outcome, regardless of whether the target sFLR was reached [49]. Contraindications to PVE include portal hypertension, tumor extension to the FLR or portal vein, coagulopathy that cannot be corrected, biliary dilatation in the FLR, and renal failure.

Two-Stage Hepatectomy

In patients with extensive, bilateral disease that cannot be resected in a single procedure while preserving sufficient remnant liver, two-stage hepatectomy, with or without preoperative PVE, has been proposed. At the University of Texas M.D. Anderson Cancer Center, we employ sequentially more aggressive treatments as a strategy to select patients with extensive hepatic disease who are likely to benefit from complete resection of multiple,

29

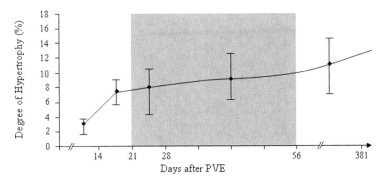

Fig. 3.2 Kinetics of future liver remnant (FLR) growth after portal vein embolization (PVE), plotted as median degree of hypertrophy. An early phase of hypertrophy occurs during the first 3 weeks after PVE, followed by a plateau phase, indicated by shaded zone, in which the increase in FLR volume is minimal. Reprinted with permission from Ribero et al. [49]

bilateral tumors (Fig. 3.3). Patients receive chemotherapy first; if their tumors respond or remain stable on chemotherapy, a minor resection of tumors in the future remnant liver is performed. Their hepatic regenerative capacity is assessed, with PVE if indicated, and a second-stage, major hepatectomy is performed. Similar to others, we found that such a step-wise approach to patients with multiple, bilateral tumor CLM results in favorable 3-year overall and disease-free survival rates of 86% and 51%, respectively [50,51].

Repeat Hepatectomy

After resection of CLM with curative intent, approximately 60–70% of patients will develop recurrent disease. Among patients who recur, one-third will have liver-only disease, of whom 10–33% with good performance status and adequate hepatic reserve are candidates for repeat hepatectomy [52, 53, 54]. Despite the technical challenges of repeat hepatectomy due to adhesions and altered hepatic anatomy, many reports show complication and survival rates after repeat hepatectomy to be similar to those after initial resections. In a study of two centers in the United States and Germany, resection of recurrent CLM resulted in a median survival of 31 months, which was comparable to that of initial resection [52].

Anesthesia and Operative Considerations

Several studies have demonstrated higher postoperative morbidity and mortality rates associated with increased blood loss and transfusion requirements [55,56]. Anesthesia and operative strategies have been developed to minimize intraoperative blood loss. Intraoperative ultrasound

(IOUS) is routinely performed to achieve margin-negative resections for both anatomic and wedge resections. The role of laparoscopic hepatectomy for CLM remains in evolution.

Anesthesia

Maintenance of low central venous pressure (CVP) and intermittent vascular inflow occlusion have resulted in significantly less intraoperative blood loss and perioperative morbidity and mortality [57]. Low CVP anesthesia reduces bleeding during parenchymal dissection and from inadvertent hepatic venous injuries. The CVP should be maintained at <5 mm Hg by limiting intravenous fluid administration until after parenchymal transection and hemostasis are secured. Intermittent vascular inflow occlusion is also used to reduce bleeding during parenchymal transection. Unlike total vascular occlusion, which is associated with a 30–60% decrease in cardiac output, inflow occlusion of the portal triad results in less hemodynamic perturbation and is better tolerated [58]. Communication between the surgeon and anesthesiologist is important, as occlusion of the portal triad results in a 5–10% decrease in cardiac output, 40% increase in systemic vascular resistance, and 15% increase in mean arterial pressure [59]. The hepatic ischemia that ensues after portal triad clamping can be tolerated in a healthy liver for up to 90 minutes and in a cirrhotic liver for up to 30 minutes.

At the University of Texas M.D. Anderson Cancer Center, most hepatic resections for CLM are performed with the use of continual thoracic epidural anesthesia, which allows for decreased intraoperative anesthetic use and optimal postoperative analgesia. Control of postoperative pain facilitates early patient mobilization and pulmonary mechanics, thereby reducing morbidity rates.

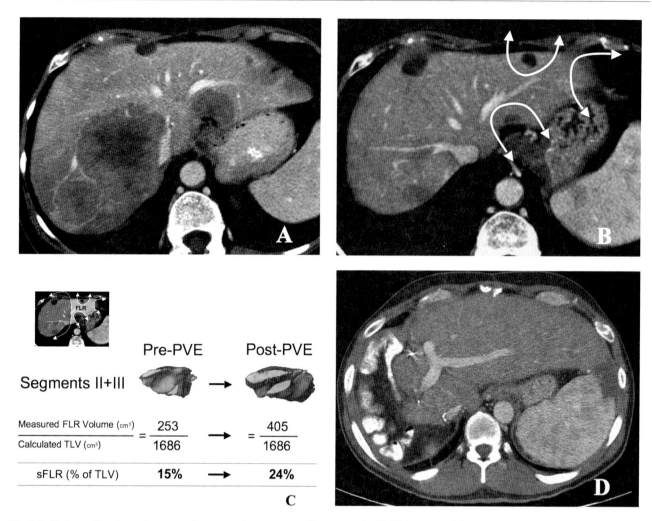

Fig. 3.3 Perioperative chemotherapy and two-stage hepatectomy. (**A**) CT of patient with multiple, bilateral CLM. (**B**) Radiographic response after six cycles of systemic therapy with 5-fluorouracil, leucovorin, and oxaliplatin. First-stage resection was performed with clearance of tumors in the future liver remnant (FLR), segments II–III (*white arrows*). (**C**) Volumetry of the FLR (*white area* in the inset) demonstrated an inadequate sFLR of 15%. Thus, PVE was performed with subsequent increase in sFLR to 24%. (**D**) CT scan performed 6 months after uneventful extended right hepatectomy and adjuvant chemotherapy showed no residual disease in the remnant liver

The use of epidural infusion also minimizes the use of narcotics during the immediate postoperative period, when liver metabolism may be compromised. Patients with uncorrectable coagulopathy should not undergo epidural catheter placement because of the risk of spinal hematoma.

Methods for Parenchymal Transection

Several devices have been developed to allow hemostatic parenchymal transection and expedite hepatic resection. These include radiofrequency and argon beam coagulators, saline-linked cautery (SLC), and ultrasonic dissectors.

At our institution, we have adopted a two-surgeon technique for hepatic transection, combining SLC with ultrasonic dissection (Fig. 3.4). In the past, we used the ultrasonic dissector for transection and suture ligatures and titanium clips for hemostasis. This was time-consuming and required the passage of multiple instruments. With the two-surgeon technique, the primary surgeon uses the ultrasonic dissector to delineate anatomy and transect the parenchyma, while the secondary surgeon uses the SLC to coagulate and divide small vessels and bile ducts, as well as for liver surface hemostasis. SLC is used for small vessels (<3 mm), while titanium clips and 3–0 silk sutures are used for medium (3–5 mm) and larger (>5 mm) vessels, respectively. Unlike monopolar electrocautery, SLC coagulates without char production. In addition, SLC not only coagulates vessels but also divides them. When patients who underwent hepatectomy using the two-surgeon technique were compared with a matched set of patients who underwent resection with

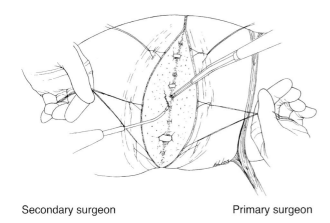

Secondary surgeon   Primary surgeon

Fig. 3.4 Two-surgeon technique for hepatic parenchymal transection. Glisson's capsule is scored with electrocautery, and 4–0 polypropylene stay sutures placed along the plane of intended transection. The primary surgeon dissects the hepatic parenchyma from the patient's *left side* using the ultrasonic dissector, while on the patient's *right side*, the secondary surgeon operates the saline-linked cautery. Reprinted with permission from Aloia et al. [60]

ultrasonic dissection alone, the two-surgeon group was found to have decreased duration of inflow occlusion, operative time, and blood loss [60].

Intraoperative Ultrasound (IOUS)

For both anatomic and nonanatomic resections, IOUS is used to guide the extent of resection by delineating the relationship of tumors to the portal triads and hepatic veins, allows continual determination of the distance between the tumor and dissection plane to ensure a negative margin, and to identify additional lesions beyond the spatial resolution of preoperative imaging studies. IOUS changes or guides the operative approach in up to 67% of procedures and detects lesions missed on preoperative imaging in up to 12% of patients [61]. A novel application of IOUS is predicting outcome based on the echogenicity of lesions. Recent studies have shown that hypoechoic metastases on IOUS, which occur in approximately 40% of cases, are associated with a shorter survival [62, 63]. One explanation for this finding is that hypoechoic hepatic metastases are more likely to be mucinous, which is an adverse prognostic factor for primary colorectal cancer.

Anatomic Versus Wedge Resection

Anatomic resection is defined as resection of one or more of Couinaud's segments according to the

Brisbane 2000 terminology of liver anatomy and resections, while wedge resection is defined as a non-anatomic resection of the tumor with a rim of normal tissue [64]. In the past, anatomic resections were recommended over wedge resections because of a lower rate of positive margins with consequent improved survival [65]. Recently, in a multi-institutional study of 72 and 181 patients who underwent wedge and anatomic resections, respectively, anatomic resection was not superior to wedge resection with respect to surgical margins, pattern of recurrence, or survival [64]. Other studies have also shown that nonanatomic resections are not associated with an increased risk of local recurrence [66]. As with all aspects of hepatic resection for CLM, the decision to perform anatomic versus wedge resection should be tailored to the patient based on tumor number, size, and anatomy, with the goal of achieving histologically negative margins while preserving adequate remnant liver.

Evolving Role of Laparoscopic Hepatectomy

Few centers have significant experience with laparoscopic hepatectomy for CLM. Laparoscopic liver resection requires surgeons with expertise in laparoscopic and hepatic surgery, as well as specialized laparoscopic equipment, including laparoscopic ultrasonography, harmonic scalpel, ultrasonic dissector, and 30-degree laparoscope. Challenges in laparoscopic hepatectomy include the inability to perform bimanual palpation and technical demands of mobilizing the liver and obtaining vascular control laparoscopically, with or without hand assistance. In addition, pneumoperitoneum may increase the risk of gas embolism, with two published cases of gas embolism with the use of the argon beam coagulator, which is now contraindicated in laparoscopic hepatectomy [67]. Although laparoscopic hemihepatectomy has been performed successfully by a handful of surgeons, the role of laparoscopy in liver resection is mainly confined to small lesions (<5 cm) located in the left lateral section or segments IV–VI. A separate, <8 cm incision in the lower abdomen or periumbilical area is needed to externalize the specimen in a protective specimen bag. The conversion rate is reported to be 10–20%, with transfusion and morbidity rates similar to those of open surgery [68]. Although long-term data are limited, oncologic outcomes, including surgical margin, disease recurrence, and survival, do not appear to be compromised. However, the advantages demonstrated in other laparoscopic surgery with regard to length of hospital stay, narcotic use, and return of bowel function have not been conclusively shown for laparoscopic liver resection [69]. Further prospective evaluation is required to assess the results of laparoscopy in the treatment of CLM [70].

Surgery in the Era of Multimodality Therapy

Over the past decade, new chemotherapeutic and biologic agents have been found with significantly increased activity against colorectal cancer. Specifically, response rates of 33% with infusional 5-fluorouracil (5-FU) and leucovorin have been increased to 50% with the addition of oxaliplatin (FOLFOX) or irinotecan (FOLFIRI). The monoclonal antibodies, bevacizumab and cetuximab, have further increased response rates. Despite the benefits of modern chemotherapy, potential hepatotoxicity should be carefully considered.

Systemic Chemotherapy for Initially Irresectable Disease

Treating patients preoperatively with oxaliplatin- or irinotecan-based chemotherapy regimens has resulted in the conversion of irresectable CLM to resectable in 13–37% of patients [26, 71]. In a study by Adam and colleagues, 138 of 1104 (12.5%) patients with initially irresectable CLM had a favorable response to preoperative chemotherapy and underwent hepatic resection [26]. Despite the presence of extensive disease, including multinodularity (> 3 metastases) in 59% of patients and extrahepatic disease in 38%, they achieved a 5-year survival of 33%, compared with 48% for patients with initially resectable disease. Effective modern chemotherapy allows not only downsizing of liver disease but also the theoretical benefit of treating micrometastatic disease early and the identification of patients whose disease progresses on chemotherapy and who would not benefit from surgery. Adam's group demonstrated that the 5-year posthepatectomy survival among patients whose disease progressed on chemotherapy was only 8% versus 37% for patients whose tumors responded to chemotherapy [72]. Finally, response to chemotherapy can guide postoperative treatment.

A few patients have a dramatic response to preoperative chemotherapy, leading to the disappearance of CLM on preoperative imaging. In a study by Benoist and colleagues of 38 patients, 66 liver metastases disappeared radiographically after chemotherapy [73]. Twenty were found at time of surgical exploration. The sites of 15 lesions not visible at surgery were resected, and of these, 12 harbored viable tumor cells. Of 31 disappeared metastases that were not resected, 23 recurred after 1 year of follow-up. Thus, until further evidence is available, hepatic resection should encompass all tumor-bearing sites seen on prechemotherapy imaging.

Systemic Chemotherapy for Initially Resectable Disease

Since most patients with CLM experience recurrence after resection, systemic chemotherapy for initially resectable disease has been advocated. In 2007, the results of the European Organization for Research and Treatment of Cancer Intergroup phase III study 40983 were presented [74]. This trial randomized patients with resectable CLM (up to four metastases, no extrahepatic disease) to surgery alone versus perioperative FOLFOX4 (oxaliplatin 85 mg/ m^2 and infusional 5-FU plus leucovorin), six cycles before and after surgery. Among the 182 patients enrolled in the chemotherapy arm, 43.9% had partial or complete response to FOLFOX4, 35.2% had stable disease, and 6.8% had progressive disease. Eight of the 12 patients with progressive disease did not undergo hepatic resection. Of 171 eligible patients in each arm, 83% underwent hepatic resection. After a median follow-up of 3.9 years, patients who received perioperative chemotherapy had a significantly better 3-year progression-free survival of 36% versus 28% for patients who underwent surgery alone. The difference was more pronounced among patients who underwent hepatic resection, with 3-year progression-free survival of 42% in the chemotherapy arm versus 33% with surgery alone. The authors concluded that perioperative FOLFOX4 improves progression-free survival over surgery alone, particularly in patients whose CLM are resected.

Chemotherapy-Induced Liver Injury

While modern systemic agents have improved survival and resectability rates in patients with CLM, the potential liver injury caused by these agents must be considered. Although most series show that perioperative morbidity and mortality are not higher after hepatectomy following chemotherapy compared with de novo resection, specific chemotherapy-related injuries can adversely affect outcomes. In addition, chemotherapy-induced hepato-toxicity is related to duration of treatment, with increased complications demonstrated after more than 3–4 months of treatment [75, 76].

Oxaliplatin-based chemotherapy has been associated with sinusoidal lesions, including sinusoidal dilatation, vascular congestion, perisinusoidal fibrosis, and venous occlusion by fibrous tissue (Fig. 3.5). These lesions are morphologically similar to those seen in sinusoidal obstruction syndrome, which occurs mainly as a complication of chemotherapy in the setting of stem cell transplantation [77]. The clinical relevance of sinusoidal dilation with respect to outcomes after hepatic resection remains uncertain. We reported no increase in morbidity and mortality after relatively short-course oxaliplatin-based chemotherapy (median 4 months), while two other studies have described an increase in blood transfusions and complications in patients treated preoperatively for more than 4 months [75, 76, 78].

Conversely, we noted a five-fold increase in steato-hepatitis in patients treated with irinotecan-based chemotherapy, which resulted in a markedly increased risk of 90-day mortality from postoperative liver failure compared with patients without steatohepatitis [78]. Although the association between irinotecan and steatohepatitis was found irrespective of body mass index (BMI), patients with BMI ≥ 25 kg/m^2 were more likely to have steatohepatitis after irinotecan-based therapy than patients with BMI <25 kg/m^2 (incidence rates 25% vs. 12%, respectively). Because of the significant risk associated with performing hepatic resection in patients with steatohepatitis, irinotecan should be administered with caution in patients with known steatosis or steatohepatitis. Since preoperative imaging cannot accurately diagnose steatohepatitis, patients with steatosis who are treated with irinotecan, particularly obese patients, should undergo laparoscopic liver biopsy before proceeding with resection.

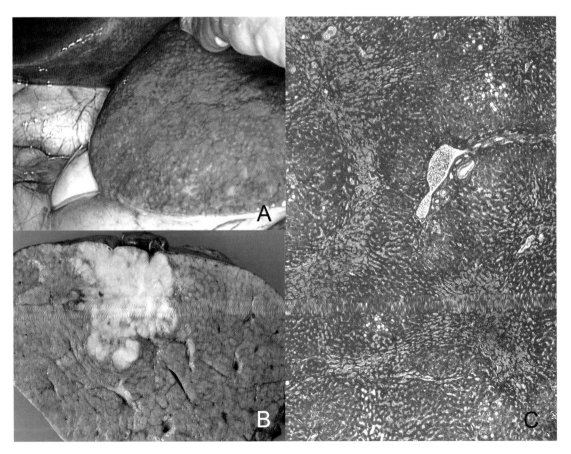

Fig. 3.5 Oxaliplatin-associated hepatic injury. (**A,B**) Gross appearance of liver with oxaliplatin-associated injury ("*blue liver*"). The distended sinusoids cause entrapment of erythrocytes, which render the liver blue in color. (**C**) Microscopic demonstration of centrilobular sinusoidal dilatation (Trichrome stain, magnification ×100). Reprinted with permission from Zorzi et al. [84]

Biologic Agents

Bevacizumab, a monoclonal antibody against vascular endothelial growth factor (VEGF), has resulted in improved response and disease-free survival rates in patients with CLM, augmenting response rates to upwards of 80% [4, 79]. However, its antiangiogenic effects have raised concerns regarding potential effects on wound healing, postoperative bleeding, and complications. Recent studies have shown that bevacizumab does not increase postoperative morbidity after hepatectomy for CLM [80, 81]. Nevertheless, given the half-life of bevacizumab of approximately 20 days, a waiting period of two half-lives (6–8 weeks) is recommended after the last dose of bevacizumab before performing liver resection [82].

In a recent study from our institution on patients undergoing hepatectomy after chemotherapy with oxaliplatin and 5-FU, bevacizumab was found to enhance the pathologic response to chemotherapy and to have liver protective effects (Fig. 3.6) [83]. Oxaliplatin and 5-FU were administered with bevacizumab in 62 patients and without bevacizumab in 43 patients. A total of 285 tumor nodules underwent pathologic review, and the addition of bevacizumab was associated with 33% residual viable tumor cells compared with 45% without bevacizumab (Fig. 3.7a). Although bevacizumab resulted in improved response, it did not increase the incidence of complete pathologic response, which was 11.3% with bevacizumab and 11.6% with oxaliplatin/5-FU alone.

In addition, the incidence and severity of sinusoidal dilation was lower in patients treated with bevacizumab (Fig. 3.7b). Oxaliplatin is hypothesized to induce sinusoidal dilatation by causing overproduction of reactive oxygen species and depletion of glutathione in endothelial cells [84]. VEGF induces matrix metalloproteinase-9 (MMP-9), which is released by endothelial cells, and promotes sinusoidal dilatation. A hypothesis for the hepato-protective mechanism of bevacizumab in patients treated with oxaliplatin is inhibition of VEGF, leading to downregulation of MMP-9 and attenuation of sinusoidal injury.

Cetuximab, a monoclonal antibody against epidermal growth factor receptor, has been shown to have activity as a single agent and to exert synergistic activity in combination with cytotoxic chemotherapy. In a recent study by Adam and colleagues, 25 patients underwent resection for CLM after stabilization or response to cetuximab combined with an irinotecan- or oxaliplatin-containing regimen [85]. Notably, cetuximab was used as second-line or higher line chemotherapy after failure of first-line chemotherapy.

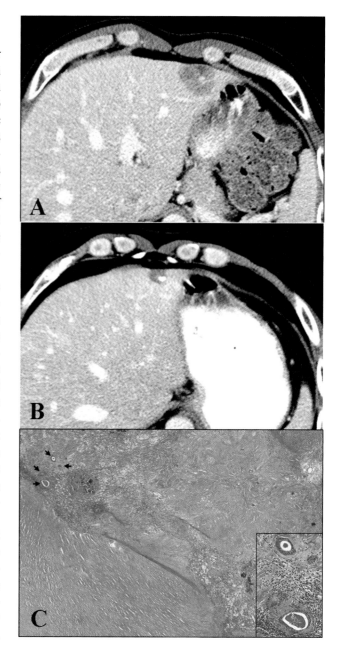

Fig. 3.6 Response to preoperative treatment with 5-FU and oxaliplatin plus bevacizumab. (**A**) Before treatment, the patient had a 3.4 cm metastasis in segment III. (**B**) Partial radiographic response to chemotherapy, with tumor downsizing to 1.5 cm. (**C**) Histologic examination after resection revealed only 1% viable tumor cells in a background of extensive fibrosis, necrosis, and inflammatory cells. (Hematoxylin and eosin stain, magnification ×20, inset ×200.) From Ribero et al. [83]. © 2007 American Cancer Society. This material is reproduced with permission of Wiley-Liss, Inc., a subsidiary of John Wiley & Sons, Inc.

After median follow-up of 16 months, median overall and progression-free survival rates of 20 and 13 months were achieved in this cohort of high-risk patients.

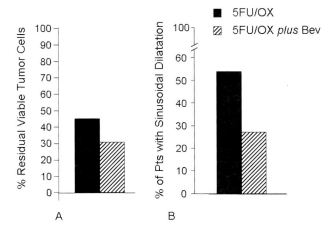

Fig. 3.7 (**A**) Significantly decreased %residual viable tumor cells in patients treated with bevacizumab (Bev) compared with 5-FU/oxaliplatin (5FU/OX) alone (33% vs. 45%, respectively). (**B**) Incidence of sinusoidal obstruction was 27% in patients treated with bevacizumab compared with 54% with 5-FU/oxaliplatin alone. (*P* < 0.05). Reprinted with permission from Ribero et al. [83]. © 2007 American Cancer Society. This material is reproduced with permission of Wiley-Liss, Inc., a subsidiary of John Wiley & Sons, Inc.

Management of Synchronous Colorectal Liver Metastases

In patients with synchronous CLM, simultaneous colorectal and minor liver resections (<3 segments) result in similar morbidity and mortality rates as staged resections [86]. However, patients who require a major hepatectomy should undergo staged resections because simultaneous procedures are associated with high morbidity and mortality rates.

Patients with synchronous presentation of advanced CLM have a poorer prognosis than patients with metachronous disease [2]. Several approaches have been advocated to improve their outcome. Patients with symptomatic primaries, such as bleeding or obstructing rectal lesions, should undergo resection of the primary tumor first. Survival in patients with asymptomatic primaries and advanced liver metastases is determined by their burden of hepatic disease and not by the primary tumor. In much patients, systemic chemotherapy before liver resection has been shown to improve survival [87]. A study by Allen and associates compared patients with synchronous CLM who underwent staged resections, with or without chemotherapy before hepatectomy [88]. Patients whose liver metastases did not progress on chemotherapy had improved survival compared with patients who did not receive chemotherapy. The advantages of preoperative systemic therapy include initial control and downsizing of liver metastases, treatment of potential micrometastases, and better selection of patients who respond to therapy and will benefit from surgery.

In Allen's study, patients underwent resection of their colorectal primary first, followed by treatment of their liver metastases. This algorithm delays treatment of liver disease, incurring the risk of tumor progression that would preclude curative liver resection, especially if complications arise after colorectal surgery. This delay is longer in patients with rectal cancer who require preoperative chemoradiation, which has been shown to be superior to postoperative chemoradiation in terms of local control and toxicity [89]. To prevent progression of liver metastases during treatment of the primary, Mentha and coworkers proposed a new strategy of delivering chemotherapy first, resection of liver metastases second, followed by chemoradiation for patients with rectal cancer, and resection of the primary last [90]. They reported in 20 patients a median survival of 46 months, which is higher than published survival rates for patients with disease of similar severity. This strategy allows early treatment of liver metastases, assessment of patient response to therapy, and delivery of preoperative chemoradiation to patients with rectal cancer without the risk of disease progression in the liver.

Conclusions

With refinements in preoperative imaging, patient selection, and surgical techniques, current 5-year overall survival rates after complete resection of CLM have reached 58%. Traditional criteria of resectability have been challenged, and the current goal of hepatic resection should be to resect all metastases with negative histologic margins while preserving sufficient functional hepatic parenchyma. Surgical strategies to increase the number of patients eligible for curative resection include PVE and two-stage hepatectomy. More active systemic chemotherapy agents are now available and are being increasingly employed as therapy before or after surgery. However, anthracinum for systemic therapy before hepatic resection should be tempered by potential risks associated with chemotherapy-induced liver injury. Despite expanding indications for resection of CLM, several studies have shown marked improvement in survival compared with historical series, and current 5-year survival rates exceed 50%. Modern treatment of CLM requires a multidisciplinary approach in an effort to increase the number of patients who may be eligible for potentially curative resection, as well as to improve patient selection and ultimately patient survival.

References

1. American Cancer Society. Cancer Facts and Figures-2007. Atlanta, Ga: ACSSR; 2007.
2. Scheele J, Stang R, Altendorf-Hofmann A, Paul M. Resection of colorectal liver metastases. World J Surg. 1995; 19(1) 59–71.
3. Venook A. Critical evaluation of current treatments in metastatic colorectal cancer. Oncologist. 2005; 10(4) 250–61.
4. Hurwitz H, Fehrenbacher L, Novotny W, et al. Bevacizumab plus irinotecan, fluorouracil, and leucovorin for metastatic colorectal cancer. N Engl J Med. 2004; 350(23) 2335–42.
5. Abdalla EK, Vauthey JN, Ellis LM, et al. Recurrence and outcomes following hepatic resection, radiofrequency ablation, and combined resection/ablation for colorectal liver metastases. Ann Surg. 2004; 239(6) 818–25; discussion 25–7.
6. Mullen JT, Ribero D, Reddy SK, et al. Hepatic insufficiency and mortality in 1,059 noncirrhotic patients undergoing major hepatectomy. J Am Coll Surg. 2007; 204(5) 854–62; discussion 62–4.
7. Belghiti J, Hiramatsu K, Benoist S, et al. Seven hundred forty-seven hepatectomies in the 1990s: An update to evaluate the actual risk of liver resection. J Am Coll Surg. 2000; 191(1) 38–46.
8. Jarnagin WR, Gonen M, Fong Y, et al. Improvement in perioperative outcome after hepatic resection: Analysis of 1,803 consecutive cases over the past decade. Ann Surg. 2002; 236(4) 397–406; discussion -7.
9. Menon KV, Al-Mukhtar A, Aldouri A, et al. Outcomes after major hepatectomy in elderly patients. J Am Coll Surg. 2006; 203(5) 677–83.
10. Hamady ZZ, Kotru A, Nishio H, Lodge JP. Current techniques and results of liver resection for colorectal liver metastases. Br Med Bull. 2004; 70: 87–104.
11. Bipat S, van Leeuwen MS, Comans EF, et al. Colorectal liver metastases: CT, MR imaging, and PET for diagnosis—meta-analysis. Radiology. 2005; 237(1) 123–31.
12. Kinkel K, Lu Y, Both M, et al. Detection of hepatic metastases from cancers of the gastrointestinal tract by using noninvasive imaging methods (US, CT, MR imaging, PET): A meta-analysis. Radiology. 2002; 224(3) 748–56.
13. Fernandez FG, Drebin JA, Linehan DC, et al. Five-year survival after resection of hepatic metastases from colorectal cancer in patients screened by positron emission tomography with F-18 fluorodeoxyglucose (FDG-PET). Ann Surg. 2004; 240(3) 438–47; discussion 47–50.
14. Rosenbaum SJ, Lind T, Antoch G, Bockisch A. False-positive FDG PET uptake—the role of PET/CT. Eur Radiol. 2006; 16(5) 1054–65.
15. Akhurst T, Kates TJ, Mazumdar M, et al. Recent chemotherapy reduces the sensitivity of [18F]fluorodeoxyglucose positron emission tomography in the detection of colorectal metastases. J Clin Oncol. 2005; 23(34): 8713–6.
16. White RR, Pappas TN. Laparoscopic staging for hepatobiliary carcinoma. J Gastrointest Surg. 2004; 8(8) 920–2.
17. Grobmyer SR, Fong Y, D'Angelica M, et al. Diagnostic laparoscopy prior to planned hepatic resection for colorectal metastases. Arch Surg. 2004; 139(12) 1326–30.
18. Charnsangavej C, Clary B, Fong Y, et al. Selection of patients for resection of hepatic colorectal metastases: Expert consensus statement. Ann Surg Oncol. 2006; 13(10) 1261–8.
19. Ballantyne GH, Quin J. Surgical treatment of liver metastases in patients with colorectal cancer. Cancer. 1993; 71(12 Suppl): 4252–66.
20. Ekberg H, Tranberg KG, Andersson R, et al. Determinants of survival in liver resection for colorectal secondaries. Br J Surg. 1986; 73(9) 727–31.
21. Pawlik TM, Abdalla EK, Ellis LM, et al. Debunking dogma: Surgery for four or more colorectal liver metastases is justified. J Gastrointest Surg. 2006; 10(2) 240–8.
22. Kokudo N, Imamura H, Sugawara Y, et al. Surgery for multiple hepatic colorectal metastases. J Hepatobiliary Pancreat Surg. 2004; 11(2) 84–91.
23. Minagawa M, Makuuchi M, Torzilli G, et al. Extension of the frontiers of surgical indications in the treatment of liver metastases from colorectal cancer: Long-term results. Ann Surg. 2000; 231(4) 487–99.
24. Hamady ZZ, Malik HZ, Finch R, et al. Hepatic resection for colorectal metastasis: Impact of tumour size. Ann Surg Oncol. 2006; 13(11) 1493–9.
25. Cady B, Jenkins RL, Steele GD Jr, et al. Surgical margin in hepatic resection for colorectal metastasis: A critical and improvable determinant of outcome. Ann Surg. 1998; 227(4) 566–71.
26. Adam R, Delvart V, Pascal G, et al. Rescue surgery for unresectable colorectal liver metastases downstaged by chemotherapy: A model to predict long-term survival. Ann Surg. 2004; 240(4) 644–57; discussion 57–8.
27. Headrick JR, Miller DL, Nagorney DM, et al. Surgical treatment of hepatic and pulmonary metastases from colon cancer. Ann Thorac Surg. 2001; 71(3) 975–9; discussion 9–80.
28. Miller G, Biernacki P, Kemeny NE, et al. Outcomes after resection of synchronous or metachronous hepatic and pulmonary colorectal metastases. J Am Coll Surg. 2007; 205(2) 231–8.
29. Inoue M, Ohta M, Iuchi K, et al. Benefits of surgery for patients with pulmonary metastases from colorectal carcinoma. Ann Thorac Surg. 2004; 78(1) 238–44.
30. Vauthey JN. Colorectal liver metastases: Treat effectively up front and consider the borderline resectable. J Clin Oncol. 2007; 25(29) 4524–5.
31. Jaeck D, Nakano H, Bachellier P, et al. Significance of hepatic pedicle lymph node involvement in patients with colorectal liver metastases: A prospective study. Ann Surg Oncol. 2002; 9(5) 430–8.
32. Elias D, Sideris L, Pocard M, et al. Results of R0 resection for colorectal liver metastases associated with extrahepatic disease. Ann Surg Oncol. 2004; 11(3) 274–80.
33. Elias D, Liberale G, Vernerey D, et al. Hepatic and extrahepatic colorectal metastases: When resectable, their localization does not matter, but their total number has a prognostic effect. Ann Surg Oncol. 2005; 12(11) 900–9.
34. Fong Y, Fortner J, Sun RL, et al. Clinical score for predicting recurrence after hepatic resection for metastatic colorectal cancer: Analysis of 1001 consecutive cases. Ann Surg. 1999; 230(3) 309–18; discussion 18–21.
35. Zakaria S, Donohue JH, Que FG, et al. Hepatic resection for colorectal metastases: Value for risk scoring systems? Ann Surg. 2007; 246(2) 183–91.
36. Iwatsuki S, Dvorchik I, Madariaga JR, et al. Hepatic resection for metastatic colorectal adenocarcinoma: A proposal of a prognostic scoring system. J Am Coll Surg. 1999; 189(3) 291–9.
37. Nordlinger B, Guiguet M, Vaillant JC, et al. Surgical resection of colorectal carcinoma metastases to the liver. A prognostic scoring system to improve case selection, based on 1568 patients. Association Francaise de Chirurgie. Cancer. 1996; 77(7) 1254–62.
38. Rubbia-Brandt L, Giostra E, Brezault C, et al. Importance of histological tumor response assessment in predicting the outcome in patients with colorectal liver metastases treated with neo-adjuvant chemotherapy followed by liver surgery. Ann Oncol. 2007; 18(2) 299–304.

39. Vauthey JN, Chaoui A, Do KA, et al. Standardized measurement of the future liver remnant prior to extended liver resection: Methodology and clinical associations. Surgery. 2000; 127(5) 512–9.

40. Shoup M, Gonen M, D'Angelica M, et al. Volumetric analysis predicts hepatic dysfunction in patients undergoing major liver resection. J Gastrointest Surg. 2003; 7(3) 325–30.

41. Kubota K, Makuuchi M, Kusaka K, et al. Measurement of liver volume and hepatic functional reserve as a guide to decision-making in resectional surgery for hepatic tumors. Hepatology. 1997; 26(5) 1176–81.

42. Ijichi M, Makuuchi M, Imamura H, Takayama T. Portal embolization relieves persistent jaundice after complete biliary drainage. Surgery. 2001; 130(1) 116–8.

43. Uesaka K, Nimura Y, Nagino M. Changes in hepatic lobar function after right portal vein embolization. An appraisal by biliary indocyanine green excretion. Ann Surg. 1996; 223(1) 77–83.

44. Abdalla EK, Barnett CC, Doherty D, et al. Extended hepatectomy in patients with hepatobiliary malignancies with and without preoperative portal vein embolization. Arch Surg. 2002; 137(6) 675–80; discussion 80–1.

45. Abdalla EK, Adam R, Bilchik AJ, Jaeck D, Vauthey JN, Mahvi D. Improving resectability of hepatic colorectal metastases: Expert consensus statement. Ann Surg Oncol. 2006; 13(10) 1271–80.

46. Abdalla EK, Hicks ME, Vauthey JN. Portal vein embolization: Rationale, technique and future prospects. Br J Surg. 2001; 88(2) 165–75.

47. Madoff DC, Abdalla EK, Vauthey JN. Portal vein embolization in preparation for major hepatic resection: Evolution of a new standard of care. J Vasc Interv Radiol. 2005; 16(6) 779–90.

48. Azoulay D, Castaing D, Smail A, et al. Resection of nonresectable liver metastases from colorectal cancer after percutaneous portal vein embolization. Ann Surg. 2000; 231(4) 480–6.

49. Ribero D, Abdalla EK, Madoff DC, et al. Portal vein embolization before major hepatectomy and its effects on regeneration, resectability and outcome. Br J Surg. 2007; 94(11) 1386–94.

50. Chun YS, Vauthey JN, Ribero D, et al. Systemic chemotherapy and two-stage hepatectomy for extensive bilateral colorectal liver metastases: Perioperative safety and survival. J Gastrointest Surg. 2007; 11(11) 1498–505.

51. Jaeck D, Oussoultzoglou E, Rosso E, et al. A two-stage hepatectomy procedure combined with portal vein embolization to achieve curative resection for initially unresectable multiple and bilobar colorectal liver metastases. Ann Surg. 2004; 240(6) 1037–49; discussion 49–51.

52. Petrowsky H, Gonen M, Jarnagin W, et al. Second liver resections are safe and effective treatment for recurrent hepatic metastases from colorectal cancer: A bi-institutional analysis. Ann Surg. 2002; 235(6) 863–71.

53. Suzuki S, Sakaguchi T, Yokoi Y, et al. Impact of repeat hepatectomy on recurrent colorectal liver metastases. Surgery. 2001; 129(4) 421–8.

54. Muratore A, Polastri R, Bouzari H, et al. Repeat hepatectomy for colorectal liver metastases: A worthwhile operation? J Surg Oncol. 2001; 76(2) 127–32.

55. Kooby DA, Stockman J, Ben-Porat L, et al. Influence of transfusions on perioperative and long-term outcome in patients following hepatic resection for colorectal metastases. Ann Surg. 2003; 237(6) 860–9; discussion 9–70.

56. Rosen CB, Nagorney DM, Taswell HF, et al. Perioperative blood transfusion and determinants of survival after liver resection for metastatic colorectal carcinoma. Ann Surg. 1992; 216(4) 493–504; discussion 5.

57. Chen H, Merchant NB, Didolkar MS. Hepatic resection using intermittent vascular inflow occlusion and low central venous pressure anesthesia improves morbidity and mortality. J Gastrointest Surg. 2000; 4(2) 162–7.

58. Walia A. Anesthetic management for liver resection. J Gastrointest Surg. 2006; 10(2) 168–9.

59. Redai I, Emond J, Brentjens T. Anesthetic considerations during liver surgery. Surg Clin North Am. 2004; 84(2) 401–11.

60. Aloia TA, Zorzi D, Abdalla EK, Vauthey JN. Two-surgeon technique for hepatic parenchymal transection of the noncirrhotic liver using saline-linked cautery and ultrasonic dissection. Ann Surg. 2005; 242(2) 172–7.

61. Zacherl J, Scheuba C, Imhof M, et al. Current value of intraoperative sonography during surgery for hepatic neoplasms. World J Surg. 2002; 26(5) 550–4.

62. DeOliveira ML, Pawlik TM, Gleisner AL, et al. Echogenic appearance of colorectal liver metastases on intraoperative ultrasonography is associated with survival after hepatic resection. J Gastrointest Surg. 2007; 11(8) 970–6; discussion 6.

63. Gruenberger T, Zhao J, King J, et al. Echogenicity of liver metastases from colorectal carcinoma is an independent prognostic factor in patients treated with regional chemotherapy. Cancer. 2002; 94(6) 1753–9.

64. Zorzi D, Mullen JT, Abdalla EK, et al. Comparison between hepatic wedge resection and anatomic resection for colorectal liver metastases. J Gastrointest Surg. 2006; 10(1) 86–94.

65. DeMatteo RP, Palese C, et al. Anatomic segmental hepatic resection is superior to wedge resection as an oncologic operation for colorectal liver metastases. J Gastrointest Surg. 2000; 4(2) 178–84.

66. Yamamoto J, Sugihara K, Kosuge T, et al. Pathologic support for limited hepatectomy in the treatment of liver metastases from colorectal cancer. Ann Surg. 1995; 221(1) 74–8.

67. Hashizume M, Takenaka K, Yanaga K, et al. Laparoscopic hepatic resection for hepatocellular carcinoma. Surg Endosc. 1995; 9(12) 1289–91.

68. Poon RT. Current role of laparoscopic surgery for liver malignancies. Surg Technol Int. 2007; 16: 73–81.

69. Vibert E, Perniceni T, Levard H, et al. Laparoscopic liver resection. Br J Surg. 2006; 93(1) 67–72.

70. Cherqui D. Laparoscopic liver resection. Br J Surg. 2003; 90(6) 644–6.

71. Alberts SR, Horvath WL, Sternfeld WC, et al. Oxaliplatin, fluorouracil, and leucovorin for patients with unresectable liver-only metastases from colorectal cancer: A North Central Cancer Treatment Group phase II study. J Clin Oncol. 2005; 23(36) 9243–9.

72. Adam R, Pascal G, Castaing D, et al. Tumor progression while on chemotherapy: A contraindication to liver resection for multiple colorectal metastases? Ann Surg. 2004; 240(6) 1052–61; discussion 61–4.

73. Benoist S, Brouquet A, Penna C, et al. Complete response of colorectal liver metastases after chemotherapy: Does it mean cure? J Clin Oncol. 2006; 24(24) 3939–45.

74. Nordlinger B, Sorbye H, Collette L, et al. Final results of the EORTC Intergroup randomized phase III study 40983 [EPOC] evaluating the benefit of peri-operative FOLFOX4 chemotherapy for patients with potentially resectable colorectal cancer liver metastases. ASCO Annual Meeting Proceedings. J Clin Oncol. 2007; 25(18S): LBA5.

75. Aloia T, Sebagh M, Plasse M, et al. Liver histology and surgical outcomes after preoperative chemotherapy with fluorouracil plus oxaliplatin in colorectal cancer liver metastases. J Clin Oncol. 2006; 24(31) 4983–90.

76. Karoui M, Penna C, Amin-Hashem M, et al. Influence of preoperative chemotherapy on the risk of major hepatectomy for colorectal liver metastases. Ann Surg. 2006; 243(1) 1–7.

77. Rubbia-Brandt L, Audard V, Sartoretti P, et al. Severe hepatic sinusoidal obstruction associated with oxaliplatin-based chemotherapy in patients with metastatic colorectal cancer. Ann Oncol. 2004; 15(3) 460–6.

78. Vauthey JN, Pawlik TM, Ribero D, et al. Chemotherapy regimen predicts steatohepatitis and an increase in 90-day mortality after surgery for hepatic colorectal metastases. J Clin Oncol. 2006; 24(13) 2065–72.

79. Kabbinavar F, Hurwitz HI, Fehrenbacher L, et al. Phase II, randomized trial comparing bevacizumab plus fluorouracil (FU)/leucovorin (LV) with FU/LV alone in patients with metastatic colorectal cancer. J Clin Oncol. 2003; 21(1) 60–5.

80. D'Angelica M, Kornprat P, Gonen M, et al. Lack of evidence for increased operative morbidity after hepatectomy with perioperative use of bevacizumab: A matched case-control study. Ann Surg Oncol. 2007; 14(2) 759–65.

81. Kesmodel SB, Ellis LM, Lin E, et al. Complication rates following hepatic surgery in patients receiving neoadjuvant bevacizumab (BV) for colorectal cancer (CRC) liver metastases. In abstracts of the 2007 Gastrointestinal Cancers Symposium; January 19–21, 2007; Orlando, FL. Abstract 234.

82. Ellis LM, Curley SA, Grothey A. Surgical resection after downsizing of colorectal liver metastasis in the era of bevacizumab. J Clin Oncol. 2005; 23(22) 4853–5.

83. Ribero D WH, Donadon M, Zorzi D, et al. Bevacizumab improves pathologic response and protects against hepatic injury in patients treated with oxaliplatin-based chemotherapy for colorectal liver metastases. Cancer. 2007; 110(12) 2761–7.

84. Zorzi D, Laurent A, Pawlik TM, et al. Chemotherapy-associated hepatotoxicity and surgery for colorectal liver metastases. Br J Surg. 2007; 94(3) 274–86.

85. Adam R, Aloia T, Levi F, et al. Hepatic resection after rescue cetuximab treatment for colorectal liver metastases previously refractory to conventional systemic therapy. J Clin Oncol. 2007; 25(29) 4593–602.

86. Reddy SK, Pawlik TM, Zorzi D, et al. Simultaneous resections of colorectal cancer and synchronous liver metastases: A multi-institutional analysis. Ann Surg Oncol. 2007; Sep 1 [Epub ahead of print].

87. Tanaka K, Shimada H, Matsuo K, et al. Outcome after simultaneous colorectal and hepatic resection for colorectal cancer with synchronous metastases. Surgery 2004; 136(3) 650–9.

88. Allen PJ, Kemeny N, Jarnagin W, et al. Importance of response to neoadjuvant chemotherapy in patients undergoing resection of synchronous colorectal liver metastases. J Gastrointest Surg. 2003; 7(1) 109–15; discussion 16–7.

89. Sauer R, Becker H, Hohenberger W, et al. Preoperative versus postoperative chemoradiotherapy for rectal cancer. N Engl J Med. 2004; 351(17) 1731–40.

90. Mentha G, Majno PE, Andres A, et al. Neoadjuvant chemotherapy and resection of advanced synchronous liver metastases before treatment of the colorectal primary. Br J Surg. 2006; 93(7) 872–8.

91. Pawlik TM, Scoggins CR, Zorzi D, et al. Effect of surgical margin status on survival and site of recurrence after hepatic resection for colorectal metastases. Ann Surg. 2005; 241(5) 715–22, discussion 722–4.

Destructive Therapies for Colorectal Cancer Metastases

4

Dan G. Blazer III, Daniel A. Anaya, and Eddie K. Abdalla

Introduction

Colorectal cancer is the third most common cancer diagnosed in men and women in the United States and is a leading cause of cancer death. It was estimated that in 2007, 52,000 people would die in the United States of cancers of the colon and rectum; the liver is the most common site of metastasis, and liver metastases are a leading cause of death from colon cancer [1, 2].

Hepatic resection of colorectal liver metastases (CLM) offers the best chance for long-term survival and remains the gold standard treatment when feasible. After resection, 5-year survival rates may be as high as 58% in selected patients and up to 71% in patients with solitary CLM [3, 4, 5, 6, 7]. Many approaches have evolved to increase the proportion of patients eligible for complete resection, including portal vein embolization (PVE), staged resections for bilateral CLM, and advances in chemotherapy [8, 9, 10, 11, 12]. The "definition" of resectability has expanded to include all patients with disease that can be resected, leaving an adequate liver remnant, regardless of size or number of lesions [13].

Despite these advances, only 10–25% of patients initially diagnosed with CLM are eligible for resection because of disease extent, severe underlying liver disease, and hepatic injury related to chemotherapy [8, 14]. Untreated liver metastases are associated with poor outcome; therefore, alternative treatment modalities are being sought. Available strategies include systemic chemotherapy, radiation therapy, hepatic-directed therapy (e.g., transarterial chemoembolization [TACE] and hepatic arterial infusion pumps), and locally ablative therapies. The latter, specifically local tumor ablation, has been extensively studied as an adjunct to surgical resection for CLM and as a stand-alone treatment with curative intent. In this chapter, ablative therapies for CLM are described and indications and limitations are reviewed. As with any treatment of CLM, the decision to pursue an ablative strategy should be made by a multidisciplinary team, including a surgeon with hepatobiliary expertise [13].

Cryoablation

Cryoablation is among the oldest of ablative therapies. The concept of hepatic cryosurgery was introduced in 1966 and its practice continues, particularly for unresectable hepatocellular carcinoma (HCC), CLM, and metastatic neuroendocrine tumors [15].

Cryoablation has been performed primarily via laparotomy although laparoscopic and percutaneous approaches are emerging. Subfreezing temperatures are delivered to the liver tumor and the surrounding parenchyma via a vacuum-insulated cryoprobe [16]. In brief, the cryoprobe is inserted into the tumor under sonographic guidance, and the probe temperature is then rapidly lowered. Freezing is generally achieved by circulating liquid nitrogen or argon gas at −196°C through the cryoprobe [17]. When temperatures lower than −20°C are reached in the surrounding tissue, ice crystals form, leading to protein denaturation and cellular dehydration, which destroy the tumor. The goal of therapy is to achieve a 5–10-mm margin of ablation. Generally, two freeze–thaw cycles are used in each area to maximize tumor destruction [16].

Cryoablation is attractive for several reasons. First, compared with other strategies, the ablation zone can be fairly accurately monitored using real-time sonography. The leading edge of the ice ball is seen on sonography as an area of increased echogenicity. Because local recurrence plagues all ablation modalities, the ability to

E.K. Abdalla (✉)
Associate Professor of Surgery, Department of Surgical Oncology, The University of Texas M.D. Anderson Cancer Center, Houston, TX, USA
e-mail: eabdalla@mdanderson.org

evaluate the treatment edge is a compelling advantage. Advocates of cryoablation also tout its ability to treat lesions close to major intrahepatic vessels, where cryotherapy can be used to destroy a tumor without permanent injury to the vessel [17, 18].

The primary contraindication to cryoablation appears to be tumor burden. Because the extent of hepatic cryotherapy contributes to the systemic effects of "cryoshock" (described in more detail below), investigators typically limit the amount of cryotherapy performed in a single setting. In addition, given that minimally invasive approaches to cryotherapy (e.g., percutaneous or laparoscopic) are still in their infancy compared with other ablative techniques, a patient's inability to tolerate laparotomy may be viewed as a relative contraindication to the use of this treatment.

The adverse effects of cryoablation can be serious. For example, myoglobinuria can lead to renal failure, and many advocate empiric alkalinization of the urine. Bile leakage, hepatic abscess, pleural effusion, consumptive coagulopathy, and thrombocytopenia can be encountered. A constellation of systemic effects of cryoablation is often described as the cryoshock phenomenon. Cryoshock is a cytokine-mediated systemic shock responsible for up to 20% of deaths associated with cryoablation [19]. The syndrome can include acute renal failure, acute respiratory distress syndrome, disseminated intravascular coagulation, and liver failure. Although the severity of cryoshock may be related to the duration of freezing, the most important risk factor is the volume of tumor treated. For this reason, treatment of a maximum of 10 cm of tumor per session is generally recommended in order to minimize morbidity.

Several studies over the past two decades have examined the role of cryoablation for the management of unresectable CLM [18, 20, 21, 22, 22]. Ravikumar et al. published one of the first series demonstrating the feasibility and safety of cryoablation and its ability to achieve an antitumor response with this technique [23]. A subsequent large series evaluated 136 patients with unresectable liver metastases [21]. Cryoablation was administered via laparotomy. A median of two tumors (range, one to seven tumors) per patient were treated. The median length of survival was 30 months for all patients; 88 patients developed recurrent disease in the liver. No 5-year survival data were published [21].

Cryoablation has also been examined as an adjunct to hepatic resection [20]. Thirty patients with unresectable CLM and no evidence of extrahepatic disease underwent cryoablation alone or as an adjunct to resection (median, two tumors per patient; range, one–seven tumors). The median length of survival was 32 months, and overall 1- and 2-year survival rates were 76% and 61%, respectively. Locoregional recurrence was reported in 6 (9%)

of 69 lesions. Again, however, the follow-up was relatively short, and no 5-year survival data were provided.

In one of the few series with 5-year survival data, Seifert and Junginger described their experience with 55 patients with CLM who underwent cryotherapy with or without concomitant resection [18]. Cryoablation was performed via laparotomy or laparoscopy after inspection for evidence of extrahepatic disease. The median length of survival was 29 months and 3- and 5-year survival rates were 44% and 26%, respectively. The locoregional recurrence rate at the cryosite for all tumors treated (including some noncolorectal lesions) was estimated to be 20%.

A study of the use of cryotherapy for lesions deemed resectable revealed a 23% local recurrence rate after ablation [19]. The corresponding median length of survival (22 months) was disappointing. Given the high incidence of local recurrence and poor survival time, the authors cautioned against the use of cryoablation for resectable disease.

In summary, cryoablation remains a popular ablative strategy worldwide for the management of unresectable CLM. Cryoablation is typically administered via laparotomy, although percutaneous and laparoscopic approaches are emerging. The ability to monitor the ablation zone with real-time sonography is a well-documented advantage to this technique. However, the advantages must be weighed against significant morbidity, most notably the cryoshock phenomenon. And finally, despite the advantages afforded by real-time monitoring, cryoablation has notable local recurrence rates, ranging from 14% to 33% [18]. Although few investigators have published long-term survival data, the data available for cryoablation do not compare favorably with resection in recent series, so this therapy is reserved for unresectable disease [18].

Radiofrequency Ablation

Over the past decade, radiofrequency ablation (RFA) has emerged as the preferred and most studied method for local ablation of liver tumors, including CLM. RFA has been compared directly with other ablation strategies such as cryoablation and seems to be equivalent in terms of local recurrence rates and survival [24]. In fact, in 2000, the U.S. Food and Drug Administration (FDA) approved RFA for ablation of unresectable CLM [13].

RFA uses heat generated by high-frequency alternating current to kill cells. Thin, partially insulated electrodes, guided with sonography, computed tomography (CT), or magnetic resonance imaging (MRI), are inserted percutaneously into the tumor; the electrodes can also be

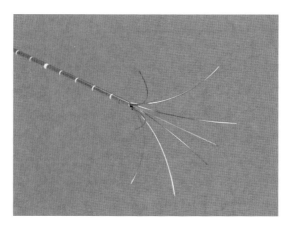

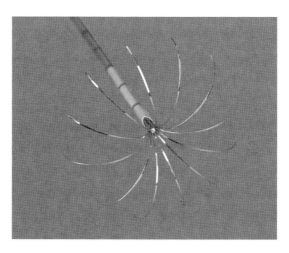

Fig. 4.1 Two commonly used radiofrequency ablation probes for the treatment of colorectal liver metastases

inserted more directly by sonographically guided laparotomy or laparoscopy. Two common probe designs are shown in Fig. 4.1. The electrode is attached to a radiofrequency generator, and alternating current is passed from the electrode tip into the tumor tissue. This current leads to ion agitation, which is converted by friction into heat. When the temperature rises above 60°C, proteins begin to denature, and cells die of coagulative necrosis. A typical RFA treatment can produce local temperatures that exceed 100°C [16]. Current and heat generation decrease in proportion to the square of the distance from the electrode, so multiple needle deployments are often necessary to treat large tumors [25]. Treatment strategies are typically designed to produce a thermal lesion incorporating the tumor and a 1-cm-wide zone of surrounding hepatic parenchyma [16]. Zones of ablation are overlapped to ensure complete destruction of the tumor with a margin of normal tissue (Fig. 4.2). Meticulous attention to creating overlapping zones is difficult due to the absence of an accurate method of monitoring ablation zones. Use of real-time MRI or sonography to monitor ablation zones is evolving.

The most common indications for RFA are unresectable HCC and metastatic liver tumors in the setting of liver-only disease. Occasionally, exceptions have been made in patients with extrahepatic disease when RFA can offer palliation of symptoms, such as in patients with metastatic functional neuroendocrine tumors [26]. RFA is often used to treat patients with tumors in locations that preclude resection for cure, such as between the inferior vena cava and the entrance of the hepatic veins into this area, although most experienced surgeons resect tumors in this location [26]. Major hepatic veins and portal branches are protected from injury caused by radiofrequency heat because they act as a heat sink that protects the endothelium from injury. Finally, RFA has been used in patients with tumor recurrence after hepatectomy, when repeat resection is not considered feasible or safe [27].

One of the primary contraindications to RFA is large tumor size. Typically, treatment is directed toward tumors less than 6 cm because of the high local recurrence rates in larger tumors [26]. In fact, in a recent consensus statement, the American Hepato-Pancreato-Biliary

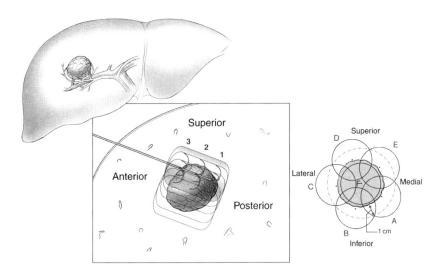

Fig. 4.2 This figure demonstrates the complexity of assuring complete ablation of a larger tumor and the geometry of overlapping ablations (here, 15 ablation regions are used to treat a 3-cm tumor). From Sielaff TD, Curley SA. Liver. In: Brunicardi FC. Schwartz's Principles of Surgery, 8th ed. New York: McGraw-Hill, 2005: 1175. Used with permission of the McGraw-Hill Companies

Association, the Society for Surgery of the Alimentary Tract, and the Society of Surgical Oncology said that "patients with tumors larger than 3 cm have high local recurrence rates and are not optimal candidates for this procedure. [13]".

In addition, RFA is typically contraindicated in tumors near the hilar plate, where the portal vein and hepatic artery enter the liver, because of the relative intolerance of large bile ducts to heat and the well-documented risk of catastrophic complications, including portal thrombosis, biloma, and biliary fistula [26].

Several studies have described percutaneous approaches for RFA, which are ideal for patients who cannot tolerate laparotomy, although open or laparoscopic RFA is recommended by the consensus panel when feasible because of the "superior probe placement with intraoperative ultrasound and the ability to detect other tumors [13]."

RFA can be performed with a low risk of complications in appropriately selected patients. Curley et al. evaluated 608 patients with malignant liver tumors that were treated with open or percutaneous RFA [28]. Early complications developed in 43 patients (7.1%) and late complications arose in 15 (2.4%). The most common early complications were symptomatic pleural effusion (1.8%) and hepatic abscess (0.8%). Other early complications included symptomatic ascites, needle track and perilesional hemorrhage, and biloma. Late complications included biliary fistula (0.3%) and biloma (1.0%). The combined overall early and late complication rate was 9.5%. Three patients died, yielding a mortality rate of 0.5%. Needle-tract seeding should not occur if the appropriate technique is used [25].

A consistently reported major limitation of RFA, which contributes significantly to decreased survival, is local recurrence, especially in larger lesions. Local

recurrence is difficult to compare across studies because investigators report it differently, some using a per-lesion rate and others using a per-patient rate. Follow-up times also vary significantly (Table 4.1) [3,6,29-34]. An early study by Lencioni et al. demonstrated incomplete ablation in 23% of lesions and a 12% local recurrence rate (per lesion) after a mean follow-up period of only 6.5 months [29]. One of the larger studies by Solbiati et al. demonstrated a local recurrence rate of 39% (in 70 of 179 lesions) by 18 months, and 55% of the patients ultimately had at least one local recurrence [30]. Livraghi et al. described patients with potentially resectable lesions and limited disease (one–three lesions, all ≤4 cm) [31]. Complete necrosis measured by CT was achieved in only 53 (60%) of 88 patients and in 85 (64%) of 134 lesions, despite small tumor size and treatment of "resectable" tumors. Local recurrence was seen despite retreatment in 35 (40%) of 88 patients [31]. Finally, in one of the most recent series, Amersi et al. looked at their ablation experience with 521 hepatic tumors in 181 patients, 74 of whom had CLM [34]. The incidence of local recurrence (per lesion) was 28% in tumors ≥3 cm and 18% (per lesion) in tumors ≤3 cm. In CLM ≥3 cm, 31% of tumors recurred [34].

The issue of incomplete necrosis and significant rates of local recurrence after RFA has been further emphasized in studies that examine both radiographic and pathologic recurrence (after explant) for HCC. Pompili et al. reported on histologic examinations of explanted livers in 40 patients with cirrhosis and HCC who underwent either percutaneous ethanol injection (PEI) or RFA as a bridge to orthotopic liver transplantation [35]. In the 30 nodules treated by RFA, complete necrosis was achieved in only 14 (47%). Even in lesions ≤3 cm, complete necrosis was achieved in only 62%. Further, Mazzaferro et al. revealed that among patients treated with

Table 4.1 Radiofrequency ablation of colorectal liver metastases

Firstauthor	Year	Number of patients	Tumor size (cm)	Tumor number	Local recurrence	Long-term survival data	Five-year survival	Median follow-up (months)
Lencioni [29]	1998	29	1.1–4.8	1–4	12%	1-yr (93%)	–	6.5 (mean)
Solbiati [30]	2001	117	0.9–9.6	1–4	39%	3-yr (46%)	–	36
Livraghi [31]	2003	88	0.6–4.0	1–3	40%	–	–	33
Oshowo [32]	2003	25	1–10	1	–	3-yr (53%)	–	37
Lencioni [33]	2004	423	0.5–5	1–4	25%	5-yr (24%)	24%	19 (mean)
Abdalla [6]	2004	57	2.5 (median)	1–8	9%	4-yr (22%)	–	21
Amersi [34]	2006	74	0.8–13.5	2.38 (mean)	≤3 cm, 18% all histologies	≤3 lesions (46%)	≤3 lesions (46%)	31
					>3 cm, 31% CLM	>3 lesions (26%)	>3 lesions (26%)	
Aloia [3]	2006	30	1–7	1	37%	5-yr 27%	27%	31*

*Only Aloia et al. [3] contain follow-up with systematic review of CT imaging post-ablation in 100% of patients.
Abbreviations: yr, year.

RFA for HCC as a bridge to transplantation, 70% appeared to have complete ablation on systematic CT (30% incomplete ablation) [36]. This radiologic response rate overestimated the true pathologic complete response rate of 55% (i.e., 45% incomplete ablation). These findings underscore the pitfalls of ablation, i.e., overestimation of efficacy of ablation by imaging, and reveal why a significant proportion of patients may recur after apparently complete RFA.

Although several groups have proposed RFA as an alternative to resection, no data have yet been reported to support the equivalence of these procedures. As shown in Table 4.1, even though a few studies have shown impressive short-term survival data, long-term survival outcomes remain disappointing.

We previously reported recurrence rates and outcomes after surgical treatment of CLM with resection and/or RFA [6]. Of the 418 patients studied, all had liver-only disease at open laparotomy. Patients underwent resection alone (*n* = 190), resection plus RFA (*n* = 101), RFA alone (*n* = 57), or no resection or ablation (*n* = 70), depending on the anatomy of the disease. The 5-year overall survival rate after resection alone was 58%; the 4-year survival rates after resection alone, resection plus RFA, and RFA alone were 65%, 36%, and 22%, respectively (*p* < 0.0001). RFA alone provided only a modest survival advantage over chemotherapy alone, and 3-year survival rates with RFA alone and resection plus ablation were comparable to those of other studies [30]. Although this study was not designed to compare resection with RFA, the groups were oncologically similar, and anatomy of disease was the predominant difference between groups.

When controlled for known risk factors for survival ≤5 years, marked differences in disease-free and overall survival rates between treatments with resection only versus any treatment involving ablation remained strikingly significant.

These findings were emphasized in our subsequent analysis of patients with solitary CLM, which included a complete follow-up imaging review [3]. One hundred and eighty patients with solitary liver metastases were studied – 150 treated by resection and 30 by RFA [3]. RFA was performed when it was perceived that the extent of resection needed would not be tolerated. Periprocedural chemotherapy use was similar in the two groups. The overall 5-year survival rate for patients who underwent resection was 71%, compared with only 27% in those treated by RFA. The local recurrence rate after resection was 5% and after RFA was 37%. Even in the treatment of tumors ≤3 cm, the local recurrence rate was 31% after RFA but only 3% after resection (median follow-up, >31 months). These striking differences in outcome would not be explained by oncologic differences in patients, but only by differences in treatment [3].

A study by Oshowo et al. is often cited as evidence of equivalence between RFA and resection [32]. In that series, 25 patients with solitary CLM were treated with RFA, and their outcomes were compared with those of 20 patients treated with liver resection. On the basis of a 3-year survival rate of 55% for resection and 53% for RFA, the authors concluded that in this selected group of patients, treatment strategies were comparable. However, a 3-year survival rate of only 55% after treatment of solitary CLM cannot be considered acceptable, given

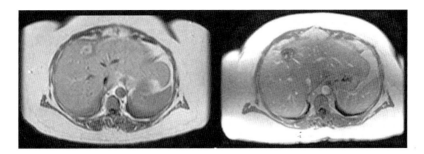

Fig. 4.3 Scans of a 5-year survivor after radiofrequency ablation (RFA) for colorectal liver metastases. The *left panel* demonstrates the pre-RFA MRI (axial T1 post-contrast) on 5/10/2002. The *right* *panel* demonstrates the post-RFA cavity on 3/13/2007. The patient remains without evidence of disease

the 71% 5-year overall survival rate reported in a much larger cohort (and in fact, no long-term survivors were reported in the Oshowo et al. study) [3, 32].

Only a randomized controlled trial of RFA versus resection for the treatment of CLM can definitively answer the question of equivalence between resection and ablation, but such a trial is unlikely to be performed because of the consistent findings of decreased rates of local recurrence and improved duration of survival in patients treated with resection. Furthermore, only a few long-term survivors after RFA for CLM have been reported; even at our institution, despite our extensive experience, we have seen only one 5-year survivor after RFA for CLM (Fig. 4.3). In this patient, severe steatohepatitis was found at laparotomy; thus, the patient underwent RFA in lieu of resection.

Because of the serious issue of local recurrence after RFA and improved survival rates with resection, we recently evaluated the utility of hepatic resection of a local recurrence after RFA for CLM in 23 patients [37]. At a median follow-up period of 29 months, the median length of overall survival was 47 months, and the median length of disease-free survival was 14 months. Of note was the common need for extended resection or resection of

adjacent structures after recurrence following RFA (in 18% and 38% of patients, respectively) and an increase in morbidity and mortality rates when resection was performed after RFA. Although the overall survival rate after salvage therapy was reasonable at early follow-up (62% at 3 years), the disease-free survival rate for this period was somewhat disappointing (only 24%) and recurrence remote from the resection site was common. Based on potential for good outcome, however, resection of RFA recurrences should be considered. One example of resection after RFA from our institution is illustrated in Fig. 4.4. This patient showed no evidence of disease recurrence after 31 months.

An important role of RFA is in the treatment of unresectable recurrences after hepatic resection. Low morbidity and mortality rates and 5-year survival rates as high as 44% in those patients eligible for potentially curative re-resection are well established, but in those patients for whom repeated hepatectomy is not feasible or safe, RFA may offer an alternative [38, 39]. Elias et al. evaluated 47 patients (29 with CLM) with liver tumors that had recurred after hepatic resection [27]. All of these patients underwent percutaneous ablation. The median follow-up period was very short (14 months). Of those 47 patients,

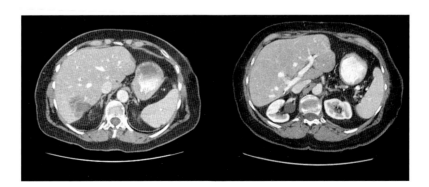

Fig. 4.4 Resection after a post-radiofrequency ablation (RFA) recurrence. The *left panel* demonstrates computed tomography (CT) evidence of a segment VIII recurrence after pre-referral RFA ablation of a small posteriorly located colorectal liver metastasis. The *right panel* is a surveillance CT image 31 months after right posterior sectionectomy. The patient has no evidence of recurrence

26 (55%) developed liver recurrences, 6 of which were considered true local recurrences. The 1- and 2-year survival rates were 88% and 55%, respectively, which suggest utility in this setting.

In summary, patients with CLM should be fully evaluated for resection of their tumor before RFA is considered [3, 6, 34]. Other strategies, including two-stage resection, PVE, and downsizing chemotherapy followed by surgery, provide outcomes that are superior to those of RFA or RFA plus resection [8, 10, 11, 12, 40]. In patients with large lesions (>4–6 cm) or lesions near the hilar plate, other local control strategies, including chemotherapy and reassessment, should definitely be considered [13].

Despite these caveats, in properly selected patients with unresectable CLM, RFA may offer a modest improvement in survival over systemic therapy alone, although as survival rates with the use of systemic chemotherapy continue to improve, this advantage may narrow further. Additional data will soon be available from a phase III randomized controlled study of RFA combined with chemotherapy versus chemotherapy alone (the Chemotherapy + LOCal ablation versus Chemotherapy [CLOCC] trial, European Organization for Research and Treatment of Cancer [EORTC] trial 40004) [13].

Microwave Coagulation Therapy

Microwave coagulation therapy (MCT) to ablate liver tumors was introduced in 1979 by Tabuse [41]. MCT has been used primarily in China and Japan; its use in the United States, however, has not yet been approved [42]. MCT was originally developed to control bleeding during hepatic resection; it was noticed, however, that the application of microwave fields to hepatic parenchyma produced rapid heating and thick coagulating layers that often provided more effective hemostasis than sutures, hemostatic agents, or even other ablative therapies such as RFA or laser surgery [43].

MCT may be administered percutaneously, laparoscopically, or via laparotomy. The microwave frequency used for surgical systems, 2.45 GHz, provides the appropriate coagulation thickness and allows the use of standard microwave oven power circuits and parts, making this technology less expensive than other ablative technologies. The rapid generation of heat produces zones of coagulative necrosis after only 30–60 seconds, more rapidly than RFA does [16].

Currently, the indications and contraindications for MCT are similar to those for RFA. MCT has been studied primarily as an ablative strategy for HCC in patients with cirrhosis who are not candidates for resection, but this technique has also been used for other unresectable metastatic liver lesions such as CLM. Some researchers have suggested that MCT may be more useful than RFA near large blood vessels. Because the technology relies less on the conduction of heat and more on the generation of a larger burn by direct heat, it may be less susceptible to the heat sink effect [42]. Just as in RFA, MCT is relatively contraindicated in large tumors. Because the rapid development of coagulative necrosis around the MCT needle produces a tissue coagulum that inhibits further dissipation of heat into the tissue, MCT produces a smaller area of ablation per needle pass than RFA does [44]. In addition, because MCT represents another form of thermal ablation, caution must be used in applying this technique near the hilar plate.

Very little has been published about the complications that occur after MCT [44]. Early concerns about microwave technology centered around the nonthermal adverse effects, most commonly, patients' extended exposure to low-level electromagnetic fields. Currently, there is no convincing evidence that microwave exposure causes any serious health hazards [43]. The effects of the thermal ablation itself are similar to those of RFA. Hepatic abscesses, bile duct fistulae, and pleural effusions have been reported [45, 46]. Thus, the available data indicate that MCT is a relatively safe technique, with caveats similar to those of RFA.

Although most of the research with MCT has focused on the treatment of unresectable HCC, a few studies have looked at the use of MCT for CLM. The first pilot study, in which 15 patients with solitary metastatic liver tumors ≤3.0 cm in diameter were targeted, used a percutaneous approach [46]. During one–three sessions, patients received 3–10 doses of microwave radiation. Complete necrosis, as determined by CT, was achieved in 13 of the 15 patients. Adverse effects were minimal. The follow-up period was short [46]. The primary contribution of this study was that it showed the safety of MCT.

Shibata et al. compared MCT with resection in patients with CLM [45]. Thirty patients with multiple metastases that were initially determined to be resectable were randomly assigned to undergo MCT ($n = 14$) or resection ($n = 16$). MCT was performed after laparotomy. Complications were comparable in the two groups and included bile duct fistula, intestinal obstruction, and hepatic abscess. No statistically significant difference in survival was seen between the MCT and resection groups. The estimated 3-year survival rates were similar (14% with MCT and 23% with resection) and the authors concluded that MCT was equivalent to resection in survival rates and represented a safer, less invasive

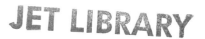

approach [45]. However, their estimated 3-year survival rate of 23% for resection was far lower than what is considered acceptable, and death from liver failure in 67% of patients after MCT (and in 58% after resection) with no survivors after 50 months further bring these data into question.

No clinical trials are ongoing in the United States for ablation of liver tumors using MCT and no studies have directly compared MCT with RFA. Much work with this promising technology remains to be done.

Other Ablation Therapies

Percutaneous Ethanol Injection (PEI)

One of the first ablative techniques described for unresectable liver tumors was PEI. Before the emergence of RFA, PEI was the most widely used minimally invasive ablative strategy for liver tumors. PEI has been well studied in unresectable HCC and can be effective for local control of small lesions (2–3 cm in diameter). Various studies have reported complete tumor necrosis in 36–80% of cases [47].

PEI is inexpensive, simple to perform, and repeatable [25]. Ninety-five percent ethanol is injected directly into the tumor under sonographic or CT guidance. The diffusion of alcohol through the tumor can be seen on sonography as echodense droplets, allowing for real-time monitoring of the injection. Ethanol causes cytoplasmic dehydration leading to coagulative necrosis and causes small-vessel thrombosis by disrupting endothelial cell integrity [16, 25]. PEI is associated with low morbidity. It is often performed in an outpatient setting for small-volume disease, but it generally must be repeated several times. Its utility for CLM is established for very small lesions but has been supplanted by more advanced flexible ablation techniques, especially RFA [48].

Interstitial Laser Photocoagulation

Interstitial laser photocoagulation (ILP) involves the direct thermal destruction of tumors using laser energy. A laser fiber or fibers are placed directly into the tumor, tumor cells are exposed to high temperatures (>55°C), and cell death is achieved by a mechanism of action similar to that of RFA [44]. In contrast to other medical laser applications, in which high-energy light is applied briefly to achieve rapid photocoagulation, ILP uses low-energy light (3–20 watts) continuously over 2–20 minutes to

avoid carbonization and vaporization of tissue adjacent to the fiber, which would limit penetration of the coagulum and expansion of the ablation zone. Despite various technical advances in ILP systems, limited ablation zones remain the primary limitation of this strategy: reproducible zones are only 10–15 mm in diameter [44]. ILP can be performed percutaneously with local anesthesia and light sedation, making it an attractive ablative strategy.

In the largest series published on the treatment of CLM, Vogl et al. performed MRI-guided ILP in 603 patients with 1801 liver metastases [49]. Patients had previously been designated ineligible for surgery. No lesions ≥5 cm were treated. Local recurrence rates at 6 months ranged from 1.9% to 4.4%. The authors maintained that no local recurrences were identified after 6 months in this patient population, but longer-term data have not been reported. The median survival time (2.9 years) and 5-year survival rate (37%) are notable, and treatment-related complications were uncommon (17/603 patients, including pleural effusion [$n = 17$], intraabdominal bleeding [$n = 2$], and liver abscess [$n = 6$]). Two patients died within 30 days of the procedure, one of jejunal perforation thought to be secondary to stress ulceration and one of sepsis of unknown origin. The overall complication rate was 1.5% [49]. Another smaller study found similar results [50].

Although more studies with longer-term follow-up are needed for ILP, advocates of this procedure highlight its low local recurrence rates compared with other ablative strategies (although no long-term data are available) and cite the benefits of using real-time MRI [49]. The best results in ILP have been seen with CT-guided needle placement followed by MRI-guided ablation, and this strategy has been advocated for best results [49]. Clearly, more studies are needed with adequate follow-up to clarify the role of ILP.

High-Intensity Focused Ultrasound

First applied clinically in the 1950s, high-intensity focused ultrasound (HIFU) has generated more interest recently as an ablative technique, with improved targeting provided by CT, MRI, and sonography [51]. HIFU uses the same principles as diagnostic sonography except that the intensity of the HIFU beam is much higher and the beam is more focused than a standard diagnostic ultrasound beam. A potential advantage of HIFU is its potential utility to treat larger lesions than other ablation modalities.

HIFU ablates target tissue via two mechanisms: heat and cavitation. The mechanical energy produced by the ultrasound wave is quickly converted to heat in the tissue, which causes irreversible cell death through coagulative necrosis. Cavitation results from small gaseous nuclei existing in subcellular organelles and fluid in tissue expanding and contracting secondary to acoustic pressure [51].

HIFU has been studied predominantly as an extracorporeal modality for liver tumors. Targeting is typically guided by sonography or MRI. Under real-time sonographic guidance, gray-scale changes during ablation can be used to estimate the extent of treatment. MRI-directed therapy relies on temperature changes in the tissue to optimize localization.

There are few published data on the efficacy of HIFU from human clinical trials, but results from the treatment of large HCC lesions have encouraged the study of this technology in other diseases [52]. A prospective nonrandomized clinical trial in the United Kingdom is under way to evaluate the safety and effectiveness of HIFU in the treatment of liver and kidney tumors [53]. Of the 30 patients enrolled, 22 have liver metastases, 18 of whom have CLM. Interim results were recently published. In the liver metastases group, 100% of the patients demonstrated some evidence of ablation. Adverse effects were minimal. Similar to the previous study described, skin toxicity was seen in eight patients, but no severe burns were noted. In this interim analysis, no recurrence data or survival data were published [53]. Clearly, these data will be important as the role of HIFU evolves in the treatment of CLM and other liver tumors.

Radiation Therapy

Finally, radiation in the form of external or internal radiation therapy has been used to "ablate" liver tumors [54, 55, 56, 57, 58]. External-beam radiation therapy (EBRT) can be delivered using conformal three- and four-dimensional (respiratory-gated) planning in selected patients so that high doses of radiation can be delivered to areas where RFA is contraindicated (e.g., centrally, without a serious risk of bile duct injury). Limitations of EBRT include the risk of radiation-induced liver disease (RILD), a clinical syndrome of anicteric hepatomegaly, pain, ascites, and increased levels of liver enzymes, and adverse effects related to treatment fields that overlap gastrointestinal mucosa or lung.

Another external beam technique introduced in 2000 by Koniaris et al. is called the interstitial point-source photon radiosurgery system (PRS) [57]. PRS delivers radiation in doses similar to those delivered in interstitial brachytherapy. In summary, limited clinical data are available to support one EBRT technique over another and all are investigational.

Radioembolic techniques have also emerged in the past few years. Selective internal radiation therapy (SIRT) has been approved by the FDA for unresectable CLM but is available in only a limited number of institutions in the United States [54]. SIRT (SIRTex Medical, Inc., Lane Cove, New South Wales, Australia) uses resin-based microspheres (SIR-Spheres, SIRTex Medical, Inc.) impregnated with yttrium-90 (^{90}Y) that are infused directly into the hepatic arterial circulation. Results from clinical trials have demonstrated the ability of SIRT to achieve local tumor control with low toxicity, but its role in the multidisciplinary management of CLM is still evolving [54]. Similar to SIR-Spheres, TheraSpheres (MDS Nordion, Inc., Ottawa, ON, Canada) are insoluble glass microspheres in which ^{90}Y is an integral constituent of the glass sphere itself. TheraSpheres are delivered in a fashion similar to SIR-Spheres. TheraSpheres have been studied primarily for the treatment of unresectable HCC, although results from one study showed some response in patients with CLM [55, 56].

In the proper settings, radioembolic techniques offer the advantage of improved targeting with less toxicity to the normal liver. However, these techniques should not be used when there is evidence of substantial lung shunting or collateral flow to the gastrointestinal tract; otherwise, radiation pneumonitis, gastritis, and/or enteritis could result [55]. As the techniques, indications, and limitations for these newer modalities are clarified, the prospects for the use of radiation therapy in the management of unresectable CLM should improve.

Conclusions

Although many ablation techniques have been used to treat CLM, RFA is the best studied in the United States and the only one approved to date by FDA. This approach clearly has a role in the treatment of unresectable CLM, but despite more than 10 years of experience, RFA has not been shown to be equivalent to resection. Advances in systemic therapy leading to responses in liver tumors and improvements in ablation technology and real-time imaging may further expand the role of these treatments.

Resection thus remains the gold standard treatment of CLM. Given novel approaches such as PVE, staged resections, and neoadjuvant chemotherapy with newer agents, the definition of resectability has greatly changed over the past decade and continues to evolve [59]. Although the indications for resection are expanding, the role of ablation is likely to persist for patients with unresectable or recurrent disease. Of paramount importance before the application of any liver-directed therapy for CLM is a thorough evaluation of the patient by a multidisciplinary team that will consider the appropriateness, sequencing, and individualization of therapy [13].

References

1. Jemal A, Siegel R, Ward E, et al. Cancer statistics, 2007. CA Cancer J Clin. 2007; 57(1): 43–66.
2. Welch JP, Donaldson GA. The clinical correlation of an autopsy study of recurrent colorectal cancer. Ann Surg. 1979; 189(4): 496–502.
3. Aloia TA, Vauthey JN, Loyer EM, et al. Solitary colorectal liver metastasis: resection determines outcome. Arch Surg. 2006; 141(5): 460–6; discussion 6–7.
4. Ercolani G, Grazi GL, Ravaioli M, et al. Liver resection for multiple colorectal metastases: influence of parenchymal involvement and total tumor volume, vs number or location, on long-term survival. Arch Surg. 2002; 137(10): 1187–92.
5. Choti MA, Sitzmann JV, Tiburi MF, et al. Trends in long-term survival following liver resection for hepatic colorectal metastases. Ann Surg. 2002; 235(6): 759–66.
6. Abdalla EK, Vauthey JN, Ellis LM, et al. Recurrence and outcomes following hepatic resection, radiofrequency ablation, and combined resection/ablation for colorectal liver metastases. Ann Surg. 2004; 239(6): 818–25; discussion 25–7.
7. Mann CD, Metcalfe MS, Leopardi LN, Maddern GJ. The clinical risk score: emerging as a reliable preoperative prognostic index in hepatectomy for colorectal metastases. Arch Surg. 2004; 139(11): 1168–72.
8. Adam R, Delvart V, Pascal G, et al. Rescue surgery for unresectable colorectal liver metastases downstaged by chemotherapy: a model to predict long-term survival. Ann Surg. 2004; 240(4) 644–57; discussion 57–8.
9. Adam R, Lucidi V, Bismuth H. Hepatic colorectal metastases: methods of improving resectability. Surg Clin North Am. 2004; 84(2): 659–71.
10. Shimada H, Tanaka K, Matsuo K, Togo S. Treatment for multiple bilobar liver metastases of colorectal cancer. Langenbecks Arch Surg. 2006; 391(2): 130–42.
11. Jaeck D, Oussoultzoglou E, Rosso E, et al. A two-stage hepatectomy procedure combined with portal vein embolization to achieve curative resection for initially unresectable multiple and bilobar colorectal liver metastases. Ann Surg. 2004; 240(6): 1037–49; discussion 49–51.
12. Abdalla EK, Barnett CC, Doherty D, et al. Extended hepatectomy in patients with hepatobiliary malignancies with and without preoperative portal vein embolization. Arch Surg. 2002; 137(6): 675–80; discussion 80–1.
13. Abdalla EK, Adam R, Bilchik AJ, et al. Improving resectability of hepatic colorectal metastases: expert consensus statement. Ann Surg Oncol. 2006; 13(10): 1271–80.
14. Fusai G, Davidson BR. Management of colorectal liver metastases. Colorectal Dis. 2003; 5(1): 2–23.
15. Cooper IS, Hirose T. Application of cryogenic surgery to resection of parenchymal organs. N Engl J Med. 1966; 274(1): 15–8.
16. Gannon CJ, Curley SA. The role of focal liver ablation in the treatment of unresectable primary and secondary malignant liver tumors. Semin Radiat Oncol. 2005; 15(4): 265–72.
17. Dick EA, Taylor-Robinson SD, Thomas HC, Gedroyc WM. Ablative therapy for liver tumours. Gut. 2002; 50(5): 733–9.
18. Seifert JK, Junginger T. Cryotherapy for liver tumors: current status, perspectives, clinical results, and review of literature. Technol Cancer Res Treat. 2004; 3(2): 151–63.
19. Bageacu S, Kaczmarek D, Lacroix M, et al. Cryosurgery for resectable and unresectable hepatic metastases from colorectal cancer. Eur J Surg Oncol. 2007; 33(5): 590–6.
20. Ruers TJ, Joosten J, Jager GJ, Wobbes T. Long-term results of treating hepatic colorectal metastases with cryosurgery. Br J Surg. 2001; 88(6): 844–9.
21. Weaver ML, Ashton JG, Zemel R. Treatment of colorectal liver metastases by cryotherapy. Semin Surg Oncol. 1998; 14(2): 163–70.
22. Ravikumar TS, Kane R, Cady B, et al. A 5-year study of cryosurgery in the treatment of liver tumors. Arch Surg. 1991; 126(12): 1520–3; discussion 3–4.
23. Ravikumar TS, Kane R, Cady B, et al. Hepatic cryosurgery with intraoperative ultrasound monitoring for metastatic colon carcinoma. Arch Surg. 1987; 122(4): 403–9.
24. Joosten J, Jager G, Oyen W, et al. Cryosurgery and radiofrequency ablation for unresectable colorectal liver metastases. Eur J Surg Oncol. 2005; 31(10): 1152–9.
25. Hong K, Georgiades CS, Geschwind JF. Technology insight: Image-guided therapies for hepatocellular carcinoma—intra-arterial and ablative techniques. Nat Clin Pract Oncol. 2006; 3(6): 315–24.
26. Curley SA. Radiofrequency ablation of malignant liver tumors. Ann Surg Oncol. 2003; 10(4): 338–47.
27. Elias D, De Baere T, Smayra T, et al. Percutaneous radiofrequency thermoablation as an alternative to surgery for treatment of liver tumour recurrence after hepatectomy. Br J Surg. 2002; 89(6): 752–6.
28. Curley SA, Marra P, Beaty K, et al. Early and late complications after radiofrequency ablation of malignant liver tumors in 608 patients. Ann Surg. 2004; 239(4): 450–8.
29. Lencioni R, Goletti O, Armillotta N, et al. Radio-frequency thermal ablation of liver metastases with a cooled-tip electrode needle: results of a pilot clinical trial. Eur Radiol. 1998; 8(7): 1205–11.
30. Solbiati L, Livraghi T, Goldberg SN, et al. Percutaneous radiofrequency ablation of hepatic metastases from colorectal cancer: long-term results in 117 patients. Radiology. 2001; 221(1): 159–66.
31. Livraghi T, Solbiati L, Meloni F, et al. Percutaneous radiofrequency ablation of liver metastases in potential candidates for resection: the "test-of-time approach." Cancer. 2003; 97(12): 3027–35.
32. Oshowo A, Gillams A, Harrison E, et al. Comparison of resection and radiofrequency ablation for treatment of solitary colorectal liver metastases. Br J Surg. 2003; 90(10): 1240–3.
33. Lencioni R, Crocetti L, Cioni D, et al. Percutaneous radiofrequency ablation of hepatic colorectal metastases: technique, indications, results, and new promises. Invest Radiol. 2004; 39(11): 689–97.
34. Amersi FF, McElrath-Garza A, Ahmad A, et al. Long-term survival after radiofrequency ablation of complex unresectable liver tumors. Arch Surg. 2006; 141(6): 581–7; discussion 7–8.
35. Pompili M, Mirante VG, Rondinara G, et al. Percutaneous ablation procedures in cirrhotic patients with hepatocellular carcinoma submitted to liver transplantation: Assessment of efficacy at explant analysis and of safety for tumor recurrence. Liver Transpl. 2005; 11(9): 1117–26.
36. Mazzaferro V, Battiston C, Perrone S, et al. Radiofrequency ablation of small hepatocellular carcinoma in cirrhotic patients awaiting liver transplantation: a prospective study. Ann Surg. 2004; 240(5): 900–9.

37. Badgwell B, Vauthey JN, Ribero D, et al. Resection of hepatic recurrence following radiofrequency ablation for liver metastases. In program and abstracts of the 2007 Annual Meeting of the American Hepato-Pancreato-Biliary Association; April 19–22, 2007; Las Vegas, NV. Abstract 243.

38. Bismuth H, Adam R, Navarro F, et al. Re-resection for colorectal liver metastasis. Surg Oncol Clin N Am. 1996; 5(2:) 353–64.

39. Adam R, Bismuth H, Castaing D, et al. Repeat hepatectomy for colorectal liver metastases. Ann Surg. 1997; 225(1): 51–60; discussion -2.

40. Chun YS, Vauthey JN, Ribero D, et al. Systemic chemotherapy and two-stage hepatectomy for extensive bilateral colorectal liver metastases: Perioperative safety and survival. J Gastrointest Surg. 2007; 11(11): 1498–504; discussion 1504–5.

41. Tabuse K. A new operative procedure of hepatic surgery using a microwave tissue coagulator. Nippon Geka Hokan. 1979; 48(2): 160–72.

42. Fox R. Equipment scarcity delays acceptance of microwave ablation. General Surgery News. April 2007; Sect. 32–3.

43. Tabuse K. Basic knowledge of a microwave tissue coagulator and its clinical applications. J Hepatobiliary Pancreat Surg. 1998; 5(2): 165–72.

44. Izzo F. Other thermal ablation techniques: microwave and interstitial laser ablation of liver tumors. Ann Surg Oncol. 2003; 10(5): 491–7.

45. Shibata T, Niinobu T, Ogata N, Takami M. Microwave coagulation therapy for multiple hepatic metastases from colorectal carcinoma. Cancer. 2000; 89(2): 276–84.

46. Seki T, Wakabayashi M, Nakagawa T, et al. Percutaneous microwave coagulation therapy for solitary metastatic liver tumors from colorectal cancer: a pilot clinical study. Am J Gastroenterol. 1999; 94(2): 322–7.

47. Giovannini M. Percutaneous alcohol ablation for liver metastasis. Semin Oncol. 2002; 29(2): 192–5.

48. Giovannini M, Seitz JF. Ultrasound-guided percutaneous alcohol injection of small liver metastases. Results in 40 patients. Cancer. 1994; 73(2): 294–7.

49. Vogl TJ, Straub R, Eichler K, et al. Colorectal carcinoma metastases in liver: laser-induced interstitial thermotherapy—local tumor control rate and survival data. Radiology. 2004; 230(2): 450–8.

50. Gillams AR, Lees WR. Survival after percutaneous, image-guided, thermal ablation of hepatic metastases from colorectal cancer. Dis Colon Rectum. 2000; 43(5): 656–61.

51. Leslie TA, Kennedy JE. High-intensity focused ultrasound principles, current uses, and potential for the future. Ultrasound Q. 2006; 22(4): 263–72.

52. Wu F, Wang ZB, Chen WZ, et al. Extracorporeal high intensity focused ultrasound ablation in the treatment of patients with large hepatocellular carcinoma. Ann Surg Oncol. 2004; 11(12): 1061–9.

53. Illing RO, Kennedy JE, Wu F, et al. The safety and feasibility of extracorporeal high-intensity focused ultrasound (HIFU) for the treatment of liver and kidney tumours in a Western population. Br J Cancer. 2005; 93(8): 890–5.

54. Welsh JS, Kennedy AS, Thomadsen B. Selective Internal Radiation Therapy (SIRT) for liver metastases secondary to colorectal adenocarcinoma. Int J Radiat Oncol Biol Phys. 2006; 66(2 Suppl): S62–73.

55. Salem R, Hunter RD. Yttrium-90 microspheres for the treatment of hepatocellular carcinoma: a review. Int J Radiat Oncol Biol Phys. 2006; 66(2 Suppl): S83–8.

56. Lewandowski RJ, Thurston KG, Goin JE, et al. 90Y microsphere (TheraSphere) treatment for unresectable colorectal cancer metastases of the liver: response to treatment at targeted doses of 135–150 Gy as measured by [18F]fluorodeoxyglucose positron emission tomography and computed tomographic imaging. J Vasc Interv Radiol. 2005; 16(12): 1641–51.

57. Koniaris LG, Chan DY, Magee C, et al. Focal hepatic ablation using interstitial photon radiation energy. J Am Coll Surg. 2000; 191(2): 164–74.

58. Dawson LA, Lawrence TS. The role of radiotherapy in the treatment of liver metastases. Cancer J. 2004; 10(2): 139–44.

59. Charnsangavej C, Clary B, Fong Y, et al. Selection of patients for resection of hepatic colorectal metastases: expert consensus statement. Ann Surg Oncol. 2006; 13(10): 1261–8.

Systemic Therapy for Non-operable Colorectal Cancer Metastases

5

Paulo M. G. Hoff and Scott Kopetz

The past decade has witnessed a substantial increase in the survival of patients diagnosed with colorectal cancer; however, almost half of the patients with this disease eventually develop metastases. Although colorectal cancer can metastasize to almost any location in the body, the most common places are the liver, lung, and peritoneum. The natural history for those patients has changed favorably but long-term survival remains elusive for most [1]. Recent advances in treatment strategies for metastatic colorectal cancer, including new cytotoxic agents and molecular-targeted therapies, aim to improve this situation when a potentially curative option, such as surgery, is not possible. In fact, for a select group of patients, the use of chemotherapy may even render disease that was initially non-operable, operable, offering an opportunity for curing it in a small subset of patients [2].

Systemic Treatment Strategies

The median survival of patients treated with the best available supportive care from the time of diagnosis of metastatic disease is only around 6 months, but the availability of new chemotherapeutics has increased overall survival to a median that is approaching 24 months. The systemic treatments currently used are usually well tolerated and the longer survival times achieved with these therapies are associated with good quality of life. After more than 50 years from its development, the major chemotherapeutic agents used in metastatic colorectal cancer remain the 5-fluorouracil (5-FU), or its oral pro-drugs, capecitabine and uracil plus tegafur (UFT). Irinotecan and oxaliplatin are the other active chemotherapy drugs, and details of the particular regimens using these

agents are given in Table 5.1. There are also three monoclonal antibodies approved for the treatment of colorectal cancer, and their development and current role will be reviewed.

Chemotherapeutic Agents

5-Fluorouracil

5-FU was developed in 1957, and remains the most commonly used chemotherapeutic agent for colorectal cancer [3]. Its effect on the cancer cells is mostly mediated through binding to the thymidylate synthetase enzyme. The most successful modulator used with 5-FU is leucovorin (folinic acid), which increases reduced folate within cancer cells, a cofactor necessary for effective inhibition of thymidylate synthetase. In a meta-analysis that compared 5-FU to 5-FU and leucovorin, the addition of leucovorin to 5-FU improved the response rate from 11% to 21% with a slight improvement in overall survival [4].

For metastatic disease, 5-FU can be delivered as a bolus or continuous infusion. The rate and dose of delivery of 5-FU influence the efficacy and toxicity profile. Bolus regimens are associated with higher rates of mucositis and neutropenia than are infusion regimens. A large meta-analysis confirmed this clinical observation: 31% of the patients given a 5-FU bolus experienced grade 3 or 4 hematologic toxicities, whereas this is seen in only 4% of those who received infusion regimens [5]. In contrast, hand–foot syndrome, or palmar-plantar erythrodysesthesia, was seen more frequently with continuous infusion than with bolus administration (34% vs. 13%) [5]. This syndrome, which is characterized by erythematous, painful swelling of the palms and soles, can occur within days of initiation of 5-FU but usually resolves within a week after discontinuation of therapy.

P.M.G. Hoff (✉)
Executive Director, Centro de Oncologia, Hospital Sirio Libanes, Sao Paulo, Brazil

J.-N. Vauthey et al. (eds.), *Liver Metastases*, DOI 10.1007/978-1-84628-947-7_5,
© Springer-Verlag London Limited 2009

Table 5.1 Commonly used chemotherapeutic agents and regimens for the treatment of patients with metastatic colorectal cancers

Regimen name	Leucovorin	Bolus 5-FU	Infusion 5-FU	Repeated
Mayo	LV 20 mg/m^2, days 1–5	5-FU 425 mg/m^2, days 1–5		Every 4–5 weeks
Roswell-Park	LV infusion 500 mg/m^2 over 2 hours	5-FU IV bolus 600 mg/m^2 weekly		Weekly ×6, with 2 weeks rest
DeGramont or LV5FU2	LV 200 mg/m^2 over 2 hours	5-FU bolus 400 mg/m^2, days 1 and 2	5-FU 600 mg/m^2 over 22 hours, days 1 and 2	Days 1 and 2, every 2 weeks
AIO	LV 500 mg/m^2 over 2 hours, day 1		5-FU 2600 mg/m^2 over 24 hours	Weekly ×6, with 2 weeks rest
IFL	LV 20 mg/m^2 over 2 hours, day 1	5-FU 425–500 mg/m^2 bolus, day 1	Irinotecan 100–125 mg/m^2, day 1	Every 4 weeks, with 2 weeks rest
FOLFIRI	LV 200 mg over 2 hours, days 1 and 2	5-FU 400 mg/m^2 bolus, days 1 and 2; 600 mg infusion over 22 hours, days 1 and 2	Irinotecan 180 mg/m^2, day 1	Every 2 weeks
FOLFOX 4	LV 200 mg IV over 2 hours, days 1 and 2	5-FU 400 mg/m^2 IV bolus, days 1 and 2; 600 mg/m^2 infusion over 22 hours, days 1 and 2	Oxaliplatin 85 mg/m^2, day 1	Every 2 weeks
FOLFOX 6	LV 400 mg IV over 2 hours, day 1	5-FU 400 mg/m^2 IV bolus, day 1; 2400–3000 mg/m^2 infusion over 46 hours	Oxaliplatin 100 mg/m^2, day 1	Every 2 weeks
Modified-FOLFOX 6	LV 400 mg IV over 2 hours, day 1	5-FU 400 mg/m^2 IV bolus, day 1; 2400–3000 mg/m^2 infusion over 46 hours	Oxaliplatin 85 mg/m^2, day 1	Every 2 weeks
FOLFOX 7 (OPTIMOX)	LV 400 mg IV over 2 hours, day 1	5-FU 400 mg/m^2 IV bolus, day 1; 2400 mg/m^2 infusion over 46 hours	Oxaliplatin 130 mg/m^2, day 1	Every 2 weeks
XELOX (CAPOX)		Capecitabine 1000 mg/m^2/day orally, twice a day, days 1–14	Oxaliplatin 130 mg/m^2 IV, day 1	Every 3 weeks

Ischemic chest pain due to coronary vasoconstriction can occur after administration of 5-FU, or the prodrug capecitabine, in patients with or without a history of cardiac problems. The presence of angina should prompt a full cardiac evaluation to rule out pre-existing coronary artery disease. If the angina is due to vasoconstriction of otherwise healthy coronary arteries, the use of nitrates has been shown to successfully control the problem in most patients [6].

The presence of severe myelosuppression, gastrointestinal toxicity, mucositis, diarrhea, alopecia and/or neurotoxicity should raise the question of whether the patient has a low level of dihydropyrimidine dehydrogenase, the main catabolic enzyme in the 5-FU catabolism pathway. Although this enzyme's activity is low in 3–5% of the population, screening is not routinely performed because of technical difficulties associated with enzyme activity assays [7]. Patients with known deficiency of dihydropyrimidine dehydrogenase should not be treated with any of the fluoropyrimidines available, and should be offered one of the other chemotherapy agents instead [8].

The use of continuous 5-FU infusion regimens can achieve protracted inhibition of thymidylate synthase, with a significant reduction on the bone marrow suppression, mucositis, and diarrhea associated with bolus administration. A meta-analysis that compared bolus and infusion regimens showed that patients who received the infusions had a better response rate (22% vs. 14%) and a small but significant prolongation of survival [5]. After a period in which American oncologists favored bolus regimens, it is clear that infusion regimens are rapidly gaining favor in clinical practice. Given the long-established benefit of 5-FU, recent advances in the treatment of metastatic colorectal cancer have added to, and not replaced, the 5-FU backbone.

Capecitabine

Capecitabine is an oral prodrug of 5-FU that is active against metastatic colorectal cancer. It is administered twice a day for an approved daily dose of 2500 mg/m^2. In a study comparing the capecitabine regimen with a bolus 5-FU regimen, capecitabine yielded a better response rate (25% vs. 15%) and a similar overall survival [9]. The combination of capecitabine plus oxaliplatin produced results similar to those of 5-FU and leucovorin plus oxaliplatin [10,11]. The toxicity profile of capecitabine is similar to that of continuously infused 5-FU, with the exception that hand–foot syndrome occurs more commonly with capecitabine. Although the results of capecitabine alone are considered inferior to those obtained with combination regimens, it is a therapeutic option for patients who wish to avoid intravenous chemotherapy.

Irinotecan

Irinotecan is a topoisomerase I inhibitor that was approved in 1997 for metastatic colorectal cancer. This approval was made on the basis of single-agent response rates of 26% in untreated patients and 13% in previously treated patients [12]. Irinotecan's efficacy is increased when it is combined with 5-FU. Two such combination regimens are in clinical use: IFL and FOLFIRI. The IFL regimen, which combines bolus 5-FU with irinotecan, has resulted in a better survival rate than 5-FU and leucovorin. However, this regimen has unacceptable toxicity: 54% grade 3 or 4 neutropenia and a 60-day mortality rate of 4.8% due to sepsis and profound diarrhea [13]. The FOLFIRI regimen, which was developed in Europe and is based on infusional 5-FU, is more effective and better tolerated than the IFL regimen [14]. As a result, the FOLFIRI regimen has become a common front-line treatment and has largely replaced IFL in clinical practice.

Diarrhea, a common side effect of irinotecan, occurs through two separate mechanisms. Early-onset diarrhea occurs within 24 hours of the infusion. It manifests as a cholinergic syndrome with flushing, abdominal cramping, miosis, diaphoresis, and excessive salivation. This is attributed to irinotecan's incidental inhibition of cholinesterase and can be treated by anticholinergic drugs such as atropine.

Late-onset diarrhea is ubiquitous after treatment with irinotecan, with grade 3 or 4 toxicity in more than 30% of patients on the IFL regimen, but less than 20% of patients on the FOLFIRI regimen. This type of diarrhea is attributed to the bowel's exposure to SN-38, the active metabolite of irinotecan. An inactive metabolite, SN-38G is excreted via the biliary system. Enzymes present in the intestinal brush border re-form the active drug SN-38, which damages the mucosal lining and induces diarrhea. Early recognition of diarrhea is critical, as early treatment with high-dose loperamide is effective in reducing the severity of diarrhea and preventing complications [15].

A recent study indicates that the use of irinotecan may be linked to the development of steatohepatitis, [16] which

may increase the risk of a postoperative complication after liver resections [16].

Oxaliplatin

Oxaliplatin is a platinum-containing agent with activity as a single agent against colorectal cancer. For reasons that are not completely clear, it has considerable synergistic activity with 5-FU, and the combination results in very high response rates [17]. A phase III trial, with 420 patients, randomized patients to receive 5-FU and leucovorin alone, or oxaliplatin (FOLFOX4 regimen), and the group given the combination had an impressive 50% response rate, with prolonged time to progression; unfortunately, there was no statistically significant improvement in overall survival [17].

A large intergroup trial with 795 patients compared front-line use of FOLFOX4, IFL, and a combination of irinotecan and oxaliplatin (IROX) [18]. The final analysis revealed a better overall survival with FOLFOX4 than with IFL or IROX (19.5 months vs. 15.0 and 17.4 months, respectively). Similarly, response rates were higher with FOLFOX (45%) than with IFL or IROX regimens (31% and 35%, respectively). A similar regimen, known as FOLFOX6, uses a smaller bolus of 5-FU and a slightly larger dose of oxaliplatin. FOLFOX6 improves the convenience than FOLFOX4 by omitting the second-day bolus of 5-FU. The efficacy of this regimen was similar to that of FOLFOX4, but patients experienced considerable neurotoxicity due to the higher dose of oxaliplatin [19]. In an effort to reduce the incidence of this neuropathy, the dose of oxaliplatin was decreased, and this so-called modified-FOLFOX6 regimen is now the most commonly used FOLFOX regimen among American oncologists.

Neuropathies seen with oxaliplatin include cold-induced pharyngolaryngeal dysesthesia and cumulative sensory neuropathies. Pharyngolaryngeal dysesthesia is a rare reaction in which patients have difficulty in breathing but show no evidence of desaturation or actual laryngospasm. The condition resolves rapidly but can be distressing if patients are not forewarned about its possibility. Patients normally begin to experience dose-limiting neuropathies after the cumulative oxaliplatin dose reaches 700–800 mg/m^2. The symptoms, which last longer after each dose of oxaliplatin, may eventually lead to discontinuation of oxaliplatin.

Similarly to what has been described for irinotecan, the use of oxaliplatin also seems to be associated with steatosis. However, it does not seem to be associated with steatohepatitis and an increase in the

use of cetuximab. In a phase III trial, the single-agent response rate was 10%, with a minor impact on progression-free survival, and no difference in overall survival [34]. After encouraging early clinical trials, panitumumab was tested in the first-line setting, in a phase III trial Panitumumab advanced colorectal cancer evaluation (PACCE), in which patients received either FOLFOX with bevacizumab, or the same combination plus panitumumab. Surprisingly, the trial was closed after an interim analysis revealed a worst survival for those patients receiving the combination of the antiVEGF and panitumumab. Whether the results will be the same for the combination of cetuximab and bevacizumab remains to be determined.

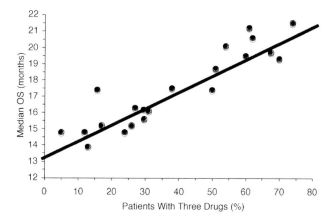

Fig. 5.2 Summary of 14 studies that correlate the percentage of patients receiving modern combination chemotherapy and the reported median overall survival (OS). Modern combination therapies were defined as 5-FU/LV plus oxaliplatin or irinotecan for first-line, or a second-line regimen including oxaliplatin or irinotecan. From Grothey A, Sargent D. Overall survival of patients with advanced colorectal cancer correlates with availability of fluorouracil, irinotecan, and oxaliplatin regardless of whether doublet or single-agent therapy is used first line. J Clin Oncol. 2005; 22: 1209–1214. Reprinted with permission from the American Society of Clinical Oncology

Recommendations for Systemic Treatments

The increase in the number of new agents available for the treatment of metastatic colorectal cancer, and the even greater number of possible combinations that can be generated make it difficult to propose a common treatment course appropriate for all patients. In general, we recommend that patients with stage IV colorectal cancer be treated with FOLFOX or FOLFIRI because these two regimens produce similar clinical benefits as first-line therapies for metastatic colorectal cancer. In one trial that supports this approach, patients were randomly assigned to one of the two regimens [35]. If their disease progressed after the first regimen, they were crossed over to the second regimen as the second-line therapy, eliminating the possible impact of exposure to different active agents. Although the trial was not designed to compare the two regimens, the response rates were similar for the two regimens, with a median overall survival time of approximately 21 months [35].

The availability of several treatment options allows personalization of the treatment course. Toxicity profiles can dictate preferred initial treatment regimens; for example, oxaliplatin-containing regimens should be avoided as first-line treatment for patients who have long-standing diabetes or neuropathy at baseline and for patients whose professions require fine motor skills. Similarly, irinotecan-containing regimens should be avoided as long as possible for patients who have Gilbert syndrome, ileostomies, or significant diarrhea at baseline.

It appears that the exact sequence or combination of agents has less impact outcomes than the ability of patients to be treated with all of the active chemotherapeutic agents. For example, a subgroup analysis of patients treated with bevacizumab plus IFL followed by a second-line oxaliplatin-containing regimen revealed a

remarkable 25-month median overall survival time. Similarly, a review of reports of several large trials found that the median overall survival is directly related to the number of active agents that a patient receives (see Fig. 5.2) [36]. For patients intolerant of intensive regimens, either capecitabine plus bevacizumab or infusional 5-FU/leucovorin plus bevacizumab is a possible therapeutic option.

Localized Treatment Strategies

Hepatic Artery Infusion

Hepatic artery infusion (HAI) is a complex treatment based on the continuous delivery of the chemotherapeutic agents from a reservoir directly into the liver. It requires surgical placement of a pump and selective cannulization of the hepatic artery. The theoretical advantage of HAI is that liver metastases are mainly perfused by the hepatic artery, whereas the normal liver is perfused predominantly by the portal vein. HAI thus allows more targeted delivery to the metastases and administration of a higher concentration of chemotherapeutic agents than can be accomplished with systemic chemotherapy. It is commonly stated that HAI could be used to convert lesions that are initially unresectable into resectable ones; however, this outcome is rather uncommon. In a retrospective review conducted at

M. D. Anderson, only a small minority of patients (22 of 383 patients) with initially unresectable hepatic metastases of colorectal cancer were able to undergo resection or ablation of their metastatic lesions after they were given HAI therapy [37]. In addition, the relapse rate was high, with only one patient disease free 1 year later, and half the patients subsequently developed extrahepatic metastases [37]. Because of this poor track record, we do not routinely advocate the use of neoadjuvant HAI for unresectable liver metastases.

The adjuvant administration of Floxuridine (FUDR) through HAI after curative resection of hepatic lesions has been evaluated in several studies, with mixed results. In one single-institution study of adjuvant systemic 5-FU with or without HAI of FUDR after liver resection, the length of progression-free survival of the patients who were also treated with FUDR by HAI was 31.2 months versus 17.2 months for those who did not receive HAI (p = 0.02) [38]. Despite this difference, however, the overall survival did not change. A recent meta-analysis that included six other studies of adjuvant 5-FU and FUDR administered by HAI found no survival benefit at 1 or 2 years [39]. The studies analyzed, however, did not compare the use of the newer systemic combination therapies with HAI. A small phase II study of 28 patients with inoperable liver metastases evaluated oxaliplatin by HAI plus systemic 5-FU. This study demonstrated a remarkable 27-month median progression-free survival [40]. Even though we do not routinely recommend the use of HAI, it remains an area of research interest.

Neoadjuvant Chemotherapy

The fact that only a small subset of patients can benefit from resection of metastatic lesions provides the rationale for using neoadjuvant chemotherapy to increase the number of patients who are candidates to surgery. Neoadjuvant chemotherapy is also useful because micrometastatic disease can theoretically be controlled early in the natural history of the disease. Additionally, patients with progressive disease despite neoadjuvant therapy may have a tumor biology that would not allow them to obtain benefit from surgery. For example, in one retrospective analysis, the response to neoadjuvant chemotherapy was evaluated in 131 patients who subsequently underwent resection [41]. The 5-year survival rates after resection were 37% for patients whose tumors had responded, 30% for those whose tumors had remained stable, and only 8% for those whose tumors had progressed [41].

Although exact numbers are difficult to obtain due to variable definitions of resectability, neoadjuvant chemotherapy may allow subsequent metastasectomy to be performed in a minority of patients whose liver metastases were initially unresectable. In one large retrospective series of patients with liver metastases only, 14% of the patients given neoadjuvant infusional 5-FU, leucovorin, and oxaliplatin as neoadjuvant therapy were able to undergo subsequent resections, with a median survival time of 4 years after the resection [2]. Although the definitions of unresectable lesions used in this study are debatable the concept of performing curative resections after neoadjuvant systemic chemotherapy has been accepted.

Conclusion

The treatment of non-operable liver metastasis has improved dramatically in the last decade, and patients can expect median survivals reaching almost 2 years. This improvement was based on the use of several new systemic drugs, and their use in combination yield relatively good response rates, with real improvements in the time for progression and in overall survival. However, even when the cancer is initially non-operable, one has to remember that the treatment of colorectal cancer is based on a multimodality approach, and that the only curative therapeutic modality is surgery. The management of metastatic colorectal cancer necessitates an understanding of both medical and surgical treatment approaches. Identifying the opportunities for metastasectomy and the means of prolonging survival when surgery is not possible requires close coordination within the oncology team.

References

1. Saad ED, Hoff PM. Chemotherapy of metastatic colorectal cancer. Curr Treat Options Gastroenterol. 2005; 8(3): 239–247.
2. Adam R, Avisar E, Ariche A, et al. Five-year survival following hepatic resection after neoadjuvant therapy for nonresectable colorectal. Ann Surg Oncol. 2001; 8(4): 347–53.
3. Heidelberger C, Chauhuri N, Dannenberg P, et al. Fluorinated pyrimidines, a new class of tumor-inhibitory compounds. Nature. 1957; 179: 663–666.
4. Thirion P, Michiels S, Pignon JP, et al. Modulation of fluorouracil by leucovorin in patients with advanced colorectal cancer: an updated meta-analysis. J Clin Oncol. 2004; 22(18): 3766–75.
5. Meta-analysis Group In Cancer. Efficacy of intravenous continuous infusion of fluorouracil compared with bolus administration in advanced colorectal cancer. Meta-analysis Group In Cancer. J Clin Oncol. 1998; 16(1): 301–8.
6. Aksoy S, Karaca B, Dincer M, Yalcin S. Common etiology of capecitabine and fluorouracil-induced coronary vasospasm in a colon cancer patient. Ann Pharmacother. 2005; 39(3): 573–4.

7. Johnson MR, Diasio RB. Importance of dihydropyrimidine dehydrogenase (DPD) deficiency in patients exhibiting toxicity following treatment with 5-fluorouracil. Adv Enzyme Regul. 2001; 41: 151–7.

8. Volk J, Reinke F, van Kuilenburg AB, et al. Safe administration of irinotecan, oxaliplatin and raltitrexed in a DPD-deficient patient with metastatic colon cancer. Ann Oncol. 2001; 12(4): 569–71.

9. Hoff PM, Ansari R, Batist G, et al. Comparison of oral capecitabine versus intravenous fluorouracil plus leucovorin as first-line treatment in 605 patients with metastatic colorectal cancer: results of a randomized phase III study. J Clin Oncol. 2001; 19(8): 2282–92.

10. Cassidy J, Tabernero J, Twelves C, et al. XELOX (capecitabine plus oxaliplatin): active first-line therapy for patients with metastatic colorectal cancer. J Clin Oncol. 2004; 22(11): 2084–91.

11. Borner MM, Bernhard J, Dietrich D, et al. A randomized phase II trial of capecitabine and two different schedules of irinotecan in first-line treatment of metastatic colorectal cancer: efficacy, quality-of-life and toxicity. Ann Oncol. 2005; 16(2): 282–8.

12. Pitot HC. US pivotal studies of irinotecan in colorectal carcinoma. Oncology. 1998; 12(8 Suppl 6): 48–53.

13. Saltz LB, Cox JV, Blanke C, et al. Irinotecan plus fluorouracil and leucovorin for metastatic colorectal cancer. Irinotecan Study Group. N Engl J Med. 2000; 343(13): 905–14.

14. Tournigand C, Andre T, Achille E, et al. FOLFIRI followed by FOLFOX6 or the reverse sequence in advanced colorectal cancer: a randomized GERCOR study. J Clin Oncol. 2004; 22(2): 229–37.

15. Rothenberg ML, Meropol NJ, Poplin EA, et al. Mortality associated with irinotecan plus bolus fluorouracil/leucovorin: summary findings of an independent panel. J Clin Oncol. 2001; 19(18): 3801–7.

16. Vauthey JN, Pawlik TM, Ribero D, et al. Chemotherapy regimen predicts steatohepatitis and an increase in 90-day mortality after surgery for hepatic colorectal metastases. J Clin Oncol. 2006; 24(13): 2065–72.

17. de Gramont A, Figer A, Seymour M, et al. Leucovorin and fluorouracil with or without oxaliplatin as first-line treatment in advanced colorectal cancer. J Clin Oncol. 2000; 18(16): 2938–47.

18. Goldberg RM, Sargent DJ, Morton RF, et al. A randomized controlled trial of fluorouracil plus leucovorin, irinotecan, and oxaliplatin combinations in patients with previously untreated metastatic colorectal cancer. J Clin Oncol. 2004; 22(1): 23–30.

19. Maindrault-Goebel F, Louvet C, Andre T, et al. Oxaliplatin added to the simplified bimonthly leucovorin and 5-fluorouracil regimen as second-line therapy for metastatic colorectal cancer (FOLFOX6). GERCOR. Eur J Cancer. 1999; 35(9): 1338–42.

20. Kohler G, Milstein C. Continuous cultures of fused cells secreting antibody of predefined specificity. Nature. 1975; 256(5517): 495–7.

21. Mellstedt H. Monoclonal antibodies in human cancer. Drugs Today (Barc). 2003; 39 Suppl C: 1–16.

22. Vaswani SK, Hamilton RG. Humanized antibodies as potential therapeutic drugs. Ann Allergy Asthma Immunol. 1998; 81(2): 105–15; quiz 115–6, 119.

23. Willett CG, Boucher Y, di Tomaso E, et al. Direct evidence that the VEGF-specific antibody bevacizumab has antivascular effects in human rectal cancer. Nat Med. 2004; 10(2): 145–7.

24. Ferrara N, Hillan KJ, Gerber HP, Novotny W. Discovery and development of bevacizumab, an anti-VEGF antibody for treating cancer. Nat Rev Drug Discov. 2004; 3(5): 391–400.

25. Kabbinavar FF, Schulz J, McCleod M, et al. Addition of bevacizumab to bolus fluorouracil and leucovorin in first-line metastatic colorectal cancer: results of a randomized phase II trial. J Clin Oncol. 2005; 23(16): 3697–705. Epub 2005 Feb 28.

26. Hurwitz H, Fehrenbacher L, Novotny W, et al. Bevacizumab plus irinotecan, fluorouracil, and leucovorin for metastatic colorectal cancer. N Engl J Med. 2004; 350(23): 2335–42.

27. Kopetz S, Glover K, Eng C, et al. Phase II study of infusional 5-fluorouracil, leucovorin, and irinotecan (FOLFIRI) plus bevacizumab as first-line treatment for metastatic colorectal cancer. J Clin Oncol. 2007; 25(18 s): 4089.

28. Giantonio BJ, Catalano PJ, Meropol NJ, et al. Bevacizumab in combination with oxaliplatin, fluorouracil, and leucovorin (FOLFOX4) for previously treated metastatic colorectal cancer: results from the Eastern Cooperative Oncology Group Study E3200. J Clin Oncol. 2007; 25(12): 1539–44.

29. Saltz L, Clarke S, Diaz-Rubio E, et al. Bevacizumab (Bev) in combination with XELOX or FOLFOX-4: updated efficacy results from XELOX-1 / N016966, a randomized phase III trial in first-line metastatic colorectal cancer J Clin Oncol. 2007; 25(18 s): 4028.

30. Cunningham D, Humblet Y, Siena S, et al. Cetuximab monotherapy and cetuximab plus irinotecan in irinotecan-refractory metastatic colorectal cancer. N Engl J Med. 2004; 351(4): 337–45.

31. Chung KY, Shia J, Kemeny NE, et al. Cetuximab shows activity in colorectal cancer patients with tumors that do not express the epidermal growth factor receptor by immunohistochemistry. J Clin Oncol. 2005; 23(9): 1803–10.

32. Van Cutsem E, Nowacki M, Lang I, et al. Randomized phase III study of irinotecan and 5-FU/FA with or without cetuximab in the first-line treatment of patients with metastatic colorectal cancer (mCRC): The CRYSTAL trial. J Clin Oncol. 2007; 25(18 s): 4000.

33. Cohenuram M, Saif MW. Panitumumab the first fully human monoclonal antibody: from the bench to the clinic. Anticancer Drugs. 2007; 18(1): 7–15.

34. Van Cutsem E, Peeters M, Siena S, et al. Open-label phase III trial of panitumumab plus best supportive care compared with best supportive care alone in patients with chemotherapy-refractory metastatic colorectal cancer. J Clin Oncol. 2007; 25(13): 1658–64.

35. Maindrault-Goebel F, Tournigand C, Andre T, et al. Oxaliplatin reintroduction in patients previously treated with leucovorin, fluorouracil and oxaliplatin for metastatic colorectal cancer. Ann Oncol. 2004; 15(8): 1210–4.

36. Grothey A, Sargent D, Goldberg RM, Schmoll HJ. Survival of patients with advanced colorectal cancer improves with the availability of fluorouracil-leucovorin, irinotecan, and oxaliplatin in the course of treatment. J Clin Oncol. 2004; 22(7): 1209–14.

37. Meric F, Patt YZ, Curley SA, et al. Surgery after downstaging of unresectable hepatic tumors with intra-arterial chemotherapy. Ann Surg Oncol. 2000; 7(7): 490–5.

38. Kemeny N, Huang Y, Cohen AM, et al. Hepatic arterial infusion of chemotherapy after resection of hepatic metastases from colorectal cancer. N Engl J Med. 1999; 341(27): 2039–48.

39. Clancy TE, Dixon E, Perlis R, et al. Hepatic arterial infusion after curative resection of colorectal cancer metastases: a meta-analysis of prospective clinical trials. J Gastrointest Surg. 2005; 9(2): 198–206.

40. Ducreux M, Ychou M, Laplanche A, et al. Hepatic arterial oxaliplatin infusion plus intravenous chemotherapy in colorectal cancer with inoperable hepatic metastases: a trial of the gastrointestinal group of the Federation Nationale des Centres de Lutte Contre le Cancer. J Clin Oncol. 2005; 23(22): 4881–7.

41. Adam R, Pascal G, Castaing D, et al. Tumor progression while on chemotherapy: a contraindication to liver resection for multiple colorectal metastases? Ann Surg. 2004; 240(6): 1052–61; discussion 1061–4.

Locoregional Chemotherapy for Hepatic Metastasis of Colorectal Cancer

Simon H. Telian, Byron E. Wright, and Anton J. Bilchik

Introduction

Colorectal cancer (CRC) is one of the most common malignancies in the United States. Over 150,000 cases are diagnosed annually, and each year there are more than 52,000 deaths from CRC [1]. This represents 10% of all cancer-related deaths in this country; only lung cancer claims more lives annually. The liver is the most common site of extranodal CRC metastasis: 25% of patients newly diagnosed with CRC will have synchronous hepatic metastasis, and an additional 25% of patients will eventually develop hepatic metastasis [2,3].

Hepatic resection has long been the only potentially curative option for patients with hepatic metastasis of CRC. Five-year survival rates reach 60% after complete resection, as compared with less than 10% for nonsurgical management [3, 4, 5]. However, because relatively few patients are candidates for complete resection of hepatic disease, effective nonsurgical adjuvant or first-line therapies are essential. Traditional systemic therapies, such as 5-fluorouracil (5-FU)-based regimens, have a modest impact on survival and recurrence after complete resection of node-positive primary CRC, but have proved disappointing for patients with unresectable hepatic metastasis [6,7]. Regional or hepatic arterial infusion (HAI) chemotherapy was developed in response to the poor results seen with systemic therapies. Because the primary blood supply for hepatic tumors is arterial rather than portal venous, high concentrations should maximize a tumor's exposure to the treating agent. In addition, localized delivery of an anti-cancer drug can produce therapeutic levels that could not be achieved by systemic infusion without excessive toxicity.

In the 5-FU era of systemic adjuvant therapy for metastatic CRC, the fluoropyrimidine FUDR (floxuridine) was the mainstay of HAI therapy. Initial studies clearly demonstrated impressive response rates but impact on overall survival was less clear [8, 9, 10]. Complications related to port placement and the therapy itself were a concern, although later studies with revised protocols and more standardized techniques demonstrated improved results [11, 12, 13]. Recent advances in systemic therapy for metastatic CRC have steered treatment away from 5-FU- and leucovorin (LVN)-based regimens. Regimens based on LVN, 5-FU, and oxaliplatin (the FOLFOX regimen) with anti-angiogenesis agents such as bevacizumab have become treatment mainstays that can produce dramatic results in patients with metastatic disease confined to the liver [4,14, 15, 16]. Patients with initially nonresectable disease may undergo several rounds of neoadjuvant chemotherapy, after which their disease is restaged; dramatic tumor regression is typical, allowing subsequent resection with or without ablation, followed by postoperative chemotherapy. The effectiveness of these newer drugs and this multimodality approach has tempered enthusiasm for regional chemotherapy. However, because many patients develop recurrence in the liver, it has been suggested that the addition of regional chemotherapy might further improve response rates and survival of patients treated with newer systemic combinations [17]. This chapter will focus on potential indications for HAI therapy, technical aspects of pump placement, and results of clinical HAI trials

Placement Technique

Any patient with CRC metastases and adequate hepatic reserve is a candidate for regional chemotherapy alone or as an adjunct to resection. Therefore, all patients should undergo a complete staging work-up that includes computed tomography (CT) of the chest, abdomen, and pelvis as well as total-body positron emission tomography

S.H. Telian (✉)
Surgical Oncology Fellow, John Wayne Cancer Institute at Saint John's Health Center, Santa Monica, CA, USA

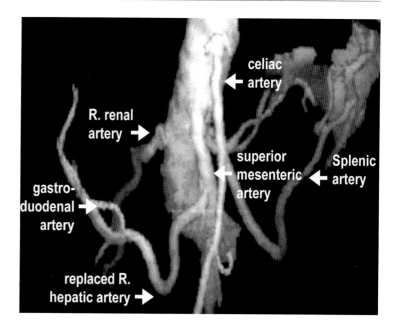

Fig. 6.1 CT angiogram showing three-dimensional image of hepatic arterial anatomy. Reprinted from: Bilchik AJ. Arterial chemotherapy as adjuvant and palliative treatment of hepatic colorectal metastases: an update. Surg Oncol Clin N Am. 2003; 12: 193–210. With permission from Elsevier

(PET) to exclude the possibility of extrahepatic disease. A thorough knowledge of both normal and aberrant hepatic arterial anatomy is critical because both replaced and/or accessory hepatic arteries are commonly seen. Although formal transfemoral angiography can be used to evaluate celiac and mesenteric arterial anatomy, CT angiography with 3-D arterial reconstruction is more common because it provides rapid and noninvasive views of the abdominal aorta and its branches (Fig. 6.1) [6]. Evidence of aberrant anatomy or incomplete hepatic perfusion may be a contraindication for HAI, as is known portal venous thrombosis; unresectable extrahepatic disease is a relative contraindication.

The traditional operative approach to HAI port placement is via a standard right subcostal incision. The upper abdomen is explored for evidence of nonhepatic metastasis and the gallbladder is then routinely removed. The common hepatic artery should be identified just medial to the common bile duct. The vessel is then mobilized back to the origin of the gastroduodenal artery (GDA). The GDA is dissected out to prevent or minimize any back perfusion of the duodenum or stomach during infusion. This is accomplished by selectively ligating any small arterial branches. The right gastric artery is also located and ligated, and the upper borders of both the stomach and duodenum are similarly skeletonized to further prevent back perfusion. Finally, the GDA is ligated distally at the point of furthest dissection.

Prior to arterial insertion, the pump is flushed with warm heparinized saline and a pocket is created on the anterior abdominal wall to accommodate the pump (Fig. 6.2) [5]. For smaller patients, a separate incision in the right lower quadrant may be optimal; alternatively, a pocket may be created through the same subcostal incision. The pump is anchored at the fascial level with suture and the catheter is passed through the fascia via a separate stab incision. The GDA is the preferred insertion site because of the tremendous collateral flow in this arterial distribution.

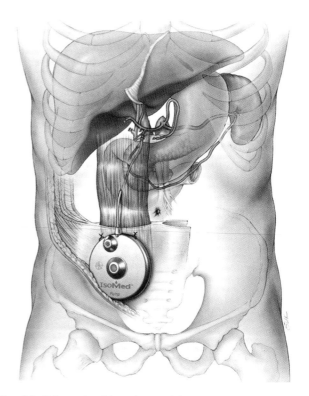

Fig. 6.2 Schematic of hepatic arterial infusion pump placement. Reprinted from: Kemeny N, Fata F. Hepatic-arterial chemotherapy. Lancet Oncol. 2001; 2: 418–428. With permission from Elsevier

The vessel is accessed and the catheter inserted utilizing standard vascular techniques. An arteriotomy is typically made on the vessel just distal to its takeoff from the common hepatic artery; after the catheter is inserted, it is secured in the vessel with ties. Bilobar hepatic perfusion is then usually confirmed with injection of 5 cc of a 10% fluorescein solution via the bolus port. Woods lamp illumination should demonstrate diffuse hepatic perfusion without illumination of the perihepatic viscera (stomach, duodenum, pancreas). Any evidence of extrahepatic perfusion should initiate a thorough search for additional side branches that require ligation. Incomplete hepatic perfusion should prompt a re-evaluation of potentially anomalous arterial anatomy as well as a reassessment of catheter placement. In the postoperative period, prior to initiation of therapy, technetium-99 macroaggregated albumin scanning is performed to mimic distribution of the planned treatment drug. Interventional embolization techniques can be used to address areas of extrahepatic perfusion.

Although this open approach to HAI port placement remains the gold standard, there are alternative techniques. Several investigators have reported the feasibility of a laparoscopic approach to port placement [18,19]. The steps of the laparoscopic technique are essentially the same as those for the open technique, except that methylene blue dye is used instead of fluorescein, to allow direct visualization of hepatic or extrahepatic perfusion. Points of potential concern include the ability to clearly visualize and inspect regional arterial anatomy, particularly complete GDA skeletonization, and also the ability to fully explore the upper abdomen to rule out extrahepatic metastases. Percutaneous positioning is another method of port placement. Early experiences with this technique were plagued by bleeding complications, problems with catheter thrombosis and high rates of extrahepatic perfusion [19]. Refinement of this technique, however, has led to a decrease in the incidence of such complications and it remains a viable alternative when an operative approach is not indicated. Because the percutaneous approach cannot be used to rule out extrahepatic disease and because it has relatively high rates of catheter migration and dislodgement, percutaneous positioning is considered only when open or laparoscopic approaches are not practical.

Historical Perspective

HAI was introduced in the 1970s, in response to disappointing results of systemic therapies for unresectable disease. Improved understanding of the biology of hepatic metastases and liver perfusion demonstrated that although the dominant blood supply to normal hepatocytes was based on portal-venous flow, metastatic deposits in the liver received primarily arterial blood flow. In addition, more effective hepatic drug delivery could be achieved with relatively isolated intra-arterial infusion and first-pass hepatic extraction, thereby markedly reducing systemic toxicity and increasing local drug levels. Early trials that used 5-FU reported high rates of systemic toxicity because first-pass hepatic extraction was only 50–55% [10,20, 21, 22]. The majority of randomized trials have utilized FUDR because its rate of first-pass hepatic extraction is 95%; this allows much higher intrahepatic concentrations without significant systemic effects.

Regional chemotherapy or HAI can be utilized in a number of different ways for the management of CRC with hepatic metastases. Many trials have assessed FUDR-based HAI for hepatic metastases: as primary therapy with and without simultaneous systemic therapy; as neoadjuvant therapy before resection/ablation; and as postresection adjuvant therapy to reduce rates of liver recurrence. The majority of initial studies showed improvements in local control but not overall survival. These early studies, however, suffered from design flaws that allowed patient crossover between treatment arms; there were also technical complications related to pump placement [8,10,20]. Later studies demonstrated response rates of 40–60% with improved outcomes over systemic therapy alone [23, 24, 25, 26].

Randomized Clinical Trials

Primary Therapy

Initial trials compared the efficacy of HAI with that of various systemic chemotherapeutic agents. Most patients in these studies had unresectable disease [8,10,16,20,22, 23, 24]. Response rates were better for HAI than for systemic treatment, but there was no significant correlation with improved overall survival (Table 6.1). Factors contributing to this finding may have been inadequate systemic chemotherapy, small study population sizes, and high rates of patient crossover to systemic chemotherapy, due to HAI toxicity. Although a meta-analysis of these studies did attribute a statistically significant survival advantage to HAI, the analysis did not account for differences in patient population, type, dose, or duration of chemotherapy. Some studies included patients with extrahepatic disease [8,22,26], whereas others used different types of drugs for systemic and regional therapy [23,24]. In a French study of

Table 6.1 Prospective randomized trials of HAI versus systemic chemotherapy for hepatic colorectal metastases. From: Bilchik AJ. Arterial chemotherapy as adjuvant and palliative treatment of hepatic colorectal metastases: an update. Surg Oncol Clin N Am. 2003; 12: 193–210. With permission from Elsevier

Group	No.of patients	Response rate HAI (%)	Systemic (%)	p	Median overall survival (months) HAI	Systemic	p
Kemeny et al. [10]	162	52	20	0.001	18	12	NS
Chang et al. [8]	64	62	17	0.003	20	11	0.03
Hohn et al. [20]	143	42	10	0.0001	17	16	NS
Martin et al. [22]	69	48	21	0.02	12.6	10.5	NS
Rougier et al. [16]	163	43	9	0.01	15	11	0.02
Allen-Mersh et al. [23]	100	50	–	–	13.5	7.5	0.03
Lorenz and Muller [24]	168	45	20	0.009	18.7	17.6	NS

Abbreviations: HAI, hepatic arterial infusion; NS, not significant.

163 patients, half of the patients in the control group did not receive systemic therapy [16].

In three of the studies, biliary sclerosis was a major complication of HAI, which resulted in insufficient doses of regional FUDR and eventual crossover to systemic therapy [10,11,16,20]. Kemeny et al. [21] demonstrated that dexamethasone significantly reduced the toxicity of FUDR. In their study, 50 patients with liver metastases received HAI of FUDR with or without dexamethasone for 14 of 28 treatment days. Although patients that received dexamethasone received higher doses of FUDR, only 9% had elevated bilirubin levels, as compared with 30% of patients who received FUDR without dexamethasone. Adding dexamethasone also increased response rates (71% vs. 40%) and improved overall survival (21 vs. 13 months).

The largest multicenter randomized study from Germany, reported by Lorenz and Muller [24], included 168 patients who had unresectable liver metastases that involved no more than 75% of the liver. There were three treatment arms: HAI with 5-FU/LV, systemic 5-FU/LV, and HAI with FUDR. Median times to disease progression were 9.2, 6.6, and 5.2 months, respectively. Median survival times were 18.7, 17.6, and 12.7 months, respectively. HAI with 5-FU/LV doubled the time to progression and improved the survival of patients with hepatic metastases in less than 25% of the liver. However, these patients had a higher rate of toxic complications than patients treated with FUDR (40% vs. 8%). Also, crossover rates between groups were high; almost one third of patients did not complete the assigned HAI regimen.

Allen-Mersh et al. [23] were the first to demonstrate that survival can be prolonged with a normal quality of life in patients with colorectal metastases. One hundred patients received either systemic 5-FU or HAI with FUDR for palliative purposes. Survival significantly improved in the HAI group with prolongation of a normal quality of life. Also, patients in the HAI group had smaller metastases and lower CEA levels than patients treated with palliative systemic 5-FU.

Secondary Therapy

When 5-FU-based chemotherapy fails, systemic treatment of liver metastases with more recent agents such as CPT-11 and oxaliplatin is associated with marginal response rates [27]. In a study comparing systemic irinotecan to best supportive care in patients that had failed a 5-FU bolus regimen, irinotecan-treated patients had a response rate of 14% and median survival time of 9.9 months [28]. The response rate was even smaller (5%) when CPT-11 was used after failure of a FOLFOX-4 regimen. A larger study that used FOLFOX-4 as second-line systemic treatment reported a response rate of nearly 10% with a median survival of 9.8 months for patients that initially failed CPT-11 [14].

Second-line systemic chemotherapies that include monoclonal antibodies against growth factor receptors have improved response rates and median overall survival. Cunningham et al. [29] reported that the combination of systemic cetuximab and irinotecan was associated with an overall response rate of 22.9% in patients that previously failed CPT-11-based treatments. In a recently reported study of patients whose hepatic metastases were refractory to CPT-11 and 5-FU, Giantonio et al. [30] found that median survival in response to a FOLFOX4 regimen was 12.9 months with bevacizumab and 10.8 months without bevacizumab.

HAI can increase response rates and median survival times of patients treated with second-line systemic chemotherapy. Kemeny et al. [31] reported a phase I study in which 38 patients received regional FUDR and systemic CPT-11. All patients had failed to respond to systemic 5-FU and/or CPT-11. Overall response rate was 74% and median survival time was 20 months. A second phase I trial investigated regional FUDR plus systemic oxaliplatin for patients that had previously been treated (74% had received systemic irinotecan) [15]. Response rates reached 85%, with a median survival of 36 months. These encouraging results for second-line locoregional and systemic chemotherapy must be confirmed by randomized control studies of older and newer biochemotherapeutic agents.

Adjuvant Therapy Postresection

High recurrence rates even after complete surgical resection have prompted evaluation of adjuvant chemotherapy regimens. In 1990, Wagman et al. [32] reported a prospective randomized study of hepatic resection with or without HAI of FUDR in patients with solitary resectable metastases. Adjuvant treatment increased time to recurrence from 9 months to 31 months but did not significantly improve overall survival (Table 6.2).

Although HAI therapy appeared to have a regional effect in controlling hepatic metastases, overall survival rates were not impressive, partly due to the appearance of extrahepatic disease. The addition of dexamethasone to HAI regimens decreased hepatotoxicity, allowing more patients to tolerate full courses of HAI therapy. Adding adjuvant systemic therapy to postoperative HAI regimens could forestall extrahepatic micrometastasis and thereby might improve survival. In 1999, Kemeny et al. [12] reported on adjuvant 5-FU-based systemic treatment with or without HAI of FUDR plus dexamethasone in 156 patients. The combination of HAI and systemic administration yielded a statistically significant increase in the overall survival rate at 2 years (86% vs. 72%) and an increase in hepatic disease-free survival (90% vs. 60%) (Fig. 6.3). In the 2006 final report, overall progression-free survival was 31 months with combined locoregional/systemic therapy versus 17 months with systemic therapy alone ($p = 0.02$) [33]. Median overall survival and 10-year overall survival were not significantly higher with locoregional/systemic therapy (68 months and 41%, respectively) than with systemic therapy alone (59 months and 27%, respectively).

A multicenter study by the Eastern Cooperative Oncology Group compared postoperative regional FUDR plus systemic 5-FU versus observation [31]. Over a 9-year accrual period, 45 patients were assigned to the observation arm and 30 patients to the adjuvant chemotherapy arm. The 4-year recurrence-free rate was 25% with postoperative observation arm and 46% with adjuvant chemotherapy ($p = 0.04$). Similarly, the 4-year liver recurrence-free rate was 43% with observation and 67% with chemotherapy ($p = 0.03$).

NSABP C-09 is a phase III clinical trial comparing systemic oxaliplatin and capecitabine with or without HAI of FUDR in patients with resected or ablated liver metastases from CRC.

Ablative Techniques

Techniques such as cryosurgical ablation (CSA) and radiofrequency ablation (RFA) are safe and effective for treatment of liver metastases that cannot be completely resected [34, 35, 36, 37]. In selected cases of metastatic colon cancer, the results of ablative techniques may be equivalent to those of surgical resection [23,38,39].

Investigators at the John Wayne Cancer Institute reported the results of ablative techniques alone or in combination with regional FUDR and systemic irinotecan for patients whose unresectable hepatic

Table 6.2 Prospective randomized trials of HAI with or without systemic 5-FU after resection of hepatic colorectal metastases. From: Bilchik AJ. Arterial chemotherapy as adjuvant and palliative treatment of hepatic colorectal metastases: an update. Surg Oncol Clin N Am. 2003; 12; 193–210. With permission from Elsevier

Group	Treatment arms	No. of patients	Overall survival		
			Median (months)	2 years (%)	5 years (%)
Wagman et al. [32]	HAI of FUDR	5	37.3	80	40
	No adjuvant therapy	6	28	67	50
Lorenz et al. [13]	HAI of 5-FU	73	44.8	60	47
	No adjuvant therapy	114	39.7	62	30
Kemeny et al. [12]	HAI of FUDR + systemic 5-FU	74	72.2	85*	68
	Systemic 5-FU	82	59.3	72*	52
Kemeny et al. [31]	HAI of FUDR + systemic 5-FU	35	63.7	80	63
	No adjuvant therapy	45	49	79	32

Abbreviations: 5-FU, 5-fluorouracil; FUDR, floxuridine; HAI, hepatic arterial infusion; NS, not significant.
*These 2-year rates were the only significant difference ($p = 0.02$) between treatment arms in all four studies.

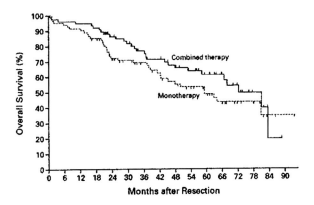
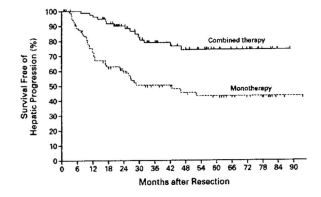

Fig. 6.3 Overall survival (*left*) and hepatic progression-free survival (*right*) after hepatic resection in patients receiving systemic 5-fluorouracil alone or in combination with hepatic arterial infusion of floxuridine. Reprinted with permission from Kemeny N, Huang Y, Cohen AM, et al. Hepatic arterial infusion of chemotherapy after resection of hepatic metastases from colorectal cancer. N Engl J Med. 1999; 341: 2039–2048. Copyright © 1999 Massachusetts Medical Society. All rights reserved

Table 6.3 Patterns of recurrence after cryosurgical ablation (cytoreduction) for hepatic metastases of CRC. From: Bilchik AJ. Arterial chemotherapy as adjuvant and palliative treatment of hepatic colorectal metastases: an update. Surg Oncol Clin N Am. 2003; 12: 193–210. With permission from Elsevier

Type of recurrence	Number of patients	
	Cytoreduction alone (114 patients)	Cytoreduction + regional floxuridine + systemic irinotecan (71 patients)
All recurrences	88 (77%)	35 (49%)*
Liver	76 (67%)	27 (38%)*
Recurrence at ablation site	14 (12%)	8 (11%)
Recurrence at different site	62 (54%)	19 (27%)*
Extrahepatic	58 (51%)	22 (31%)*
Progression-free survival	10 months	19 months**

* $p<0.05$; * * $p<0.001$.

metastases did not respond to systemic 5-FU therapy. Between 1992 and 1999, 185 patients who experienced CRC progression during systemic 5-FU treatment underwent ablation with or without hepatic resection [40]. All patients had complete treatment of all identifiable sites of disease. Patients then received FUDR/dexamethasone via HAI and irinotecan via systemic infusion. Of the 185 patients, 114 underwent ablation alone and 71 underwent ablation followed by regional FUDR and systemic irinotecan; 67 (36%) patients underwent concurrent liver resection. Median time to progression was 10 months after ablation alone, as compared with 19 months after ablation plus adjuvant therapy ($p<0.001$; [Table 6.3]). Respective overall rates of recurrence were 77% and 49% ($p<0.005$), and respective rates of hepatic recurrence were 38% and 67% ($p<0.01$). As a result, the median survival of patients treated with ablation plus adjuvant therapy was 30.6

months, as compared with 10 months for those treated with ablation alone ($p<0.007$) (Table 6.4); corresponding rates of 2-year survival were 75% and 35% ($p<0.01$). This survival benefit was independent of the type of ablative procedure. This study confirms that adjuvant HAI with FUDR can significantly lower rates of recurrence and increase survival times in patients whose hepatic metastases of CRC fail to respond to 5-FU. The addition of systemic irinotecan may be effective in decreasing the recurrence of extrahepatic disease in an adjuvant setting.

Newer Agents Via HAI

Adjuvant systemic administration of irinotecan and oxaliplatin has improved outcomes in patients with CRC.

Table 6.4 Survival of patients undergoing cryosurgical ablation (cytoreduction) with or without regional floxuridine and systemic irinotecan. From: Bilchik AJ. Arterial chemotherapy as adjuvant and palliative treatment of hepatic colorectal metastases: an update. Surg Oncol Clin N Am. 2003; 12: 193–210. With permission from Elsevier

	Median survival, months	
Characteristics	Cytoreduction alone (114 patients)	Cytoreduction + irinotecan + floxuridine (71 patients)
Location		
Unilobar	21.7	33.0*
Bilobar	19.5	29.0*
Detection		
Synchronous	24.8	32.0*
Metachronous	22.1	28.3*
Number		
Less than 3	23.5	32.5*
More than 3	20.0	27.0*
Size		
Less than 4 cm	23.0	35.0*
More than 4 cm	20.0	27.0*

* $p < 0.05$

Fig. 6.4 Role of hepatic arterial infusion (HAI) for the treatment of isolated colorectal metastases in the liver. Surgery includes resection and/or ablative techniques

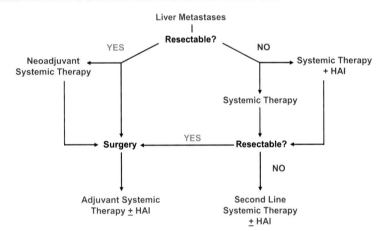

Combined with other standard chemotherapy agents, FOLFOX and FOLFIRI regimens have become widely accepted adjuvant treatments [15,41,42]. As a result, locoregional infusion of these newer agents has been the focus of recent research.

In a phase II study from France [43], locoregional oxaliplatin was combined with systemic 5-FU and LVN for treatment of isolated nonresectable liver metastases from CRC. Response rates and disease-free survival were 64% and 27 months, respectively. Recently introduced biological agents, mainly bevacizumab and cetuximab, also have become important components of primary and secondary treatment regimens for patients with CRC [29]. In a 2007 study from Greece [44, 32] patients with synchronous bilobar hepatic metastases were initially treated with a combination of portal vein branch ligation and microwave ablation followed by three cycles of biochemotherapy with bevacizumab via

HAI. Patients then underwent hepatic resection followed by adjuvant HAI with biochemotherapy. In a 31-month follow-up period, 2-year survival rate was 80%. Further studies of locoregional infusion of these agents are underway.

Summary

There has been a paradigm shift in the treatment of patients with unresectable metastatic CRC isolated to the liver. Early studies incorporated HAI with 5-FU-based chemotherapy regimens mainly to improve palliation. However, newer biological and chemotherapeutic regimens for aggressive treatment of initially unresectable liver metastases show promise for increasing the number of candidates for ablation and/or resection. Figure 6.4

presents an algorithm for use of HAI in patients with isolated hepatic metastases. Surgical therapy can include resection and/or ablative techniques. Patients with isolated resectable metastases should undergo surgical resection without neoadjuvant treatment whenever possible. If neoadjuvant systemic therapy is considered for patients with resectable disease, patients must be closely followed for signs of hepatotoxicity. Hepatic dysfunction caused by neoadjuvant therapy reportedly can jeopardize possible curative resection [45].

The addition of postsurgical adjuvant HAI may play an important role in increasing the time to local recurrence and increasing survival, but at present these results need validation in large multicenter clinical trials.

Acknowledgement This work was supported by funding from the Davidow Foundation, Los Angeles, California and the Rod Fasone Memorial Cancer Fund, Los Angeles, California.

References

1. Jemal A, Siegel R, Ward E, et al. Cancer statistics, 2007. CA Cancer J Clin. 2007; 57: 43–66.
2. Fong Y, Blumgart L. Hepatic colorectal metastases: current status of surgical therapy. Oncology 1998; 12: 1489–98.
3. Fong Y, Cohen A, Fortner J, et al. Liver resection for colorectal metastases. J Clin Oncol. 1997; 15: 938–46.
4. Fong Y, Salo J. Surgical therapy of hepatic colorectal metastases. Semin Oncol. 1999; 26: 514–23.
5. Kemeny N, Fata F. Hepatic-arterial chemotherapy. Lancet. Oncol. 2001; 2: 418–28.
6. Bilchik AJ. Arterial chemotherapy as adjuvant and palliative treatment of hepatic colorectal metastases: an update. Surg Oncol Clin N Am. 2003; 12: 193–210.
7. Kemeny N, Gonen M, Sullivan D, et al. Phase I study of hepatic arterial infusion of floxuridine and dexamethasone with systemic irinotecan for unresectable hepatic metastases from colorectal cancer. J Clin Oncol. 2001; 19: 2687–95.
8. Chang AE, Schneider PD, Sugarbaker PH, et al. A prospective randomized trial of regional versus systemic continuous 5-fluorodeoxyuridine chemotherapy in the treatment of colorectal liver metastases. Ann Surg. 1987; 206: 685–93.
9. Grosso M, Scarrone A, Pedrazzini F, et al. Intra-arterial hepatic chemotherapy: management of liver tumors by percutaneous port-a-cath positioning. J Exp Clin Cancer Res. 2003; 22: 171–5.
10. Kemeny N, Daly J, Reichman B, et al. Intrahepatic or systemic infusion fluorodeoxyuridine in patients with liver metastases from colorectal carcinoma. A randomized trial. Ann Intern Med. 1987; 107: 459–65.
11. Kemeny N, Conti J, Cohen A, et al. Phase II study of hepatic fluorouridine, leucovorin and dexamethasone for unresectable liver metastases from colorectal carcinoma. J Clin Oncol. 1994; 12: 2288–95.
12. Kemeny N, Huang Y, Cohen AM, et al. Hepatic arterial infusion of chemotherapy after resection of hepatic metastasis from colorectal cancer. N Engl J Med. 1999; 341: 2039–48.
13. Lorenz M, Muller HH, Schramm H, et al. Randomized trial of surgery versus surgery followed by adjuvant hepatic arterial infusion with 5-fluorouracil and folic acid for liver metastases of colorectal cancer. German Cooperative on Liver Metastases. Ann Surg. 1998; 228: 756–62.
14. Chung KY, Kemeny N. Regional and systemic chemotherapy for primary hepatobiliary cancer and for colorectal cancer metastatic to the liver. Semin Radiat Oncol. 2005; 15: 284–98.
15. Kemeny N, Jarnagin W, Paty P, et al. Phase I trial of systemic oxaliplatin combination chemotherapy with hepatic arterial infusion in patients with unresectable liver metastases from colorectal cancer. J Clin Oncol. 2005; 23: 4888–96.
16. Rougier P, Laplanche A, Huguier M, et al. Hepatic arterial infusion of floxuridine in patients with liver metastases from colorectal carcinoma: long term results of a prospective randomized trial. J Clin Oncol. 1992; 10: 1112–8.
17. Kemeny N. Current approaches for liver-only metastases in colorectal cancer. Commun Oncol. 2006; 3: 26–35.
18. Franklin ME Jr, Gonzalez J Jr. Laparoscopic placement of hepatic artery catheter for regional chemotherapy infusion: technique, benefits, and complications. Surg Laparosc Endosc Percutan Tech. 2002; 12: 398–407.
19. Franklin M, Trevino J, Hernandez-Oaknin H, et al. Laparoscopic hepatic artery catheterization for regional chemotherapy: is this the best current option for liver metastatic disease? Surg Endosc. 2006; 20: 554–8.
20. Hohn DC, Stagg RJ, Friedman MA, et al. A randomized trial of continuous intravenous versus hepatic intraarterial floxuridine in patients with colorectal cancer metastatic to the liver: the Northern California Oncology Group trial. J Clin Oncol. 1989; 7: 1646–54.
21. Kemeny N, Seiter K, Niedzwiecki D, et al. A randomized trial of intrahepatic infusion of fluorodeoxyuridine with dexamethasone versus fluorodeoxyuridine alone in the treatment of metastatic colorectal cancer. Cancer. 1992; 69: 327–34.
22. Martin JK, O'Connell MJ, Wieand HS, et al. Intra-arterial floxuridine vs. systemic fluorouracil for hepatic metastases from colorectal cancer. Arch Surg. 1990; 125: 1022–27.
23. Allen-Mersh TG, Earlam S, Fordy C, et al. Quality of life and survival with continuous hepatic artery floxuridine infusion for colorectal liver metastases. Lancet. 1994; 344: 1255–60.
24. Lorenz M, Muller HH. Randomized, multi-center trial of fluorouracil plus leucovorin administered either via hepatic arterial or intravenous infusion versus fluorodeoxyuridine administered via hepatic arterial infusion in patients with nonresectable liver metastases from colorectal carcinoma. J Clin Oncol. 2000; 18: 243–54.
25. Rothbarth J, Pijl ME, Vahrmeijer AL, et al. Isolated hepatic perfusion with high-dose melphalan for the treatment of colorectal metastasis confined to the liver. Br J Surg. 2003; 90: 1391–7.
26. Rougier P, Van Cutsem E, Bajetta E, et al. Randomized trial of irinotecan versus fluorouracil by continuous infusion after fluorouracil failure in patients with metastatic colorectal cancer. Lancet. 1998; 352: 1407–13.
27. Shimada Y, Yoshino M, Wakui A, et al. Phase II study of CPT-11, a new camptothecin derivative, in metastatic colorectal cancer. CPT-11 Gastrointestinal Cancer Study Group. J Clin Oncol. 1993; 11: 909–13.
28. Cunningham D, Pyrhonen S, James R, et al. Randomized trial of irinotecan plus supportive care versus supportive care alone after fluorouracil failure in patients with metastatic colorectal cancer. Lancet. 1998; 352: 1413–8.
29. Cunningham D, Humblet Y, Siena S, et al. Cetuximab monotherapy and cetuximab plus irinotecan in irinotecan-refractory metastatic colorectal cancer. N Engl J Med. 2004; 351: 337–45.

30. Giantonio BJ, Catalano PJ, Meropol NJ, et al. Bevacizumab in combination with oxaliplatin, fluorouracil, and leucovorin (FOLFOX4) for previously treated metastatic colorectal cancer: results from the Eastern Cooperative Oncology Group Study E3200. J Clin Oncol. 2007; 25: 1539–44.

31. Kemeny MM, Adak S, Gray B, et al. Combined modality treatment for resectable metastatic colorectal carcinoma to the liver: surgical resection of hepatic metastases in combination with continuous infusion of chemotherapy—an intergroup study. J Clin Oncol. 2002; 20: 1499–1505.

32. Wagman LD, Kemeny MM, Leong L, et al. A prospective, randomized evaluation of the treatment of colorectal cancer metastatic to the liver. J Clin Oncol. 1990; 8: 1885–93.

33. Kemeny N, Niedzwiecki D, Hollis D, et al. Hepatic arterial infusion versus systemic therapy for hepatic metastases from colorectal cancer; a randomized trial of efficacy, quality of life, and molecular markers. J Clin Oncol. 2006; 24: 1395–403.

34. Bilchik AJ, Wood TF, Allegra D, et al. Cryosurgery and radiofrequency ablation for unresectable hepatic malignancies: a proposed algorithm. Arch Surg. 2000; 135: 657–62.

35. Curley SA, Izzo F, Delrio P, et al. Radiofrequency ablation of unresectable primary and metastatic hepatic malignancies: results in 123 patients. Ann Surg. 2000; 230: 1–8.

36. Scaife CL, Curley SA, Izzo F, et al. Feasibility of adjuvant hepatic arterial infusion of chemotherapy after radiofrequency ablation with or without resection in patients with hepatic metastases from colorectal cancer. Ann Surg Oncol. 2003; 10: 332–3.

37. Wood TF, Rose DM, Chung M, et al. Radiofrequency ablation of 231 unresectable hepatic tumors: indications, limitations, and complications. Ann Surg Oncol. 2000; 7: 593–600.

38. Weaver M, Ashton J, Zemel R. Treatment of colorectal liver metastases by cryotherapy. Semin Surg Oncol. 1998; 14: 163–70.

39. Yan TD, Padang R, Morris DL. Long term results and prognostic indicators after cryotherapy and hepatic arterial chemotherapy with or without resection for colorectal liver metastases in 224 patients: long term survival can be achieved in patients with multiple bilateral liver metastases. J Am Coll Surg. 2006; 202: 100–11.

40. Bilchik AJ, Wood TF, Chawla SP, et al. Systemic irinotecan or floxuridine chemotherapy prolongs survival after hepatic cryosurgery in patients with metastatic colon cancer refractory to 5-fluorouracil. Clin Colorectal Cancer. 2001; 1: 36–42.

41. Kemeny N, Jarnagin W, Gonen M, et al. Phase I/II study of hepatic arterial therapy with floxuridine and dexamethasone in combination with intravenous irinotecan as adjuvant treatment after resection of hepatic metastases from colorectal carcinoma. J Surg Oncol. 2005; 91: 97–101.

42. Litvak D, Wood T, Tsioulias G, Chung M, et al. Systemic irinotecan and regional floxuridine after hepatic cytoreduction in 185 patients with unresectable colorectal cancer metastases. Ann Surg Oncol. 2002; 9: 148–55.

43. Ducreux M, Ychou M, Laplanche A, et al. Hepatic arterial oxaliplatin infusion plus intravenous chemotherapy in colorectal cancer with inoperable hepatic metastases: a trial of the gastrointestinal group of the Federation Nationale des Centres de Lutte Contre le Cancer. J Clin Oncol. 2005; 23: 4881–7.

44. Lygidakis NJ, Bhagat AD, Vrachnos P, et al. Challenges in everyday surgical practice: synchronous bilobar hepatic colorectal metastases—newer multimodality approach. Hepatogastroenterology. 2007; 54: 1020–4.

45. Bilchik AJ, Poston G, Curley SA, et al. Neoadjuvant chemotherapy for metastatic colon cancer: a cautionary note. J Clin Oncol. 2005; 23: 9073–8.

Robbert J. de Haas, Dennis A. Wicherts, and René Adam

Introduction

Metastases frequently occur in the liver and this organ is often the only site of metastatic spread. As an example, over half of patients with colorectal cancer will develop liver metastases, either synchronous or metachronous [1]. With the increasing incidence of colorectal cancer cases each year, colorectal liver metastases are a major health issue.

Hepatic resection is well established as the only treatment option providing long-term survival for patients with colorectal metastases (reported 5-year survival ranging between 15% and 67%) as well as for selected patients with liver metastases from other noncolorectal nonendocrine cancers [2, 3]. Therefore, the most important issue to appreciate in case of liver metastases is resectability.

With currently used criteria, curative hepatectomy can only be offered to 10–20% of patients that present with colorectal liver metastases. A variety of therapeutic approaches have been proposed for the majority of patients with unresectable metastases, including chemotherapy, radiofrequency ablation (RFA), and cryotherapy. However, none of these therapies can individually achieve long-term survival comparable to that of radical surgery. Nevertheless, when used in combination with surgery, efficient treatment strategies can be created to achieve curative treatment in patients previously judged inoperable.

This chapter will describe the currently available methods to improve resectability, thereby offering patients with liver metastases from colorectal and other cancers a chance of long-term survival.

Definition of Unresectability

Negative prognostic factors for survival have been previously used to exclude patients from hepatic resection. For patients with colorectal metastases, these factors included high number and large size of metastases, and the presence of extrahepatic disease [4, 5]. The same considerations have been made regarding the width of the resection margin [4, 5]. Empirically, a resection margin of 1 cm or more was used as one of the important selection criteria for hepatic resection of colorectal metastases.

Regardless the fact that extensive tumor involvement is associated with unfavorable outcome, long-term survival can be achieved in a large number of patients when complete resection is performed of both intrahepatic and extrahepatic tumor deposits. In addition, it has been shown that a tumor-free resection margin is of more prognostic importance than its width [6].

The improved knowledge of the influence of prognostic factors and of the established impact of complete resection on long-term outcome has resulted in a pragmatic definition of unresectability. In current practice, a liver remnant that is too small in relation to the extent of the resection needed to achieve radicality is the only remaining indicator of unresectability. Patients are considered resectable as long as all liver metastases can be completely resected with tumor-free margins, while leaving at least 25–30% of remnant liver volume to prevent postoperative liver insufficiency [7]. In general, resection margins of >1 cm are recommended, but it should not limit hepatic resection as long as it can be macroscopically complete. Additionally, the presence of resectable extrahepatic disease is no longer considered as a contraindication for surgery. The main causes that are responsible for technical unresectability are therefore multinodularity, large metastases, vascular-ill location of metastases, and extensive extrahepatic disease.

R. Adam (✉)
Professor, Centre Hépato-Biliaire, AP-HP, Hôpital Paul Brousse, Villejuif, France

J.-N. Vauthey et al. (eds.), *Liver Metastases*, DOI 10.1007/978-1-84628-947-7_7,
© Springer-Verlag London Limited 2009

In practice, patients with liver metastases can be divided into three categories:

1. *Easily resectable.* In this group, liver metastases can be completely resected with adequate oncological margins of normal parenchyma. In general, no need exists to improve resectability of the metastases before proceeding to surgery.
2. *Marginally resectable.* These patients present with more extensive hepatic disease, limiting the possibilities of upfront surgery. Surgery may be limited by difficulties in achieving tumor-free margins due to large tumor involvement. Furthermore, the need for major hepatectomy might endanger a required remnant liver volume of 25–30%. Finally, patients with limited hepatic disease and concomitant resectable extrahepatic disease can also be ascribed to this group. Different methods may be used for these patients to reduce tumor load and to improve "curativity" of resection.
3. *Definitely unresectable.* This group represents a subset of patients with widespread hepatic disease with extensive concomitant extrahepatic disease, usually disseminated over multiple metastatic sites. In most cases, both upfront chemotherapy treatment and intraoperative strategies are mandatory to control and downsize the metastatic disease and to technically enable curative surgery in these patients.

Obviously, the chance of further resectability decreases from group 1 to group 3. However, owing to the increasing efficacy of chemotherapy, some patients will be switched to complex and/or sequential surgery, even when presenting initially as "definitely" unresectable.

Improving Resectability

Downstaging with Preoperative Chemotherapy

Chemotherapy treatment for metastatic colorectal cancer has made great progress during the last years. Response rates to 5-fluorouracil (5-FU) and leucovorin (LV) have been significantly increased by combining them with oxaliplatin and irinotecan. Response rates up to 66% can now be achieved with associated median survivals up to 21 months [8, 9]. More importantly, the increase in response rates has offered the possibility for an increasing number of patients to undergo curative resection of their initially unresectable metastases. Initially described with chronotherapy regimens [10, 11], surgery after

downsizing by chemotherapy has been extensively reported after different chemotherapy regimens, independent of the type of delivery.

Conversion to Resectability

The high response rates of combination chemotherapy regimens have led to the possibility of curative hepatectomy for patients with unresectable metastases by switching them to a resectable state after tumor downstaging. After our first reports on the concept of proposing surgery to 13–16% of patients with initially unresectable liver metastases who responded to chemotherapy [12, 13], different studies have further reported resectability rates between 10% and 54% after tumor downsizing by chemotherapy (Table 7.1) [13, 14, 15, 16, 17, 18, 19, 20]. The wide range of resectability rates is related to differences in patient selection caused by unequal definitions of unresectability between centers and by the inclusion of selected (liver only) or unselected (both intra- and extrahepatic disease) patients. Overall, 5-year survival after secondary hepatic resection ranges from 33% to 58% for unselected and selected patients, respectively [13, 15]. Similar results of long-term survival have never been reported for chemotherapy alone.

The probability of individual patients to benefit from this treatment strategy can be based on four preoperatively available prognostic factors of survival. We recently proposed a predictive model that included the presence of a primary rectal cancer, more than three liver metastases, a maximum tumor size of more than 10 cm, and a preoperative carbohydrate antigen (CA) 19.9 level of more than 100 IU/l as independent factors [13]. Adjusted 5-year survival rates ranged from 59% to 0% according to the presence of none to all factors.

A critical point to address concerning preoperative chemotherapy is that secondary liver resection can only offer long-term survival when the metastatic disease is well controlled by preoperative chemotherapy. We have previously shown that progression of colorectal liver metastases during chemotherapy treatment was independently associated with decreased survival after hepatectomy [21]. Five-year survival for these patients was only 8%, which is significantly lower than that seen with patients whose disease responded to, or was stabilized by chemotherapy. Therefore, response to chemotherapy can be used to select patients that may benefit the most from hepatic resection. Also, prolonged chemotherapy should be avoided when the metastases become resectable to minimize the risk of reprogression after an initial control of the disease.

Table 7.1 Resection rates after conventional chemotherapy in patients with initially unresectable colorectal liver metastases

Author	Year	No. of Patients	Regimen	Resection rate (%)
Unselected patients[a]				
Adam [13]	2004	1104	Variable	12.5
Masi [14]	2006	74	FOLFIRIFOX	25.7
Selected patients[b]				
Giacchetti [15]	1999	151	FOLFOX	38.4
Pozzo [16]	2004	40	FOLFIRI	32.5
de la Camara [17]	2004	212	FOLFIRIFOX	43
Quenet [18]	2004	26	FOLFIRIFOX	54
Alberts [19]	2005	42	FOLFOX4	33.3
Ho [20]	2005	40	FOLFIRI	10

[a] Patients with concomitant extrahepatic disease were also included.
[b] Patients with only intrahepatic disease.

Chemotherapy Combined with Biological Agents

The fact that the majority of patients with unresectable metastases still do not respond sufficiently to conventional chemotherapy to become resectable, has driven the development of more effective therapies. The use of monoclonal antibodies like cetuximab and bevacizumab has recently been shown to be of particular value in increasing response rates in patients with colorectal metastases.

Cetuximab is a monoclonal antibody that binds with high affinity to epidermal growth factor receptor (EGFR) and blocks endogenous ligand binding. This binding results in inhibition of cell proliferation and angiogenesis and stimulation of apoptosis, hereby preventing metastases outgrowth [22]. Bevacizumab is directed against vascular endothelial growth factor (VEGF), which is an important regulator of pathologic angiogenesis. When combined with conventional chemotherapy, response rates up to 70% have been reported in first-line treatment for both cetuximab and bevacizumab [23, 24].

However, the associated rate by which unresectable patients can be switched to resectability is a more important endpoint to consider than response rate alone. After cetuximab-containing regimens in first line treatment, 21–24% of patients with metastatic colorectal disease may become amenable for liver resection (Table 7.2) [23, 25, 26]. Driven

by these encouraging results after first-line treatment, we recently evaluated resection rates in patients with unresectable disease refractory to conventional regimens [27]. Interestingly, 7% of unselected patients treated at our institution with cetuximab after failure of conventional therapy experienced a treatment response that allowed for potentially curative hepatectomy. These results indicate that the addition of cetuximab to chemotherapy in second or higher lines can increase the number of patients who become eligible for curative resection by nearly 50%.

When bevacizumab is added to conventional chemotherapy as first-line treatment in unresectable patients, 15% of them may become secondarily resectable as reported in a recent publication (Table 7.2) [28].

Risks Related to Preoperative Chemotherapy

While representing the best means for increasing resectability, chemotherapy may be deleterious in cases of overtreatment or hepatic toxicity.

A potential pitfall of preoperative chemotherapy is the development of a complete clinical response, i.e., a complete radiological disappearance of all lesions. Although infrequent, this situation has recently attracted the attention as one of the major objectives of chemotherapy.

Table 7.2 Resection rates after conventional chemotherapy combined with monoclonal antibodies in patients with initially unresectable colorectal liver metastases

Author	Year	No. of Patients	Regimen	Line	Resection rate (%)
Peeters [25]	2005	42	Cetuximab + FOLFIRI	First	24
Cervantes [26]	2005	42	Cetuximab + FOLFOX4	First	21
Folprecht [23]	2006	21	Cetuximab + FOLFIRI	First	24
Adam [27]	2007	27	Cetuximab + variable agents	≥Second	7
Emmanouilides [28]	2007	53	Bevacizumab + FOLFOX	First	15

However, it has been shown to be of limited value for predicting total tumor necrosis. A recent study showed that for 83% of metastases with a complete clinical response, active tumor cells still persisted or in situ recurrence occurred within 1 year postoperatively [29]. Therefore, all previous sites of metastases should be resected, if possible, and the complete disappearance of metastases on imaging should not be a non-indication for surgery. As complete clinical response might seem an attractive outcome for oncologists, it represents a difficult surgical situation because of the inability to localize previous metastatic lesions and therefore achieve a curative situation. Contrarily, complete pathological response might be much more clinically relevant than complete clinical response but remains largely unexplored in the literature. We previously showed that complete pathological response occurred in only 6% of patients who responded strongly to chemotherapy, in such a way that they were switched to liver resection while initially unresectable [13].

Chemotherapy has anecdotally been associated with changes in the macroscopic appearance of the liver, increased fragility, and poor hemostasis. In addition, during the last few years interesting data have become available regarding the relationship between preoperative chemotherapy, histologic changes of the parenchyma, and postoperative outcome. Some reports have suggested that preoperative chemotherapy, especially the use of oxaliplatin, is related to vascular lesions [30, 31]. Likewise, preoperative use of irinotecan has been associated with steatohepatitis, which is related to an increased 90-day mortality [32]. In our experience, vascular lesions were significantly associated with the use of oxaliplatin, and severe vascular lesions were related to increased intraoperative transfusion requirements [33]. To minimize these adverse events of prolonged chemotherapy, liver surgery should be proposed as soon as a potentially curative resection becomes possible.

Increasing Resectability with Specific Techniques

Even in patients having a good response, chemotherapy may not be sufficient to allow complete resection of the metastases, either because of too small future remnant liver, multinodularity or a close contact with vascular structures. To cope with these situations, some technical refinements are used to allow further surgery.

Portal Vein Embolization (PVE)

Postoperative liver failure is still the most important cause of death following liver surgery. The risk of liver insufficiency exists especially after resection of more than 60–70% of liver parenchyma, leaving less than 25–30% of normal functioning hepatocytes in place. For this reason, patients needing a liver resection exceeding the removal of more than 70% of liver parenchyma to be curative were historically deemed unresectable.

In 1986 it was observed that obstruction or narrowing of portal veins by hilar carcinomas led to segmental atrophy, while the unaffected contralateral side with patent portal veins hypertrophied [34]. In the same year, the use of PVE was described in patients with hepatocellular carcinoma [35]. In 1990, Makuuchi and colleagues described the technique of preoperative PVE in patients with hilar bile duct carcinoma to reduce the risk of postoperative liver failure [36].

Currently, PVE is a widely used technique to extend resectability rates in patients needing a major hepatectomy. The concept consists of embolization of one side of the portal venous system, thereby inducing atrophy of the embolized liver lobe and compensatory hypertrophy of the contralateral liver lobe, i.e., the future remnant liver. PVE is indicated when hepatic resection is estimated to comprise more than 70% of liver volume, thereby leaving less than 25–30% of normal functioning liver parenchyma. However, in case of underlying liver disease or previous treatment with intensive chemotherapy, an estimated remnant liver volume of 40% should be pursued.

Embolization of the portal veins can be performed by two different techniques: transileocolic or percutaneous transhepatic portal embolization. Besides these two techniques, embolization and ligation of a portal branch can be performed directly during laparotomy.

With percutaneous PVE, performed under local or general anesthesia, a branch of the portal vein is punctured under ultrasound guidance, followed by a control venous portography. If the catheter is correctly positioned, embolization can be performed using several agents, such as fibrin glue, ethanol, gel foam, metal coils, and cyanoacrylate, with none of them being superior to the others.

The transileocolic approach consists of direct cannulation of the ileocolic vein through a short laparotomy. After passing through the superior mesenteric vein, the portal branch is selectively embolized under fluoroscopic guidance.

Computed tomography volumetric analysis is used to monitor changes in hepatic volume after PVE, enabling determination of the degree of compensatory hypertrophy of the future remnant liver as well as to re-evaluate tumoral disease. Generally, a period of 4–6 weeks after PVE is sufficient to allow adequate hypertrophy enabling safe hepatic resection. During the period between PVE and hepatic resection, systemic chemotherapy and/or local treatment modalities can be used to prevent accelerated outgrowth of tumoral disease in the non-embolized hemiliver after PVE.

In our institute, PVE has shown to be a safe technique with no mortality within 2 months and a morbidity rate of only 3% [37]. A significant increase of future remnant liver volume of up to 43% was achieved, allowing hepatic resection in 63% of patients treated by PVE [37]. Actuarial survival rates after PVE are close to that of patients who did not undergo PVE prior to hepatectomy. This technique has also been used in combination with intra-arterial hepatic chemotherapy with promising results [38].

In summary, PVE is a safe method to cause compensatory hypertrophy of the future remnant liver and thereby increasing resectability rates, with similar survival rates as in patients not treated by PVE prior to hepatectomy.

Local Treatment Modalities

When numerous liver metastases are present which cannot be treated curatively by resection alone, local destructive treatment modalities, like RFA or cryotherapy, can be indicated.

Treatment by RFA can be performed percutaneously or during laparoscopy or laparotomy. A multiple array needle electrode is deployed and positioned in the tumor, allowing a high frequency (400–500 kHz) alternating current to be delivered. The delivered energy is turned into heat ($>60^{\circ}C$), leading to tissue destruction. Currently, metastatic lesions of up to 3 cm in diameter can be treated by RFA.

Cryotherapy is based upon the application of extremely low temperatures ($-196^{\circ}C$) to the tumor, causing in situ tumor destruction. The mechanism of tumoral destruction comprises direct cellular freezing, cellular dehydration, interruption of microcirculation, anoxia, and cellular necrosis. The effect of cryotherapy depends on the rapidity and duration of freezing, and extent of hypothermia.

RFA and cryotherapy combined with hepatic resection are reported to be safe treatment modalities showing similar results as hepatic resection alone with a possibility of long-term survival [39, 40], and therefore can be a valuable addition to the treatment armamentarium for patients with initially unresectable liver metastases. In general, local treatment is indicated for up to three lesions no larger than 3 cm.

Two-Stage Hepatectomy

When a single hepatectomy, even when combined with local treatment modalities, cannot be curative, because of bilateral involvement of multiple large liver metastases necessitating removal of more than 70% of liver parenchyma, a two-stage hepatectomy might be indicated.

The two-stage procedure consists of two subsequent hepatectomies, with the objective of the first hepatectomy to make the second hepatectomy potentially curative. The main principle of the two-stage procedure is liver regeneration between the two hepatectomies, allowing a safe second hepatectomy by which all remaining liver metastases are resected, leaving at least 30% of normal functioning liver parenchyma. To promote liver regeneration after the first hepatectomy, PVE of the portal branch supplying the liver lobe that will be removed during the second hepatectomy can be performed, thereby inducing adequate hypertrophy of the future remnant liver. To prevent tumor progression caused by growth factors involved in liver regeneration after resection and PVE, systemic chemotherapy is usually administered between both hepatic resections. Chemotherapy should be started 2–3 weeks after the first hepatic resection, to minimize interference with early liver regeneration.

Our institute published the first results of the two-stage procedure in 2000 [41]. Sixteen patients with multinodular intrahepatic tumor spread from colorectal metastases were scheduled for a two-stage procedure after a partial response or stabilization of their liver disease after chemotherapy. Both hepatectomies could be performed in 13 (81%) of these patients. The other three patients were ineligible for the second-stage resection because of disease-progression after the first hepatectomy. Other studies have reported comparable completion rates between 76% and 100% [42, 43]. No patients died within 2 months after the first hepatectomy, compared with two perioperative deaths after the second hepatectomy (15%). Morbidity rates were 31% after the first hepatectomy and 45% after the second hepatectomy. Three-year overall survival for patients who completed the two-stage procedure was 35%. Afterwards, similar results were reported by others [42, 43]. Jacek achieved a 3-year survival rate of 54% with 0 mortality and morbidity rates of 15% and 56% after the first and second hepatectomy, respectively [42]. A 45% 3-year survival rate was reported by Togo in a group of 11 patients with only 2 cases of morbidity after the second procedure [43].

Two-stage hepatectomy combined with chemotherapy can offer long-term survival for patients with initially unresectable multinodular liver metastases. However, this treatment strategy can only be applied to a highly selected patient group.

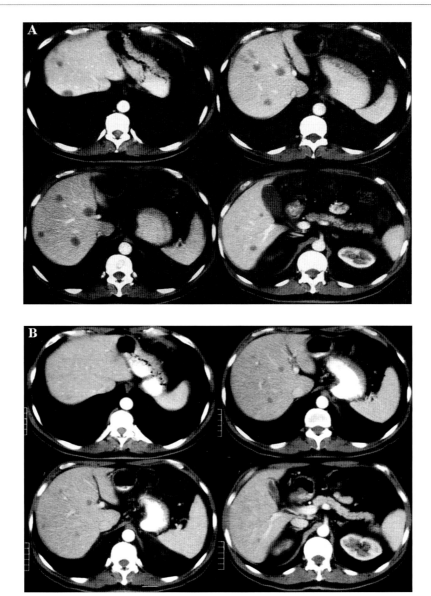

Fig. 7.2 A. Multiple bilateral liver metastases from a left colonic adenocarcinoma in a 59-year-old patient. **B.** Partial regression of more than 50% was observed for all metastases after seven cycles of chemotherapy (FOLFOX) enabling curative hepatectomy combined with radiofrequency ablation

chemotherapy treatment, five bilateral metastases remained, necessitating both a right hepatectomy and a left lobectomy to achieve a curative resection (Fig. 7.4). Since this strategy would result in a resection of more than 70% of the total liver volume, it was decided to attempt a curative resection by performing a two-stage procedure.

During the first step, a left lobectomy was performed, combined with embolization and ligature of the right branch of the portal vein. At histopathologic examination, three nodules were found with a maximum diameter of 12 mm. Postoperatively, chemotherapy treatment was continued.

Two months after PVE, the future remnant liver volume (i.e., segments I and IV) showed a sufficient hypertrophy to enable a safe second step of the two-stage procedure (Fig. 7.5A,B). The second step consisted of a right hepatectomy (Fig. 7.5C). Histopathologically, four remaining metastases were identified (maximum diameter: 55 mm).

Postoperatively, adjuvant chemotherapy was administered, consisting of a FOLFOX-regimen. After eight cycles, a solitary pulmonary lesion was diagnosed located in the left upper lobe. Chemotherapy was switched to a regimen containing 5-FU, LV, and irinotecan (FOLFIRI), and after three cycles the pulmonary lesion was

Fig. 7.3 Computed tomographic images 2 months after hepatectomy and radiofrequency ablation showing four lesions compatible with radiofrequency treatment. No other suspect nodules are visualized

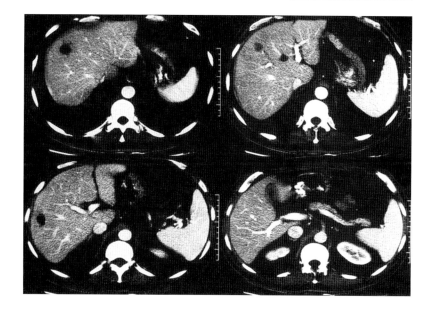

Fig. 7.4 Bilateral liver metastases in a 50-year-old male necessitating a left lobectomy as well as a right hepatectomy to achieve curative resection

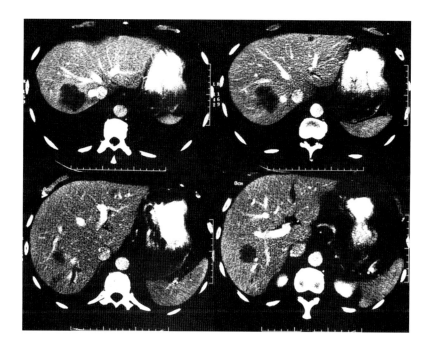

stabilized, and pulmonary resection was undertaken. Four months after pulmonary resection, a solitary liver recurrence appeared in segment IV. Partial hepatectomy was performed, followed by adjuvant chemotherapy consisting of FOLFIRI combined with cetuximab. After five cycles, an endobiliary recurrence was observed, and chemotherapy was furthermore changed into a regimen of FOLFOX combined with bevacizumab.

At last follow-up, 4 years and 4 months after the second hepatectomy, recurrences are observed in the lungs as well as in the liver.

Case Report: Two-Stage Hepatectomy, Portal Vein Embolization, and Radiofrequency Ablation

A 55-year-old woman, presenting an asymptomatic adenocarcinoma of the sigmoid colon and multiple synchronous bilateral liver metastases, was referred to our hospital (Fig. 7.6). At diagnosis, carcinoembryonic antigen (CEA) level was 500 ng/ml ($N < 5$ ng/ml), and CA 19.9 level was 510 IU/ml ($N < 37$ IU/ml). Chemotherapy treatment consisted of 5-FU, LV, and oxaliplatin

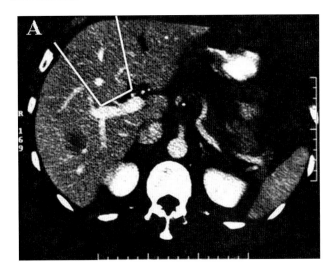
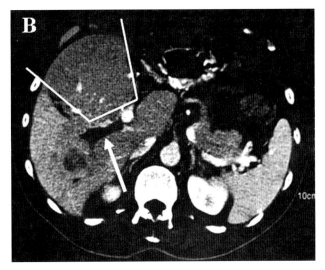

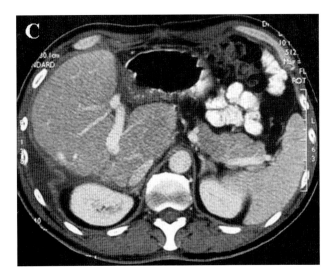

Fig. 7.5 After left lobectomy and embolization of the right branch of the portal vein, compensatory hypertrophy of segments I and IV allowed a safe right hepatectomy. **A**: Before left lobectomy and portal embolization. **B**: After left lobectomy and portal embolization (notice the absence of contrast injection of the right portal branch [*arrow*]). **C**: Final situation after the second stage right hepatectomy

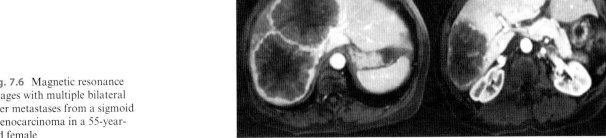

Fig. 7.6 Magnetic resonance images with multiple bilateral liver metastases from a sigmoid adenocarcinoma in a 55-year-old female

Fig. 7.7 Computed tomographic images after chemotherapy treatment (FOLFOX), showing a partial response of more than 50%

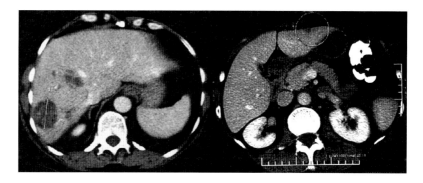

Fig. 7.8 Compensatory hypertrophy of the left liver lobe after embolization of the right branch of the portal vein, enabling an extended right hepatectomy. A: Before portal vein embolization; B: after portal vein embolization

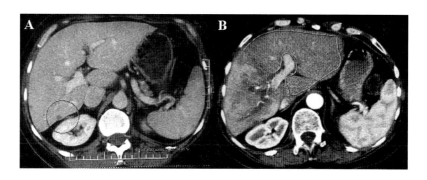

(FOLFOX), resulting in a partial radiological response (>50%) (Fig. 7.7), and a decrease of tumor markers with a CEA level of 25 ng/ml and a CA 19.9 level of 31 IU/ml.

Because of multinodularity and bilateral distribution of liver metastases identified by intraoperative ultrasound, it was decided to perform a two-stage procedure. The first step consisted of five partial resections in the left liver lobe

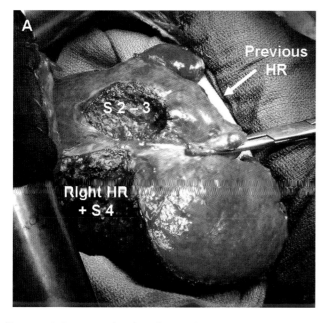

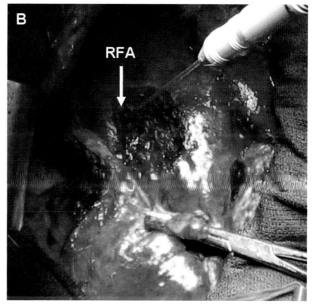

Fig. 7.9 A. Intraoperative view after multiple partial resections in the left liver lobe during the first step and an extended right hepatectomy and partial resection of segments II and III during the second step of a two-stage procedure. (Abbreviations: HR = hepatectomy; S = segment.) B. Radiofrequency ablation (RFA) of a nodule deeply situated in segment II, performed during the second step of a two-stage procedure

and segment IV, combined with embolization of the right branch of the portal vein, followed by a left colectomy during the same operation. Histopathologic examination revealed a T3N1 adenocarcinoma of the sigmoid. Five liver metastases were identified with a maximum size of 13 mm, and free surgical resection margins.

Postoperatively, oxaliplatin (FOLFOX) was replaced by irinotecan (FOLFIRI) because of neurotoxicity for a total of three cycles. Three months after the first operation, the left part of the liver had hypertrophied sufficiently, enabling a safe resection of the right liver (Fig. 7.8).

The second step of the procedure consisted of a right hepatectomy, combined with partial resections of segments II, III, and IV, and RFA of another lesion in segment II (Fig. 7.9A,B). Two years after the second hepatectomy, the patient died of disease progression.

References

1. Steele G, Ravikumar TS. Resection of hepatic metastases from colorectal cancer: biologic perspectives. Ann Surg. 1989; 210: 127–38.
2. Simmonds PC, Primrose JN, Colquitt JL, et al. Surgical resection of hepatic metastases from colorectal cancer: a systematic review of published studies. Br J Cancer. 2006; 94: 982–99.
3. Adam R, Chiche L, Aloia T, et al. Hepatic resection for non-colorectal nonendocrine liver metastases. Ann Surg. 2006; 244: 524–35.
4. Fong Y, Fortner J, Sun RL, et al. Clinical score for predicting recurrence after hepatic resection for metastatic colorectal cancer: analysis of 1001 consecutive cases. Ann Surg. 1999; 230: 309–18.
5. Nordlinger B, Guiguet M, Vaillant JC, et al. Surgical resection of colorectal carcinoma metastases to the liver. A prognostic scoring system to improve case selection, based on 1568 patients. Association Française de Chirurgie. Cancer. 1996; 77: 1254–62.
6. Pawlik TM, Scoggins CR, Zorzi D, et al. Effect of surgical margin status on survival and site of recurrence after hepatic resection for colorectal metastases. Ann Surg. 2005; 241: 715–22.
7. Vauthey JN, Chaoui A, Do KA, et al. Standardized measurement of the future liver remnant prior to extended liver resection: methodology and clinical associations. Surgery. 2000; 127: 512–9.
8. Levi F, Zidani R, Brienza S, et al. A multicenter evaluation of intensified, ambulatory, chronomodulated chemotherapy with oxaliplatin, 5-fluorouracil, and leucovorin as initial treatment of patients with metastatic colorectal carcinoma. International Organization for Cancer Chronotherapy. Cancer. 1999; 85: 2532–40.
9. Tournigand C, André T, Achille E, et al. FOLFIRI followed by FOLFOX6 or the reverse sequence in advanced colorectal cancer: a randomized GERCOR study. J Clin Oncol. 2004; 22: 229–37.
10. Levi F, Misset JL, Brienza S, et al. A chronopharmacologic phase II clinical trial with 5-fluorouracil, folinic acid, and oxaliplatin using an ambulatory multichannel programmable pump. High antitumor effectiveness against metastatic colorectal cancer. Cancer. 1992; 69: 893–900

11. Levi F, Zidani R, Misset JL. Randomised multicentre trial of chronotherapy with oxaliplatin, fluorouracil, and folinic acid in metastatic colorectal cancer. International Organization for Cancer Chronotherapy. Lancet. 1997; 350: 681–6.
12. Bismuth H, Adam R, Levi F, et al. Resection of nonresectable liver metastases from colorectal cancer after neoadjuvant chemotherapy. Ann Surg. 1996; 224: 509–22.
13. Adam R, Delvart V, Pascal G, et al. Rescue surgery for unresectable colorectal liver metastases downstaged by chemotherapy: a model to predict long-term survival. Ann Surg. 2004; 240: 644–57.
14. Masi G, Cupini S, Marcucci L, et al. Treatment with 5-fluorouracil/folinic acid, oxaliplatin, and irinotecan enables surgical resection of metastases in patients with initially unresectable metastatic colorectal cancer. Ann Surg Oncol. 2006; 13: 58–65.
15. Giacchetti S, Itzhaki M, Gruia G, et al. Long-term survival of patients with unresectable colorectal cancer liver metastases following infusional chemotherapy with 5-fluorouracil, leucovorin, oxaliplatin and surgery. Ann Oncol. 1999; 10: 663–9.
16. Pozzo C, Basso M, Cassano A, et al. Neoadjuvant treatment of unresectable liver disease with irinotecan and 5-fluorouracil plus folinic acid in colorectal cancer patients. Ann Oncol. 2004; 15: 933–9.
17. de la Camera J, Rodriguez J, Rotellar F. Triplet therapy with oxaliplatin, irinotecan, 5-fluorouracil and folinic acid within a combined modality approach in patients with liver metastases from colorectal cancer. Proc Am Soc Clin Oncol. 2004; 23: Abstract 3593.
18. Quenet F, Nordlinger B, Rivoire M. Resection of previously unresectable liver metastases from colorectal cancer (LMCRC) after chemotherapy (CT) with CPT-11/L-OHP/LV5FU (Folfirinox): a prospective phase II trial. Proc Am Soc Clin Oncol. 2004; 23: Abstract 3613.
19. Alberts SR, Horvath WL, Sternfeld WC, et al. Oxaliplatin, fluorouracil, and leucovorin for patients with unresectable liver-only metastases from colorectal cancer: a North Central Cancer Treatment Group phase II study. J Clin Oncol. 2005; 23: 9243–9.
20. Ho WM, Ma B, Mok T, et al. Liver resection after irinotecan, 5-fluorouracil, and folinic acid for patients with unresectable colorectal liver metastases: a multicenter phase II study by the Cancer Therapeutic Research Group. Med Oncol. 2005; 22: 303–12.
21. Adam R, Pascal G, Castaing D, et al. Tumor progression while on chemotherapy: a contraindication to liver resection for multiple colorectal metastases? Ann Surg. 2004; 240: 1052–61.
22. Baselga J. The EGFR as a target for anticancer therapy—focus on cetuximab. Eur J Cancer. 2001; 37 Suppl 4: S16–22.
23. Folprecht G, Lutz MP, Schoffski P, et al. Cetuximab and irinotecan/5-fluorouracil/folinic acid is a safe combination for the first-line treatment of patients with epidermal growth factor receptor expressing metastatic colorectal carcinoma. Ann Oncol. 2006; 17: 450–6.
24. Kopetz S, Abbruzzese JL, Eng C, et al. Preliminary results from a phase II study of infusional 5-FU, leucovorin, and irinotecan (FOLFIRI) plus bevacizumab as first-line treatment for metastatic colorectal cancer (mCRC). Journal of Clinical Oncology 2006 ASCO Annual Meeting Proceedings Part I; 24: Abstract 3579.
25. Peeters M, Raoul J, van Laethem J, et al. Cetuximab in combination with irinotecan/5-fluorouracil (5-FU)/folinic acid (FA) (FOLFIRI) in the first-line treatment of metastatic colorectal cancer (mCRC). Eur J Cancer. 2005; 3(suppl): 188.
26. Cervantes A, Casado E, van Cutsem E, et al. Cetuximab plus oxaliplatin/5-fluorouracil (5-FU)folinic acid (FA) (FOLFOX4)

for the epidermal growth factor receptor (EGFR)-expressing metastatic colorectal cancer (mCRC) in the first-line setting: a phase II study. Eur J Cancer. 2005; 3(suppl): 181–2.

27. Adam R, Aloia T, Levi F, et al. Hepatic resection following rescue cetuximab treatment for colorectal liver metastases previously refractory to conventional systemic therapy. J Clin Oncol. 2007; 25(29): 4593–602.

28. Emmanouilides C, Sfakiotaki G, Androulakis N, et al. Front-line bevacizumab in combination with oxaliplatin, leucovorin and 5-fluorouracil (FOLFOX) in patients with metastatic colorectal cancer: a multicenter phase II study. BMC Cancer. 2007; 7: 91.

29. Benoist S, Brouquet A, Penna C, et al. Complete response of colorectal liver metastases after chemotherapy: does it mean cure? J Clin Oncol. 2006; 24: 3939–45.

30. Karoui M, Penna C, Amin-Hashem M, et al. Influence of preoperative chemotherapy on the risk of major hepatectomy for colorectal liver metastases. Ann Surg. 2006; 243: 1–7.

31. Rubbia-Brandt L, Audard V, Sartoretti P, et al. Severe hepatic sinusoidal obstruction associated with oxaliplatin-based chemotherapy in patients with metastatic colorectal cancer. Ann Oncol. 2004; 15: 460–6.

32. Vauthey JN, Pawlik TM, Ribero D, et al. Chemotherapy regimen predicts steatohepatitis and an increase in 90-day mortality after surgery for hepatic colorectal metastases. J Clin Oncol. 2006; 24: 2065–72.

33. Aloia T, Sebagh M, Plasse M, et al. Liver histology and surgical outcomes after preoperative chemotherapy with fluorouracil plus oxaliplatin in colorectal cancer liver metastases. J Clin Oncol. 2006; 24: 4983–90.

34. Takayasu K, Muramatsu Y, Shima Y, et al. Hepatic lobar atrophy following obstruction of the ipsilateral portal vein from hilar cholangiocarcinoma. Radiology. 1986; 160: 389–93.

35. Kinoshita H, Sakai K, Hirohashi K, et al. Preoperative portal vein embolization for hepatocellular carcinoma. World J Surg. 1986; 10: 803–8.

36. Makuuchi M, Thai BL, Takayasu K, et al. Preoperative portal embolization to increase safety of major hepatectomy for hilar bile duct carcinoma: a preliminary report. Surgery. 1990; 107: 521–7.

37. Azoulay D, Castaing D, Smail A, et al. Resection of nonresectable liver metastases from colorectal cancer after percutaneous portal vein embolization. Ann Surg. 2000; 231: 480–6.

38. Selzner N, Pestalozzi B.C., Kadry Z, et al. Downstaging colorectal liver metastases by concomitant unilateral portal vein ligation and selective intra-arterial chemotherapy. Br J Surg. 2006; 93: 587–92.

39. Elias D, Baton O, Sideris L, et al. Hepatectomy plus intraoperative radiofrequency ablation and chemotherapy to treat technically unresectable multiple colorectal liver metastases. J Surg Oncol. 2005; 90: 36–42.

40. Rivoire M, De Cian F, Meeus P, et al. Combination of neoadjuvant chemotherapy with cryotherapy and surgical resection for the treatment of unresectable liver metastases from colorectal carcinoma. Cancer. 2002; 95: 2283–92.

41. Adam R, Laurent A, Azoulay D, et al. Two-stage hepatectomy: A planned strategy to treat irresectable liver tumors. Ann Surg. 2000; 232: 777–85.

42. Jaeck D, Oussoultzoglou E, Rosso E, et al. A two-stage hepatectomy procedure combined with portal vein embolization to achieve curative resection for initially unresectable multiple and bilobar colorectal liver metastases. Ann Surg. 2004; 240: 1037–49.

43. Togo, S, Nagano Y, Masui H, et al. Two-stage hepatectomy for multiple bilobular liver metastases from colorectal cancer. Hepatogastroenterology. 2005; 52: 913–9.

44. Heaney JP, Stanton WK, Halbert DS, et al. An improved technic for vascular isolation of the liver: experimental study and case reports. Ann Surg. 1966; 163: 237–41.

45. Bismuth H, Castaing D, Garden OJ. Major hepatic resection under total vascular exclusion. Ann Surg. 1989; 210: 13–9.

46. Iwatsuki S, Todo S, Starzl TE. Right trisegmentectomy with a synthetic vena cava graft. Arch Surg. 1988; 123: 1021–2.

47. Cherqui D, Malassagne B, Colau PI, et al. Hepatic vascular exclusion with preservation of the caval flow for liver resections. Ann Surg. 1999; 230: 24–30.

48. Huguet C, Gavelli A, Chieco PA, et al. Liver ischemia for hepatic resection: where is the limit? Surgery. 1992; 111: 251–9.

49. Azoulay D, Eshkenazy R, Andreani P, et al. In situ hypothermic perfusion of the liver versus standard total vascular exclusion for complex liver resection. Ann Surg. 2005; 241: 277–85.

50. Azoulay D, Andreani P, Maggi U, et al. Combined liver resection and reconstruction of the supra-renal vena cava: the Paul Brousse experience. Ann Surg. 2006; 244: 80–8.

Adjuvant Chemotherapy

Christophe Penna and Bernard Nordlinger

Introduction

Approximately 50% of patients with colorectal cancer develop liver metastases at some point during the course of their disease [1, 2]. Surgical resection remains the only treatment that can, to date, ensure long-term survival in 25–40% of the patients [3, 4].

Thus tumor relapse occurs in up to 60% of patients who underwent curative resection after a median of only 9–12 months. Various attempts are being made to reduce this risk including more aggressive surgical techniques, new methods of ablation such as cryotherapy, radiofrequency ablation, and laser hyperthermia or better selection of patients in whom surgery is considered. Probably the most promising way to improve outcome after resection of liver metastases and to cure more patients is to combine surgery with chemotherapy. Chemotherapy is effective on unresectable liver metastases as well as adjuvant treatment for stage III colon cancer. Therefore it is rational to propose its use in adjuvant treatment for resectable liver metastases. Adjuvant chemotherapy can be delivered as intravenous infusion after curative resection of liver metastases but it can also be delivered before surgery and is then referred as neoadjuvant chemotherapy. After hepatic resection chemotherapy can also be given directly into the liver via a catheter left in place in the hepatic artery.

In this review, we will summarize the current data on the rationale, the potential benefits and complications and the results of adjuvant and neoadjuvant chemotherapy for the treatment of resectable colorectal liver metastases.

C. Penna (✉)
Professor of Surgery, Department of Digestive Surgery
and Oncology, Ambroise Pare Hospital, Boulogne, France

Adjuvant Chemotherapy

The rationale for using adjuvant chemotherapy after curative surgery for colorectal liver metastases is based on studies showing survival benefit of adjuvant chemotherapy in stage III patients. Adjuvant chemotherapy after resection of colorectal metastases can be delivered intravenously, by hepatic arterial infusion (HAI) or both.

Hepatic Arterial Infusion of Chemotherapy with or Without Systemic Chemotherapy After Resection of Hepatic Metastases

An explanation of intrahepatic recurrence following curative liver resection is the growth of dormant liver metastases. These lesions are smaller than a few millimeters and therefore are undetectable by conventional imaging techniques, including perioperative ultrasonography. However, if their diameter is larger than 1 mm their blood supply is mainly derived from the hepatic artery, as opposed to the healthy liver, whose blood supply comes chiefly from the portal vein. This forms the rationale for the use of adjuvant HAI of chemotherapy. Seven randomized trials comparing HAI with systemic therapy in patients with unresectable hepatic metastases have shown that response rates were higher in patients receiving HAI [5, 6, 7]. Fluoropyrimidine analogs such as floxuridine are extracted in the liver, resulting in decreased extrahepatic concentration of the drug. HAI of floxuridine may therefore result in a significant increase of exposure of tumor to the drug with reduced systemic side effects.

HAI has also limitations. Extrahepatic progression is observed in 50–70% of patients with unresectable metastases treated with HAI because only the liver receives a sufficient amount of the drug [6]. This suggests that HAI should be combined with systemic chemotherapy. In a randomized multicenter trial in patients with non-resectable liver metastases HAI with floxuridine combined with intravenous 5 FU and folinic acid was superior to HAI with floxuridine only for time to progression and overall survival [8]. The second limit of HAI is the risk of severe side effects including biliary toxicity almost exclusively observed with floxuridine [6], and technical problems precluding the use of the intrahepatic catheter.

Adjuvant HAI after curative hepatic resection has been tested in several phase III trials with or without systemic chemotherapy.

A prospective randomized trial including 226 patients from 26 German hospitals between 1991 and 1996 compared resection of liver metastases followed by adjuvant HAI of 5-fluorouracil (5-FU) plus folinic acid every 28 days during 6 months or liver resection alone [9]. Patients had a maximum of six resectable liver metastases without extrahepatic or primary residual disease and were stratified by the number of metastases and the site of the primary tumor. A total of 113 patients were assigned to each group. Twenty-four patients in the HAI group and 13 in the control group did not receive the assigned treatment. The first planned intention-to-treat interim analysis showed a median survival of 34.5 months for patients with adjuvant HAI therapy versus 40.8 months for control patients. Grade 3 and 4 toxicities occurred in 25.6% of cycles and 63% of patients receiving HAI. According to this interim analysis the chance of detecting an expected 50% improvement in survival by the use of HAI was only 5% and the patient accrual was terminated. A study from the Memorial Sloan-Kettering Cancer Center compared six cycles of HAI with floxuridine and dexamethasone plus intravenous fluorouracil with or without leucovorin, or 6 weeks of similar systemic therapy alone [10]. Among 156 patients who underwent complete resection of hepatic metastases 74 were randomly assigned to receive HAI plus systemic chemotherapy and 82 were assigned to receive systemic therapy alone. There were no significant differences between the two groups with respect to base-line characteristics. The toxic effects of chemotherapy were similar in both groups. In the combined therapy group six patients never received HAI, 66% received more than three cycles of HAI but only 26% received more than 50% of the planned dose of floxuridine. Sixteen complications were related to the pump or catheter use for HAI. The actuarial rate of overall survival at 2 years was 86% in the HAI group and 72% in the group given systemic therapy alone ($p = 0.03$). After 2 years the rates of survival free of hepatic recurrence were 90% in the combined therapy group and 60% in the monotherapy group ($p < 0.001$). At 2 years the risk ratio for death was 2.34 among patients treated

with systemic therapy alone compared with patients who received combined therapy (95% CI 1.1–4.98; $p = 0.027$).

Another trial organized by the Eastern Cooperative Oncology Group evaluated HAI with floxuridine plus intravenous continuous infusion of 5-FU or no further treatment after liver resection [11]. Randomization before surgery was chosen but resulted in a high proportion of patients (26.6%) who were ineligible at surgery because of the perioperative discovery of previously unsuspected extrahepatic disease. Moreover, because more than 25% of the patients do not receive the treatment to which they were allotted because of eligibility criteria or technical problems results were analyzed according to treatment actually delivered instead of an intention to treat analysis. Conclusions of the study were that HAI combined with intravenous continuous 5-FU reduced the risk of recurrence when compared with surgery alone but resulted in no benefit in overall survival.

In summary, HAI alone is not sufficient as adjuvant treatment for liver metastases. HAI associated with systemic chemotherapy can reduce the risk of recurrences after surgery but this potential benefit is counterbalanced by a significant increase in side effects. A widespread use of HAI as adjuvant treatment after hepatectomy is also limited by technical reasons precluding catheter placement, availability of floxuridine, high cost of infusion pumps, and risks of catheter thrombosis. Since these trials were designed, chemotherapy has evolved and new effective drugs are available. Ongoing trials investigate adjuvant treatments with HAI of floxuridine and new combinations of systemic chemotherapy: capecitabine (NSABP C09), capecitabine plus oxaliplatin (NCCTG) or irinotecan. Meanwhile, impressive results have been reported with the use of HAI with oxaliplatin in patients with unresectable liver metastases [12] and this new approach certainly deserve to be tested in an adjuvant setting.

Systemic Chemotherapy After Resection of Hepatic Metastases

Although the effectiveness of systemic chemotherapy has been well demonstrated for unresectable colorectal metastases, very few studies have addressed the question of adjuvant systemic chemotherapy after complete resection of liver metastases. A small randomized study showed no survival difference between surgery alone or followed by systemic chemotherapy with fluorouracil and folinic acid [13]. In the multicenter trial reported by

Portier et al. [14] 173 patients with completely resected hepatic metastases from colorectal cancer were randomly assigned over a 10-year period to observation (87 patients) or 6 months of systemic chemotherapy with a fluorouracil and folinic acid monthly regimen (86 patients). The primary endpoint was disease-free survival. The median duration of follow-up was 87 months and was similar in both groups. The total number of recurrence was 52 in the chemotherapy group and 55 in the observation group. There was no statistically significant difference between both groups for 5–year disease-free survival (33.5% for the chemotherapy group vs. 26.7% for the control group) or overall survival (81% vs. 82% at 2 years and 51% vs. 42% at 5 years for chemotherapy and control group, respectively). Cox multivariate analysis showed a statistically significant positive effect of chemotherapy on disease-free survival (odds ratio for recurrence or death, 0.66; 95% CI, 0.46–0.96; $p = 0.028$) leading the authors to conclude to the beneficial effect of postoperative chemotherapy despite the lack of statistical difference observed for the primary endpoint.

Another phase III multicenter trial (EORTC/NCIC/GIVIO) which tested fluorouracil plus I-leucovorin versus observation after potentially curative resection of liver metastases from colorectal cancer also failed to show any significant difference between both groups for progression-free survival (PFS) and overall survival despite a trend in favor of the chemotherapy arm [15]. However, this trial was prematurely closed after the randomization of 129 patients in 4 years because of slow accrual.

Both trials showed a non-significant trend for improvement in PFS and overall survival for patients treated with chemotherapy and a lack of power may explain these results. Therefore a pooled analysis based on individual data from these trials with very similar design has been done and recently reported [16]. Two hundred and seventy-eight patients were included (surgery: 138, chemotherapy: 140). The observed improvement in median PFS was almost but not statistically significant ($p = 0.059$) and the improvement in overall survival was not significant ($p = 0.125$).

In summary, randomized trials have failed to demonstrate a survival benefit of adjuvant systemic chemotherapy after complete resection of liver metastases from colorectal cancer. Several reasons may explain this result. A very low accrual rhythm led to stop the inclusions in both studies resulting in a lack of power. The chemotherapy regimens used, which were the standard regimens at the time when the studies began, were not optimal and newer drug combinations including oxaliplatin or irinotecan are probably more efficient as demonstrated in adjuvant treatment of stage III colon cancer. Recurrences in both arms were treated by second-line chemotherapy or by repeat liver resection, which influence the natural history of the disease and affect overall survival in both arms. Whatsoever, currently available data support that adjuvant systemic chemotherapy may have a beneficial impact but are no sufficient to propose, to date, this treatment as a standard. Several trials are currently ongoing testing the association of LV5FU plus irinotecan or LV5FU plus irinotecan and oxaliplatin after complete resection of liver metastases.

Neoadjuvant Chemotherapy

Another area of clinical research to improve the prognosis of resected colorectal liver metastases is to deliver the chemotherapy before the resection. This approach is supported by several arguments and the results of randomized trials testing neoadjuvant chemotherapy are currently available.

The Rationale for Neoadjuvant Chemotherapy in Patients with Resectable Liver Metastases

The administration of chemotherapy before a planned resection of resectable liver metastases has several potential advantages. Neoadjuvant chemotherapy can in theory be effective on micrometastatic disease allowing eradication of dormant cancer cells in the liver. Neoadjuvant chemotherapy may induce tumor shrinkage. In this setting, even if the tumor deposits were resectable, the downsizing may help to obtain better resection margin or even to realize less extended liver resections thus decreasing postoperative morbidity [17]. Chemoresponsiveness to neoadjuvant treatment is useful to determine which treatment should be given after resection [18]. Finally, two recent studies have shown that response to preoperative chemotherapy is an important prognostic factor and may be helpful to select good candidates for surgical resection [19, 20]. In one study [19], the outcomes of patients referred for resection of synchronous colorectal liver metastases with or without previous chemotherapy were compared. Patients and tumor-related variables were similar in both groups. Five-year survival was similar in both groups, but the subgroup of patients with stable disease or disease responding to chemotherapy had a better survival when compared to patients who did not receive chemotherapy (85% vs. 35%, $p = 0.03$). In another study [20], 131 patients who became candidates for liver resection after systemic chemotherapy (5-FU and leucovorin plus oxaliplatin or irinotecan) were divided into three groups according to the response to chemotherapy: patients with an objective response, tumor stabilization or with tumor progression. Patients with tumor progression had a lower 5-year survival when compared with patients with objective response and stabilization (8% vs. 37% and 30%), suggesting that tumor progression while on chemotherapy is a poor prognostic factor and could even be considered as a contraindication for surgery.

The Potential Drawbacks of Neoadjuvant Chemotherapy

Complete Response Before Surgery

Following the administration of few cycles of chemotherapy, some small liver metastases can be no longer detectable with pre and perioperative imaging techniques. A major question is to know whether the sites of metastases that have disappeared should be resected or if they can be left in place and considered as cured. This is particularly important when the disappearance of lesions allows the surgeon to perform a minor instead of a major resection with a lower operative risk. In a recently published study [21] we have shown that cancer persisted in more than 80% of the cases at the initial site of liver metastases that had disappeared on imaging, suggesting that resection of the sites of initial metastases was necessary. In such cases, it may be difficult or even impossible for the surgeon to identify where the metastases were located and thus to decide what type of resection is mandatory. One risk of neoadjuvant chemotherapy is therefore to preclude surgical resection in some patients with initially resectable liver metastases because of the absence of residual visible tumor. Response to neoadjuvant chemotherapy should be closely monitored in order to avoid such situations, keeping in mind that complete response is not an endpoint of chemotherapy for resectable liver metastases.

Chemotherapy-Associated Hepatotoxicity

Chemotherapy administered before liver resection may induce hepatic damage which could increase the risks of surgery and even preclude liver resection. There are now accumulating data showing that preoperative chemotherapy is associated with pathologic changes of liver parenchyma [22, 23, 24, 25, 26, 27, 28, 29]. The question is whether these hepatic damages can be observed after neoadjuvant chemotherapy.

Two main types of chemotherapy-associated liver injuries have been reported: vascular changes and chemotherapy-associated steatohepatitis. The vascular changes include sinusoidal dilation with erythrocytes congestion, occasionally accompanied by perisinusoidal fibrosis and fibrotic venular occlusion, which could result in severe cases in sinusoidal obstruction syndrome as observed in veno-occlusive disease [22]. Steatohepatitis is defined by the association of severe steatosis, lobular inflammation, and ballooning [27]. Few studies have evaluated the correlation between the type of liver injury and the preoperative chemotherapy regimen. The liver damage that can result from systemic therapy is not restricted to the current generation of chemotherapies and it has been reported that even 5-FU can be associated with an increased risks of severe steatosis but not of steatohepatitis [30]. Oxaliplatin-based combination regimen is associated with an increased risk of vascular lesions of the liver [22, 27, 28] and irinotecan-containing regimens have been associated with increased risks of steatosis and steatohepatitis [23, 24, 27]. It is possible that specific chemotherapy regimens do not automatically predispose to steatosis, but can aggravate it when it already exists [25].

That chemotherapy can be associated with liver injury is now well recognized. The main question is whether collective damages to the liver induced by preoperative chemotherapy have any clinical significance. The safety data of European Organization for Research and Treatment of Cancer (EORTC) study 40983, comparing perioperative chemotherapy with 5FU, leucovorin, and oxaliplatin (six cycles before surgery and six cycles after) to surgery alone in 364 patients, were presented in 2005 [31]. The results showed that mortality rate was very low (close to 1%) in the two treatment arms and the rate of reversible complications was acceptable. Thus, administration of six cycles of FOLFOX before surgery appears feasible. Another report from our institution brought another insight into the relation between duration of preoperative chemotherapy and perioperative morbidity, and showed that administration of more than six cycles of preoperative systemic chemotherapy increased morbidity after major liver resection but did not increase mortality [26]. Furthermore, it has been reported that patients with more than 12 cycles of preoperative chemotherapy had a higher risk of reoperation and a longer hospital stay [28].

Some studies have looked at the relationship between the type of lesions induced by chemotherapy and their potential clinical consequences. Steatosis is associated with increased overall and infective complications but does not have a significant impact on mortality [23]. Sinusoidal injury increases the risk of operative bleeding but does not increase perioperative morbidity and mortality [27, 28]. Finally, steatohepatitis is the most severe injury, since it increases overall postoperative mortality and specifically death from postoperative liver failure [27]. Consequently, the use of neoadjuvant therapy including the choice of chemotherapy regimens and the duration of treatment should be carefully considered because the risk of hepatotoxicity is significant. Preoperative liver biopsy has been suggested in patients who have received prolonged systemic chemotherapy to evaluate the degree of chemotherapy-induced liver injury [25]. The interest of such an approach is uncertain, given the problems with intra- and interobserver variations in the evaluation of chemotherapy-induced injury [27] and the heterogeneity of lesions due to chemotherapy in the liver. Using such information to deny resection of resectable liver metastases, based only on the results of biopsies, may not prove easy. The best alternative would be to be able to identify other factors which could predict, before start of treatment, which patients are at risk of developing chemotherapy-induced liver injury.

Concerning targeted agents, there are only few data describing the potential toxicity of anti-vascular endothelial growth factor (VEGF) therapy such as bevacizumab. Bevacizumab has been considered responsible for increased risk of organ perforation [32] and might affect wound healing and liver regeneration. In a case matched study realized at the Memorial Sloan-Kettering Cancer Center [33] comparing 32 patients receiving bevacizumab before or after hepatic resection to 32 patients who underwent liver resection without bevacizumab and matched for age, gender, type of hepatectomy, number and size of liver metastases, and risk factors there was no statistical difference between groups for postoperative morbidity. In a pilot study of 34 liver resection for metastases following six cycles of chemotherapy with 5-FU, oxaliplatin, and bevacizumab, 82% of the patients had a complete (5/34) or a partial (23/34) response. There was no postoperative liver insufficiency or perioperative bleeding. Hepatic regeneration measured 3 months after liver resection on CT-scan does not seem to be altered by preoperative treatment [34].

The questions raised by the use of bevacizumab on liver parenchyma and function are still unanswered but if a 6–8–week interval between the last administration of bevacizumab and surgery is respected it is likely that a neoadjuvant chemotherapy with bevacizumab does not increase the risks of hepatectomy.

Results of Neoadjuvant Chemotherapy in Patients with Resectable Liver Metastases

The feasibility and the benefits of neoadjuvant chemotherapy have been suggested in phase II studies. In a first study [35], 20 patients with initially resectable liver metastases received three cycles of combination neoadjuvant chemotherapy with weekly high-dose of 5-FU as 24-hour infusion, folinic acid, and oxaliplatin. The curative resectability rate was 80%, the operative mortality and morbidity rates were 0 and 25%, and toxicity grade 3–4 was observed in 30% of patients. The 2-year disease-free survival rate was 52% and the 2-year cancer-related survival rate was 80%. In another study [36], liver resection was performed after six cycles of LV5FU plus oxaliplatin and followed by six cycles of LV5FU plus irinotecan in 22 patients. The curative resection rate was 91% and grade 3–4 toxicity was observed in 30% of patients. The 2-year overall and disease-free survival rates were 89% and 47%, respectively. Other phase II studies evaluating neoadjuvant chemotherapy with irinotecan or bevacizumab regimens for resectable liver metastases are also ongoing.

Progression-free and overall survival rates reported in these phase II studies are promising but survival benefit of neoadjuvant chemotherapy for resectable colorectal liver metastases can only be demonstrated by a phase III clinical trial. To demonstrate that chemotherapy combined with surgery is a better treatment than surgery alone the EORTC has conducted a phase III trial comparing pre and postoperative oxaliplatin-based chemotherapy versus no chemotherapy [37]. Patients with potentially resectable liver metastases of colorectal cancer with up to four deposits on CT-scan and no extrahepatic disease nor previous chemotherapy with oxaliplatin were randomized between surgery alone or surgery preceded by six cycles of LV5FU plus oxaliplatin and followed by six cycles of the same chemotherapy. The primary endpoint was to demonstrate a 40% increase in median PFS with perioperative chemotherapy. Three hundred and sixty-four patients (182 in each arm) were included between September 2000 and July 2004. Both groups were comparable for age, gender, Tumor Node Metastasis (TNM) status of the primary and mean number of liver metastases on CT-scan. In the chemotherapy group 171 patients received preoperative chemotherapy and 143 received six cycles. Toxicity of the regimen was low with 8% grade 3 diarrhea, 2.3% sensory neuropathy grade 3 and 18% grade 3–4 neutropenia. There was no toxic death due to preoperative chemotherapy and no grade 4 digestive or neurologic toxicity. The median size of liver deposits (sum of the largest diameters) was 45 mm before preoperative chemotherapy (5–255) and 30 mm after preoperative chemotherapy (0–230), the relative decrease in size was 29.5%. Following preoperative chemotherapy, response according to Response Evaluation Criteria in solid tumours (RECIST) criteria was evaluable in 156 patients. Complete response was observed in 7 patients (3.8%), partial response in 73 (40.1%), stable disease in 64

(35.2%) and progression in 12 (6.6%) of whom 4 were resected. In the chemotherapy group 22 patients were not operated mainly for more advanced disease, refusal or poor general condition and 8 were not resected. In the surgery group 8 patients were not operated and 18 were not resected, mainly because of the perioperative discovery of more advanced disease. Postoperative complication rate was significantly higher in the preoperative chemotherapy arm (25.2% vs. 15.9%, $p = 0.04$) due to an increase in intraabdominal infection and biliary fistula. There was one postoperative death in the chemotherapy group and two in the surgery alone group. Postoperative chemotherapy was delivered to 115 patients and 80 completed six cycles. After a median follow-up of 48 months, with 171 patients eligible in each group the difference in PFS was significantly better in the perioperative group (%absolute difference in 3-year PFS + 8.1% [28.1–36.2%], $p = 0.041$). The difference was even more significant for resected patients ($+9.2\%$, $p = 0.025$). This large randomized study demonstrated that perioperative chemotherapy with LV5FU plus oxaliplatin improves PFS in patients with resectable metastases. This treatment should be proposed as the new standard for these patients.

Neoadjuvant Therapies Including Targeted Agents

Given the positive results of perioperative adjuvant chemotherapy, a promising way to improve outcome in patients with resectable liver metastases is the administration of regimens combining cytotoxic drugs and novel-targeted agents. The addition of bevacizumab to chemotherapy improves objective response and prolongs survival in both first- and second-line therapies [34]. To date, the role of targeted agents to render patients with initially unresectable liver metastases resectable has only been reported in few preliminary trials. These results are promising with response rate ranging from 46% to 78%, but do not allow comparison with chemotherapy regimens using only cytotoxic agents because of the heterogeneity of study populations and the lack of long-term data. The conclusion we can deduct from these preliminary trials is that targeted agents combined with cytotoxic regimens are associated with high tumor response rates, which are likely to translate into high resection rates and improved long-term survival. An ongoing study conducted by EORTC will evaluate the feasibility and safety of liver surgery for metastases in patients who had received neoadjuvant chemotherapy with 5FU, oxaliplatin, and cetuximab, with or without bevacizumab.

Conclusions

We have now learned that neoadjuvant chemotherapy has both positive and negative impacts and we must deal with both. Thus, the drugs and the duration of treatment must be decided with care.

For patients with resectable metastases, neoadjuvant chemotherapy can be considered pending the results of EORTC study 40983, but these patients also should not be over-treated, to avoid chronic and progressive chemotherapy-induced liver damage, which could preclude curative surgery.

In the fast-moving field of combined treatment of patients with colorectal cancer liver metastases, multidisciplinary discussion and repeated evaluations are more indispensable than ever. If neoadjuvant chemotherapy is well chosen and well monitored and surgery planned at the right moment, liver metastases can be resected safely.

References

1. Jemal A, Murray T, Ward E, et al. Cancer statistics, 2005. CA Cancer J Clin. 2005; 55: 10–30.
2. Stangl R, Altendorf-Hofmann A, Charnley RM, Scheele J. Factors influencing the natural history of colorectal liver metastases. Lancet. 1994; 343: 1405–10.
3. Nordlinger B, Jaeck D, Guiguet M, et al. Surgical resection of hepatic metastases. Multicentric retrospective study by the French Association of Surgery. In: Nordlinger B, Jaeck D, eds. Treatment of Hepatic Metastases of Colorectal Cancer. Paris: Springer-Verlag; 1992: 129–146.
4. Fong Y, Fortner J, Sun RL, et al. Clinical score for predicting recurrence after hepatic resection for metastatic colorectal cancer: analysis of 1001 consecutive cases. Ann Surg. 1999; 230: 309–18.
5. Hohn DC, Stagg RJ, Friedman MA, et al. A randomized trial of continuous intravenous versus hepatic intraarterial floxuridine in patients with colorectal cancer metastatic to the liver: the Northern California Oncology Group trial. J Clin Oncol. 1989; 7: 1646–54.
6. Rougier P, Laplanche A, Huguier M, et al. Hepatic arterial infusion of floxuridine in patients with liver metastases from colorectal carcinoma: long term results of a prospective randomized trial. J Clin Oncol. 1992; 10: 1112–8.
7. Allen-Mersh TG, Earlam S, Fordy C, et al. Quality of life and survival with continuous hepatic-artery floxuridine infusion for colorectal liver metastases. Lancet. 1994; 344: 1255–60.
8. Lorenz M, Muller HH. Randomized, multicenter trial of fluorouracil plus leucovorin administered either via hepatic arterial or intravenous infusion versus fluorodeoxyuridine administered via hepatic arterial infusion in patients with non resectable liver metastases from colorectal carcinoma. J Clin Oncol. 2000; 18: 243–54.
9. Lorenz M, Muller HH, Schramm H, et al. Randomized trial of surgery versus surgery followed by adjuvant hepatic arterial infusion with 5-fluorouracil and folinic acid for liver metastases of colorectal cancer. German Cooperative on Liver Metastases. Ann Surg. 1998; 228: 756–62.

10. Kemeny N, Huang Y, Cohen AM, et al. Hepatic arterial infusion of chemotherapy after resection of hepatic metastases from colorectal cancer. N Engl J Med. 1999; 341: 2039–48.

11. Kemeny MM, Adak S, Gray B, et al Combined-modality treatment for resectable metastatic colorectal carcinoma to the liver: surgical resection of hepatic metastases in combination with continuous infusion of chemotherapy-an intergroup study. J Clin Oncol. 2002; 20: 1499–1505.

12. Ducreux M, Ychou M, Laplanche A, et al. Hepatic arterial oxaliplatin infusion plus intravenous chemotherapy in colorectal cancer with inoperable hepatic metastases: a trial of the gastrointestinal group of the Federation Nationale des Centres de Lutte Contre le Cancer. J Clin Oncol. 2005; 23: 4881–7.

13. Lopez-Ladron A, Salvador AJ, Bernabe R, et al. Observation versus postoperative chemotherapy after resection of liver metastases in patients with advanced colorectal cancer. Proc Am Soc Clin Oncol. 2003; 22: 373 (abstr 1497).

14. Portier G, Elias D, Bouche O, et al. Multicenter randomized trial of adjuvant fluorouracil and folinic acid compared with surgery alone after resection of colorectal liver metastases: FFCD ACHBTH AURC 9002 trial. J Clin Oncol. 2006; 24: 4976–82.

15. Langer B, Bleiberg H, Labianca R. Fluorouracil (FU) plus l-leucovorin (1-LV) versus observation after potentially curative resection of liver or lung metastases from colorectal cancer (CRC): results of the ENG (EORTC/NCIC CTG/GIVIO) randomized trial. J Clin Oncol. 2002; 20: 149a (abstr 592).

16. Mitry E, Fields A, Bleiberg H, et al. Adjuvant chemotherapy after potentially curative resection of metastases from colorectal cancer. A meta-analysis of two randomized trials. J Clin Oncol. 2006; 24: 18S (abst 3524).

17. Tanaka K, Adam R, Shimada H, et al. Role of neoadjuvant chemotherapy in the treatment of multiple colorectal metastases to the liver. Br J Surg. 2003; 90: 963–9.

18. Leonard GD, Brenner B, Kemeny NE. Neoadjuvant chemotherapy before liver resection for patients with unresectable liver metastases from colorectal carcinoma. J Clin Oncol. 2005; 23: 2038–48.

19. Allen PJ, Kemeny N, Jarnagin W, et al. Importance of response to neoadjuvant chemotherapy in patients undergoing resection of synchronous colorectal liver metastases. J Gastrointest Surg. 2003; 7: 109–15.

20. Adam R, Pascal G, Castaing D, et al. Tumor progression while on chemotherapy: a contraindication to liver resection for multiple colorectal metastases? Ann Surg. 2004; 240: 1052–61.

21. Benoist S, Brouquet A, Penna C, et al. Complete response of colorectal liver metastases after chemotherapy: does it mean cure? J Clin Oncol. 2006; 24: 3939–45.

22. Rubbia-Brandt L, Audard V, Sartoretti P, et al. Severe hepatic sinusoidal obstruction associated with oxaliplatin-based chemotherapy in patients with metastatic colorectal cancer. Ann Oncol. 2004; 15: 460–6.

23. Kooby DA, Fong Y, Suriawinata A, et al. Impact of steatosis on perioperative outcome following hepatic resection. J Gastrointest Surg. 2003; 7: 1034–44.

24. Fernandez FG, Ritter J, Goodwin JW, et al. Effect of steatohepatitis associated with irinotecan or oxaliplatin pretreatment on resectability of hepatic colorectal metastases. J Am Coll Surg. 2005; 200: 845–53.

25. Bilchik AJ, Poston G, Curley SA, et al. Neoadjuvant chemotherapy for metastatic colon cancer: a cautionary note. J Clin Oncol. 2005; 23: 9073–8.

26. Karoui M, Penna C, Amin-Hashem M, et al. Influence of preoperative chemotherapy on the risk of major hepatectomy for colorectal liver metastases. Ann Surg. 2006; 243: 1–7.

27. Vauthey JN, Pawlik TM, Ribero D, et al. Chemotherapy regimen predicts steatohepatitis and an increase in 90-day mortality after surgery for hepatic colorectal metastases. J Clin Oncol. 2006; 24: 2065–72.

28. Aloia T, Sebagh M, Plasse M, et al. Liver histology and surgical outcomes after preoperative chemotherapy with fluorouracil plus oxaliplatin in colorectal cancer liver metastases. J Clin Oncol. 2006; 24: 4983–90.

29. Nordlinger B, Benoist S. Benefits and risks of neoadjuvant therapy for liver metastases. J Clin Oncol. 2006; 24: 4954–5.

30. Peppercorn PD, Reznek RH, Wilson P, et al. Demonstration of hepatic steatosis by computerized tomography in patients receiving 5-fluorouracil-based therapy for advanced colorectal cancer. Br J Cancer. 1998; 77: 2008–11.

31. Nordlinger B, Sorbye H, Debois M, et al. Feasibility and risks of pre-operative chemotherapy with FOLFOX 4 and surgery for resectable colorectal liver metastases. Interim results of the EORTC intergroup randomized phase III study 4093. J Clin Oncol. 2005; 23: 253 s (abstr 3528).

32. Hurwitz H, Fehrenbacher L, Novotny W, et al. Bevacizumab plus irinotecan, fluorouracil, and leucovorin for metastatic colorectal cancer. N Engl J Med. 2004; 350: 2335–42.

33. D'Angelica M, Kornprat P, Gonen M, et al. Lack of evidence for increased operative morbidity after hepatectomy with perioperative use of bevacizumab: A matched case-control study. Ann Surg Oncol. 2006; 14: 759–65.

34. Gruenberger T, Sorbye H, Debois M, et al. Tumor response to pre-operative chemotherapy with FOLFOX-4 for resectable colorectal cancer liver metastases. Interim results of EORTC intergroup randomized phase III study 40983. J Clin Oncol. 2006; 24: 146s (abstr 3500).

35. Wein A, Riedel C, Bruckl W, et al. Neoadjuvant treatment with weekly high-dose 5-Fluorouracil as 24-hour infusion, folinic acid and oxaliplatin in patients with primary resectable liver metastases of colorectal cancer. Oncology. 2003; 64: 131–8.

36. Taieb J, Artru P, Paye F, et al. Intensive systemic chemotherapy combined with surgery for metastatic colorectal cancer: results of a phase II study. J Clin Oncol. 2005; 23: 502–9.

37. Nordlinger B, Sorbye H, Collette L, et al. Final results of the EORTC Intergroup randomized phase III trial study 40983 [EPOC] evaluating the benefit of peri-operative FOLFOX4 chemotherapy for patients with potentially resectable colorectal cancer liver metastases. J Clin Oncol. 2007; 25: 18S (abstr LBA5).

Gunnar Folprecht

Antibodies and other inhibitors of specific signaling pathways—often called "biologicals"—have been investigated in the treatment of colorectal cancer and several other tumors. Some drugs, such as antibodies against the epidermal growth factor receptor (EGFR) and vascular endothelial growth factor (VEGF), have reached clinical practice and will be discussed in detail, while other compounds, i.e., tyrosine kinase inhibitors of the same pathways are not (or not yet) proven to be of therapeutic value in colorectal cancer.

Treatment with the EGFR antibody cetuximab has been shown to increase response rates in multiple chemotherapeutical combinations and to increase the probability of liver resection. Efficacy of EGFR antibodies seems to be limited to patients without *k-ras* mutations. Bevacizumab induces a longer progression-free survival, while data with bevacizumab with respect to response rates and resection rates are less conclusive. Additionally, some concerns remain regarding wound healing complications after pretreatment with bevacizumab.

EGFR-Targeted Therapy

Deregulation of EGFR tyrosine kinase activity has been identified in many different human tumors including colorectal carcinoma (CRC), head and neck squamous cell carcinoma, and non-small cell lung cancer [1]. Overexpression of EGFR, or increased tyrosine kinase activity arising from mutations that cause its constitutive activation, or over-expression of EGFR natural ligands (epidermal growth factor or transforming growth factor alpha), can lead to cell proliferation, increased motility, and protection against apoptosis, while inhibition of the

EGFR pathway induces apoptosis and cell-cycle arrest and inhibits angiogenesis, tumor cell invasion, and metastasis [2]. Preclinical studies showed that cetuximab reduced EGFR-dependent tumor cell proliferation in colon cancer tumor models [3, 4] and found that the addition of cetuximab to several chemotherapeutic agents demonstrated significant synergistic effect [5, 6, 7].

EGFR Antibodies in Pretreated Patients with Metastatic Colorectal Cancer

Currently, most data available was obtained with the use of cetuximab (Erbitux®) a chimeric IgG1 antibody. A second antibody, panitumumab (Vectibix®, a human IgG2 antibody), was recently approved as a monotherapy for previously treated patients with colorectal cancer. Other EGFR antibodies are currently in clinical testing.

Cetuximab is active against metastatic colorectal cancer after failure of irinotecan-based therapy. In irinotecan pretreated patients, cetuximab given as a single agent has yielded response rates of around 10% [8, 9] and was shown to improve overall survival in comparison to best supportive care [10]. However, the combination cetuximab/irinotecan is more active in the same patient population, with an increase in response rate (23% vs. 10%) and progression-free survival (4.5 months vs. 1.5 months) when compared to monotherapy with cetuximab [8]. The combination of cetuximab plus irinotecan is therefore preferred when using cetuximab in pretreated patients.

In patients pretreated with oxaliplatin/5-FU (FOLFOX), the combination of cetuximab and irinotecan is more active than irinotecan given as a monotherapy [15]. The combination induced more frequent tumor responses, and a longer progression-free survival, but without a substantial effect on overall survival, probably due to the fact that every second patient in the control group received cetuximab after progressing with irinotecan.

G. Folprecht (✉)
Medical Department I, University Hospital Carl Gustav Carus, Dresden, Germany

J.-N. Vauthey et al. (eds.), *Liver Metastases*, DOI 10.1007/978-1-84628-947-7_9,
© Springer-Verlag London Limited 2009

Panitumumab was initially investigated in pretreated patients. A randomized comparison to best supportive care demonstrated response rates of 10% and a superior progression-free survival (Table 9.1) [11–17]. However, in that study, patients on the best supportive care arm were allowed to receive panitumumab after disease progression, and it is possible that, for that reason, the study failed to demonstrate a difference in overall survival between the two study arms [16]. Mature data on combination therapy with panitumumab are still lacking.

Toxicity of EGFR Antibodies

The typical toxicity of EGFR antibodies is an acne-like rash which occurs in most patients in any grade (80%) and is severe in 8% of patients [8]. Occurrence and intensity of the rash are associated with efficacy and overall survival [18]. In irinotecan refractory patients, the response rate is 55% in patients with severe skin toxicity, but only 6% in patients without any skin toxicity [8]. Dose escalation of cetuximab in patients without or with only mild skin toxicity was investigated and showed promising results with regard to tumor response, but should still be regarded as experimental [19]. With longer treatment duration, dry skin, paronychia, and hair changes may occur with anti-EGFR treatment. In addition to skin toxicity, infusional reactions, hypomagnesemia, and—in combination with chemotherapy—slightly increased rates of diarrhea are common findings with EGFR antibodies.

Data on perioperative morbidity of patients pretreated with cetuximab are rare.

Preclinical Markers for Efficacy

The initial trials with cetuximab in colorectal cancer had been restricted to patients with tumors that had a positive EGFR immunohistochemistry. However, it is now quite clear that EGFR staining intensity, or the proportion of EGFR "positive" cells is not predictive for efficacy [8, 17].

Important is the absence of k-ras mutations. Mutations of the EGFR receptor downstream effector molecule k-ras result in a constitutional activation of the ras-pathway and occur in ca 40% of the patients [17, 56, 57]. In a trial comparing panitumumab with best supportive care, panitumumab was ineffective if k-ras mutation existed in the tumor. By contrast, panitumumab monotherapy induced responses in 17% of patients without k-ras mutations; the progression-free survival was 12.3 weeks versus 7.3 weeks (hazard ratio 0.45, $p < 0.0001$) [17]. These data are in accordance to a number of studies describing the lacking efficacy of EGFR antibodies in pretreated patients with k-ras mutant tumors [20, 21, 22, 23], and were confirmed in patients with first-line therapy (Table 9.1) [56].

Further predictive markers for response to anti-EGFR treatment are EGFR amplification/gene copy number [23, 24], and the levels of EGFR ligands [22], but these markers require still more confirmatory investigations and cannot be recommended for routine use.

EGFR Antibodies in Untreated Patients

In first-line treatment, several phase II studies demonstrated high response rates (>65%) when cetuximab was combined with standard chemotherapy, with high observed resection rates, although all trials were planned for treatment of metastatic colorectal cancer patients and did not have a neoadjuvant focus [25, 26]. The improvement in response rates was confirmed in the CRYSTAL trial, a randomized phase III study [11], and in other randomized studies [12, 13] (see Table 9.1). The benefit of adding an EGFR antibody was limited to patients without k-ras mutations. In these patients with k-ras wild type, the response rates were increased from 37%–43% to 59%–61% [56, 57].

Interestingly, the effect of cetuximab on efficacy was more pronounced in patients with isolated liver metastases; in combination with FOLFOX, the response rates were 54% with cetuximab/FOLFOX and 36% with chemotherapy alone (data for patients not selected for k-ras wild-type). For the comparison FOLFIRI/cetuximab versus FOLFIRI, response rates increased from 50% to 77% in patients with k-ras wildtype and liver metastases only [56]. In both studies, higher rates of curative liver resection were found with the cetuximab-containing treatment (see Table 9.1) [11, 12].

Based on the available data, cetuximab-containing combination therapy is one of the most active regimens for downsizing metastases in patients without k-ras mutations.

EGFR Tyrosine Kinase Inhibitors in Metastatic Colorectal Cancer

In contrast to EGFR antibodies, a benefit for the use of EGFR tyrosine kinase inhibitors in metastatic colorectal cancer has not been proven so far.

EGFR tyrosine kinase inhibitors such as erlotinib (Tarceva[R]) and gefitinib (Iressa[R]) bind to the intracellularly located tyrosine kinase. However, in contrast to non-small cell lung cancer, the efficacy of these drugs as single agents in metastatic colorectal cancer is limited and resulted in objective response rate of ≤4% [27, 28, 29]. Although a limited number of phase II studies of the combination of gefitinib/FOLFOX have reported encouraging results with response rates of 74–77% as first-line therapy [30, 31] and 33% in pretreated patients [32], other trials have been less successful. Several studies have failed to achieve full doses of chemotherapy in combination with the recommended doses of the tyrosine kinase inhibitors, have shown an unfavorable safety

Table 9.1 Randomized trials with EGFR antibodies

Schedule	N	Response rate	PFS/TTP	Overall survival	Liver resections
First-line therapy					
CRYSTAL [11]					
Cetuximab + FOLFIRI	602	46.9%**	8.9 mo*	19.9 mo	4.3%**
FOLFIRI	600	38.7%	8.0 mo	18.6 mo	1.5%
			HR 0.85 (95% CI 0.73–0.99)		
Subgroup: k-ras wild-type [56]§					
Cetuximab + FOLFIRI	172	59.3%**	9.9 mo*	24.9 mo	
FOLFIRI	176	43.2%	8.7 mo	21.0 mo	
			HR 0.68		
OPUS [12]					
Cetuximab + FOLFOX	169	45.6%	7.2 mo		4.7%
FOLFOX	168	35.7%	7.2 mo		2.4%
Subgroup: k-ras wild-type [57]§					
Cetuximab + FOLFOX	61	60.7%*	7.7 mo*		
FOLFOX	73	37.0%	7.2 mo		
			HR 0.57		
CALGB-80203 [13]					
Cetuximab + Chemotherapy+	108	52%*	8.5 mo		
Chemotherapy+	116	38%	9.4 mo		
SAKK [14]					
Cetuximab + CapOx	37	46%*			
CapOx	37	36%			
Pretreated patients					
BOND [8]					
Pretreatment with irinotecan-containing schedule					
Cetuximab + irinotecan	218	22.9%**	4.1 mo***	8.6 mo	
Cetuximab	111	10.8%	1.5 mo	6.9 mo	
			HR 0.54 (0.42–0.71)	HR 0.91 (0.68–1.21)	
EPIC [15]					
Second line treatment following FOLFOX					
Cetuximab + irinotecan	648	16.4%***	4.0 mo***	10.7 mo	
Irinotecan	650	4.2%	2.6 mo	10.0 mo	
			HR 0.69 (0.62–0.78)	HR 0.98 (0.85–1.11)†	
NCIC CTG C0.17 [10]					
Pretreatment with irinotecan, oxaliplatin, and 5-FU§					
Cetuximab + BSC	287	6.6%***	1.9 mo**	6.1 mo**	
Best supportive care	285	0%	1.8 mo	4.6 mo	
			HR 0.68 (0.58–0.80)	HR 0.77 (0.64–0.92)	

Table 9.1 (continued)

Schedule	N	Response rate	PFS/TTP	Overall survival	Liver resections
Pretreatment with irinotecan, oxaliplatin, and 5-FU [16]					
Panitumumab + BSC	231	10%***	HR 0.54 (0.44–0.66)***	HR 1.0 (0.82–1.22)†	
Best supportive care	232	0%			
Subgroup: k-ras wild-type [17]§					
Panitumumab + BSC	124	17%	12.3 weeks	8.1 mo	
Best supportive care	119	0%	7.3 weeks	7.6 mo	
			HR 0.45 (95%CI 0.34–0.59)	HR 0.99 (0.75–1.29)†	

All trials were performed in a population not selected for the k-ras mutation status.
+ FOLFOX or FOLFIRI.
$ Are not suitable for treatment with irinotecan, oxaliplatin, and 5-FU.
† Cross-over was allowed for patients randomized in the arm without EGFR antibody.
§ k-ras status was not known for all patients in the trial.
*$p<0.05$.
**$p<0.01$.
***$p<0.001$.

profile, and/or—more importantly—have not suggested higher efficacy results than those obtained with chemotherapy alone [33, 34, 35, 36, 37, 38, 39, 40, 41, 42, 43, 44]. Therefore, the value of the available EGFR tyrosine kinase inhibitors is rather questionable as a therapy for metastatic colorectal cancer.

Anti-Angiogenetic Therapy

Formation of new blood vessels is essential for tumor growth, invasion, and metastasis. While tumors < 1 mm³ can be supplied with oxygen and nutrients by diffusion, new blood vessels are necessary for tumors growing beyond that size. Among other factors, the VEGF and its receptors play an important role in the regulation of that complex process. Besides the mitotic effect, VEGF increases the vascular permeability. Preclinical models showed that inhibition of the VEGF pathway normalized the vessel architecture and decreased the interstitial pressure which may lead to an improved supply with oxygen (and drugs) during the early treatment course [45, 46].

VEGF Antibody

Bevacizumab (Avastin®) is a humanized antibody to VEGF and has been demonstrated to improve the progression-free survival in various combinations [47, 48, 49]. In combination with the irinotecan/5-FU bolus/FA

regimen IFL, overall survival was improved when bevacizumab was added (Table 9.2) [49, 50, 51]. Based on these results, bevacizumab-containing schedules became widely used in most parts of the world, as one of the standard regimens for palliative treatment of metastatic colorectal cancer. In contrast to the increased efficacy regarding progression-free survival, the influence of bevacizumab on response rates was less consistent. In a large randomized trial comparing oxaliplatin-based chemotherapy with or without bevacizumab in first-line treatment of metastatic colorectal cancer, a difference in response rate was not observed, resulting in a similar rate of liver resections in both study arms (see Table 9.2) [50].

Hypertension, proteinuria, arterial thromboembolic events, and gastrointestinal perforations are more frequently observed when bevacizumab is added to chemotherapy. More important for perioperative treatment are observations of wound healing complications with bevacizumab. Scappaticci et al analyzed the registration trials with bevacizumab and found that the rate of wound healing complications was not increased if bevacizumab is administered postoperatively (1.3% vs. 0.5% with bevacizumab of placebo, respectively). However, if an emergency surgery was performed during bevacizumab-containing treatment, the complication rate was 13% (10/75 pts.) compared to 3.4% (1/29 pts.) [52]. Although some series reported no increased perioperative morbidity with preoperative bevacizumab [53, 54, 58], increased complication rates are not completely excluded. Kesmodel and coworkers analyzed 125 patients with preoperative treatment and liver surgery and found 23 complications in 44 patients without bevacizumab pretreatment, but

Table 9.2 Randomized trials with bevacizumab

Schedule	N	Response rate	PFS/TTP	Overall survival	Liver resections
First-line therapy					
AVF2107 [47]					
Bevacizumab + IFL[‡]	402	44.8 %**	10.6 mo***	20.3 mo***	<2%
IFL[‡]	411	34.8%	6.2 mo	15.6 mo	
			HR 0.54	HR 0.66	
N016966 [49,50]					
Bevacizumab + chemotherapy[+]	699	47%	9.4 mo**	21.3 mo	8.4%
Chemotherapy[+]	701	49%	8.0 mo	19.9 mo	6.1%
			HR 0.83	HR 0.89	
			(95% CI 0.72–0.95)	(95% CI 0.76–1.03)	
[48]					
Bevacizumab + 5-FU/FA	108	26%	9.2 mo***	16.6 mo	
5-FU/FA	116	15%	5.5 mo	12.9 mo	
			HR 0.50	HR 0.79	
			(95% CI 0.34–0.73)	(95% CI 0.56–1.10)	
Pretreated patients					
E3200 [51]					
Bevacizumab[$] + FOLFOX	286	22.7%***[§]	7.3 mo***[§]	12.9 mo*[§]	
FOLFOX	291	8.6%	4.7	10.8	
Bevacizumab[$]	243	3.3%	2.7	10.2	
			HR 0.61	HR 0.75	

[‡] IFL: irinotecan/5-FU (bolus)/folinic acid.
[+] Chemotherapy: FOLFOX or capecitabine/oxaliplatin.
[$] Bevacizumab 10 mg/kg.
[§] Comparing Bev./FOLFOX to FOLFOX.
* $p<0.05$.
** $p<0.01$.
*** $p<0.001$.

58 complications in 81 with neoadjuvant treatment with bevacizumab [55]. Further investigations are necessary to exclude an increased risk with neoadjuvant bevacizumab treatment.

If bevacizumab is used for neoadjuvant therapy, it is currently recommended that this antibody is stopped at least 6 weeks prior to any elective surgery and that it is not to be restarted before 4 weeks after the Procedure.

VEGFR and Multiple Tyrosine Kinase Inhibitors

Vatalanib (PTK 787/ZK 222584), an oral tyrosine kinase inhibitor of vascular endothelial growth factor receptor (VEGFR), Platelet-derived growth factor receptor (PDGFR), and c-Kit, was investigated in combination with FOLFOX in first- and second-line treatments of metastatic colorectal cancer. Both studies failed to demonstrate a meaningful improvement in efficacy for the entire patient population. Although there was an interesting improvement for progression-free survival in patients with high lactate dehydrogenase (LDH), development of the drug is in question at this time.

Further compounds directed against angiogenesis, such as VEGF trap and tyrosine kinase inhibitors (i.e. sunitinib and sorafenib) are in clinical testing.

References

1. Nicholson RI, Gee JM, Harper ME. EGFR and cancer prognosis. Eur J Cancer. 2001; 37(Suppl 4): S9–15.
2. Mendelsohn J, Baselga J. Status of epidermal growth factor receptor antagonists in the biology and treatment of cancer. J Clin Oncol. 2003, 21(14), 2787–2799.
3. Feng RL, Wild R, Dong H, et al. Pharmacokinetics and pharmacodynamics of ERBITUX (cetuximab), an anti-epidermal growth factor receptor antibody, in nude mice bearing the GEO human colon carcinoma xenograft. Proc Am Assoc Cancer Res. 2003; 44: 173.
4. Ciardiello F, Bianco R, Damiano V, et al. Antiangiogenic and antitumor activity of anti-epidermal growth factor receptor C225 monoclonal antibody in combination with vascular endothelial growth factor antisense oligonucleotide in human GEO colon cancer cells. Clin Cancer Res. 2000; 6(9): 3739–3747.
5. Prewett M, Hooper AT, Bassi R, et al. Growth inhibition of human colorectal carcinoma xenografts by anti-EGF receptor monoclonal antibody IMC-C225 in combination with 5-fluorouracil or irinotecan. Proc Am Assoc Cancer Res. 2001; 42: 287.

6. Prewett MC, Hooper AT, Bassi R, et al. Enhanced antitumor activity of anti-epidermal growth factor receptor monoclonal antibody IMC-C225 in combination with irinotecan (CPT-11) against human colorectal tumor xenografts. Clin Cancer Res. 2002; 8(5): 994–1003.

7. Prewett M, Hooper AT, Bassi R, et al. Enhanced antitumor activity of anti-epidermal growth factor receptor monoclonal antibody cetuximab (IMC-C225) in combination with irinotecan (CPT-11), 5-FU, and leucovorin against human colorectal carcinoma xenografts. Eur J Cancer. 2002; 38(S7): abstr 501.

8. Cunningham D, Humblet Y, Siena S, et al. Cetuximab monotherapy and cetuximab plus irinotecan in irinotecan-refractory metastatic colorectal cancer. N Engl J Med. 2004; 351(4): 337–345.

9. Saltz LB, Meropol NJ, Loehrer PJ Sr, et al. Phase II trial of cetuximab in patients with refractory colorectal cancer that expresses the epidermal growth factor receptor. J Clin Oncol. 2004; 22(7): 1201–1208.

10. Jonker D, Karatis CS, Moore M, et al. Randomized phase III trial of cetuximab monotherapy plus best supportive care (BSC) versus BSC alone in patients with pretreated metastatic epidermal growth factor receptor (EGFR)-positive colorectal carcinoma: a trial of the National Cancer Institute of Canada Clinical Trials Group (NCIC CTG) and the Australasian Gastro-Intestinal Trials Group (AGITG). Program and abstracts of the American Association for Cancer Research Annual Meeting, April 14–18, 2007; Los Angeles, California.

11. Van Cutsem E, Nowacki MP, Lang I, et al. Randomized phase III study of irinotecan and 5-FU/FA with or without cetuximab in the first-line treatment of patients with metastatic colorectal cancer (mCRC): the CRYSTAL trial. J Clin Oncol. 2007; 25(18S): 4000.

12. Bokemeyer C, Staroslawska E, Makhson A, et al. Cetuximab plus 5-FU/FA/oxaliplatin (FOLFOX-4) versus FOLFOX-4 in the first-line treatment of metastatic colorectal cancer (mCRC): OPUS, a randomized phase II study. Eur J Cancer. 2007; Supplements 5(4): 236 (abstract 3004).

13. Venook A, Niedzwiecki D, Hollis D, et al. Phase III study of irinotecan/5FU/LV (FOLFIRI) or oxaliplatin/5FU/LV (FOL-FOX) {+/−} cetuximab for patients (pts) with untreated metastatic adenocarcinoma of the colon or rectum (MCRC): CALGB 80203 preliminary results. ASCO Meeting Abstracts. 2006;24 (18 suppl): 3509.

14. Borner M, Mingrone W, Koeberle D, et al. The impact of cetuximab on the capecitabine plus oxaliplatin (XELOX) combination in first-line treatment of metastatic colorectal cancer (MCC): A randomized phase II trial of the Swiss Group for Clinical Cancer Research (SAKK). ASCO Meeting Abstracts. 2006; 24(18 suppl): 3551.

15. Sobrero A, Fehrenbacher L, Rivera F, et al. Randomized phase III trial of cetuximab plus irinotecan versus irinotecan alone for metastatic colorectal cancer in 1298 patients who have failed prior oxaliplatin-based therapy: the EPIC Trial. Proc Am Ass Can Res. 2007; abstract LB2.

16. Van Cutsem E, Peeters M, Siena S, et al. Open-label phase III trial of panitumumab plus best supportive care compared with best supportive care alone in patients with chemotherapy-refractory metastatic colorectal cancer. J Clin Oncol. 2007; 25(13): 1658–1664.

17. Amado RG, Wolf M, Peeters M, et al. Wild-type kras is required for panitumumab efficacy in patients with metastatic colorectal cancer. J Clin Oncol. 2008; 26(10): 1026–1034.

18. Lacouture ME. Mechanisms of cutaneous toxicities to EGFR inhibitors. Nat Rev Cancer. 2006; 6(10): 803–812.

19. Van Cutsem E, Humblet Y, Gelderblom H, et al. Cetuximab dose-escalation study in patients with metastatic colorectal cancer (mcrc) with no or slight skin reactions on cetuximab standard dose treatment (everest): preliminary pk and efficacy data of a randomized study. Ann Oncol. 2006; 17(S9): LBA4.

20. Benvenuti S, Sartore-Bianchi A, Di, Nicolantonio F, et al. Oncogenic activation of the RAS/RAF signaling pathway impairs the response of metastatic colorectal cancers to anti-epidermal growth factor receptor antibody therapies. Cancer Res. 2007; 67(6): 2643–2648.

21. Di Fiore F, Blanchard F, Charbonnier F, et al. Clinical relevance of KRAS mutation detection in metastatic colorectal cancer treated by Cetuximab plus chemotherapy. Br J Cancer. 2007; 96(8): 1166–1169.

22. Khambata-Ford S, Garrett CR, Meropol NJ, et al. Expression of epiregulin and amphiregulin and K-ras mutation status predict disease control in metastatic colorectal cancer patients treated with cetuximab. J Clin Oncol. 2007; 25(22): 3230–3237.

23. Finocchiaro G, Cappuzzo F, Janne PA, et al. EGFR, HER2 and Kras as predictive factors for cetuximab sensitivity in colorectal cancer. ASCO Meeting Abstracts. 2007; 25(18_suppl): 4021.

24. Moroni M, Veronese S, Benvenuti S, et al. Gene copy number for epidermal growth factor receptor (EGFR) and clinical response to antiEGFR treatment in colorectal cancer: a cohort study. Lancet Oncol. 2005; 6(5): 279–286.

25. Folprecht G, Lutz M, Schöffski P, et al. Cetuximab and irinotecan/5-fluorouracil/folinic acid is a safe combination for the first-line treatment of patients with epidermal growth factor receptor expressing metastatic colorectal carcinoma. Ann Oncol. 2006; 17(2): 450–456.

26. Diaz-Rubio E, Tabernero J, Van Cutsem E, et al. Cetuximab in combination with oxaliplatin/5-fluorouracil (5-FU)/folinic acid (FA) (FOLFOX-4) in the first-line treatment of patients with epidermal growth factor receptor (EGFR)-expressing metastatic colorectal cancer: an international phase II study. Proc Amer Soc Clin Oncol. 2005; 24: abstract 3535.

27. Rothenberg ML, LaFleur B, Levy DE, et al. Randomized phase II trial of the clinical and biological effects of two dose levels of gefitinib in patients with recurrent colorectal adenocarcinoma. J Clin Oncol. 2005; 23(36): 9265–9274.

28. Mackenzie MJ, Hirte HW, Glenwood G, et al. A phase II trial of ZD1839 (Iressa) 750 mg per day, an oral epidermal growth factor receptor-tyrosine kinase inhibitor, in patients with metastatic colorectal cancer. Invest New Drugs. 2005; 23(2): 165–170.

29. Keilholz U, Arnold D, Niederle N, et al. Erlotinib as 2nd and 3rd line monotherapy in patients with metastatic colorectal cancer. Results of a multicenter two-cohort phase II trial. J Clin Oncol. 2005; 23(16s): 3575.

30. Fisher GA, Kuo T, Cho CD, et al. A phase II study of gefitinib in combination with FOLFOX-4 (IFOX) in patients with metastatic colorectal cancer. J Clin Oncol. 2004; 22(14s): 3514.

31. Zampino MG, Magni E, Massacesi C, et al. First clinical experience of orally active epidermal growth factor receptor inhibitor combined with simplified FOLFOX6 as first-line treatment for metastatic colorectal cancer. Cancer. 2007; 110(4): 752–758.

32. Kuo T, Cho CD, Halsey J, et al. Phase II study of gefitinib, fluorouracil, leucovorin, and oxaliplatin therapy in previously treated patients with metastatic colorectal cancer. J Clin Oncol. 2005; 23(24): 5613–5619.

33. Hartmann JT, Kroening H, Bokemeyer C, et al. Phase I study of gefitinib in combination with oxaliplatin and weekly 5-FU/FA (FUFOX) for second-/third-line treatment in patients (pts) with

metastatic colorectal cancer (CRC). J Clin Oncol. 2005; 23(16 s): 3154.

34. Delord JP, Beale P, Van Cutsem E, et al. A phase 1b dose-escalation trial of erlotinib, capecitabine and oxaliplatin in metastatic colorectal cancer (MCRC) patients. J Clin Oncol. 2004; 22(14 s): abstract 3585.

35. Spigel DR, Hainsworth J, Burris HA, et al. Phase II study of FOLFOX4, bevacizumab, and erlotinib as first-line therapy in patients with advanced colorectal cancer. Proc Gastrointest Canc Symp (ASCO/AGA/ASTRO/SSO). 2006; abstract 238.

36. Messersmith WA, Laheru DA, Senzer NN, et al. Phase I trial of irinotecan, infusional 5-fluorouracil, and leucovorin (FOLFIRI) with erlotinib (OSI-774): early termination due to increased toxicities. Clin Cancer Res. 2004; 10(19): 6522–6527.

37. Hochhaus A, Hofheinz R, Heike M, et al. Gefitinib in combination with 5-fluorouracil (5-FU)/folinic acid and irinotecan in patients with 5-FU/oxaliplatin – refractory colorectal cancer: a phase I/II study of the Arbeitsgemeinschaft für Internistische Onkologie (AIO). Onkologie. 2006; 29(12): 563–567.

38. Redlinger M, Kramer A, Flaherty K, et al. J. A phase II trial of gefitinib in combination with 5-FU/LV/irinotecan in patients with colorectal cancer. J Clin Oncol. 2004; 22(14s): 3767.

39. Arnold D, Constantin C, Seufferlein T, et al. Phase I study of gefitinib in combination with capecitabine and irinotecan for 2nd- and/or 3rd-line treatment in patients with metastatic colorectal cancer. J Clin Oncol. 2005; 23(16s): 3691.

40. Meyerhardt JA, Stuart K, Fuchs C, et al. Phase II study of FOLFOX, bevacizumab and erlotinib as first-line therapy for patients with metastastic colorectal cancer. Ann Oncol. 2007; 18(7): 1185–1189.

41. Meyerhardt JA, Zhu AX, Enzinger PC, et al. Phase II study of capecitabine, oxaliplatin, and erlotinib in previously treated patients with metastastic colorectal cancer. J Clin Oncol. 2006; 24(12): 1892–1897.

42. Veronese ML, Sun W, Giantonio B, et al. A phase II trial of gefitinib with 5-fluorouracil, leucovorin, and irinotecan in patients with colorectal cancer. Br J Cancer. 2005; 92(10): 1846–1849.

43. Tejpar S, Van Cutsem E, Gamelin E, et al. Phase 1/2a study of EKB-569, an irreversible inhibitor of epidermal growth factor receptor, in combination with 5-fluorouracil, leucovorin, and oxaliplatin (FOLFOX-4) in patients with advanced colorectal cancer (CRC). J Clin Oncol. 2004; 22(14S): abstract 3579.

44. Folprecht G, Tabernero J, Köhne CH, et al. Phase I pharmacokinetic/pharmacodynamic study of EKB-569—an irreversible inhibitor of the epidermal growth factor receptor (EGFR) tyrosine kinase—in combination with irinotecan, 5-fluorouracil and leucovorin (FOLFIRI) in first-line treatment of patients with metastatic colorectal cancer. Clin Cancer Res. 2008; 14(1): 215–223.

45. Hicklin DJ, Ellis LM. Role of the vascular endothelial growth factor pathway in tumor growth and angiogenesis. J Clin Oncol. 2005; 23(5): 1011–1027.

46. Jain RK, Normalization of tumor vasculature: an emerging concept in antiangiogenic therapy. Science. 2005; 307(5706): 58–62.

47. Hurwitz H, Fehrenbacher L, Novotny W, et al. Bevacizumab plus irinotecan, fluorouracil, and leucovorin for metastatic colorectal cancer. N Engl J Med. 2004; 350(23): 2335–2342.

48. Kabbinavar FF, Schulz J, McCleod M, et al. Addition of bevacizumab to bolus fluorouracil and leucovorin in first-line metastatic colorectal cancer: results of a randomized phase II trial. J Clin Oncol. 2005; 23(16): 3697–3705.

49. Cassidy J, Clarke S, Diaz-Rubio E, et al. First efficacy and safety results from XELOX-1/N016966, a randomised 2×2 factorial phase III trial of XELOX vs.FOLFOX4 / bevacizumab or placebo in first-line metastatic colorectal cancer (MCRC). Ann Oncol. 2006; 17(S9): LBA3.

50. Saltz LB, Clarke S, Diaz-Rubio E, et al. Bevacizumab (Bev) in combination with XELOX or FOLFOX4: efficacy results from XELOX-1/N016866, a randomized phase III trial in the first-line treatment of metastatic colorectal cancer (MCRC). Proc Gastrointest Canc Symp (ASCO/AGA/ASTRO/SSO). 2007; abstract 238.

51. Giantonio BJ, Catalano PJ, Meropol NJ, et al. Bevacizumab in combination with oxaliplatin, fluorouracil, and leucovorin (FOLFOX4) for previously treated metastatic colorectal cancer: results from the Eastern Cooperative Oncology Group Study E3200. J Clin Oncol. 2007; 25(12): 1539–1544.

52. Scappaticci FA, Fehrenbacher L, Cartwright T, et al. Surgical wound healing complications in metastatic colorectal cancer patients treated with bevacizumab. J Surg Oncol. 2005; 91(3): 173–180.

53. D'Angelica M, Kornprat P. Gonen M, et al. Lack of evidence for increased operative morbidity after hepatectomy with perioperative use of bevacizumab: a matched case-control study. Ann Surg Oncol. 2007; 14(2): 759–765.

54. Gruenberger T, Gruenberger B, Scheithauer W. Neoadjuvant therapy with bevacizumab. J Clin Oncol. 2006; 24(16): 2592–2593.

55. Kesmodel SB, Ellis LM, Lin E, et al. Complication rates following hepatic surgery in patients receiving neoadjuvant bevacizumab (BV) for colorectal cancer (CRC) liver metastases. Proc Gastrointest Canc Symp (ASCO/AGA/ASTRO/SSO). 2007; abstract 234.

56. Van Cutsem E, Lang I, D'Haens et al. KRAS status and efficacy in the CRYSTAL study: 1st-line treatment of patients with metastatic colorectal cancer (mCRC) receiving with FOLFIRI with or without cetuximab. Ann oncol. 2008; 19(S19): abstract 71.

57. Bokemeyer C, Bondarenko I, Hartmann J et al. KRAS status and efficacy of first-line treatment of patients with metastatic colorectal cancer (mCRC) with FOLFOX with or without cetuximab: The OPUS experience, J Clin Oncol. 2008; 26(15S): abstract 4000.

58. Reddy SK, Morse MA, Hurwitz HI et al. Addition of bevacizumab to irinotecan- and oxaliplatin-based preoperative chemotherapy regimens does not increase morbidity after resection of colorectal liver metastases. J Am Coll Surg. 2008; 206(1): 96–106.

Internal Radiation for the Treatment of Liver Metastases

10

Douglas M. Coldwell and Andrew S. Kennedy

Introduction

Tumors in the liver are commonly treated by either a local method, i.e., one tumor at a time, or a regional method, i.e., a lobe of the liver or the entire liver as the treatment field. Local ablative therapies include radiofrequency ablation (RFA) and laser-induced interstitial thermotherapy (LITT). RFA uses "ionic agitation" which is produced when electric current is applied in the tissue within the tumor. Depending on the charge, the current moves ions either toward or away from the RFA probe in the tumor, creating heating up to $100\,^{\circ}$C due to inter-atomic friction [1]. LITT also uses heat to cause coagulation necrosis with the energy generated from a neodymium:yttrium-aluminum-garnet (Nd:YAG) laser [2, 3]. Lesions treated with these local therapies are localized with computed tomography (CT) [3] or magnetic resonance imaging (MRI), [2] and may be monitored for completeness of ablation with MRI [2]. At 6 months post-treatment with a total of 640 patients from 2 reported series, selected liver metastases fitting established number, size, and distribution criteria reached local tumor control of over 90% [2, 3]. Yet another variation of heat-induced cytocide, reported with impressive results from one institution, is to combine the known synergy of heat with ionizing radiation via brachytherapy and LITT. Still, despite these efforts, many patients will die of liver disease and additional approaches are needed.

Radiotherapy is effective in destroying tumors, typically with combined chemotherapy – usually 5-fluorouracil (5-FU) – at doses above 50 Gy. Using traditional permanent interstitial seed brachytherapy, ^{125}I has been successful in controlling selected colorectal liver metastases [4], and high-dose afterloading of ^{192}Ir with ultrasound or CT guidance [3, 5]. Because of significant technologic advances in radiation treatment planning and delivery, there has been renewed interest in using external beam radiotherapy. This offers the promise that three-dimensional radiotherapy [2, 6, 7, 8, 9, 10, 11, 12], intensity-modulated radiotherapy [13], and stereotactic radiotherapy [14, 15, 16, 17, 18, 19] may benefit an increasing number of patients with liver metastases. The key limitation in this treatment is the tolerance of normal liver parenchyma to radiation; the maximum acceptable dose to the whole liver of 35 Gy is far below that which is required to destroy adenocarcinoma metastases, estimated at ≥ 70 Gy.

The conundrum ensues that one must apply a much higher dose for tumoricidal effect than is tolerated by the normal hepatic parenchyma. This problem can be addressed by the use of an alternate approach by implantation of radiation sources into the tumor, i.e., brachytherapy. ^{90}Y-microspheres combines brachytherapy with the unique blood supply of the liver. Since the portal vein supplies normal parenchyma and the hepatic artery supplies tumor, selective delivery of chemotherapeutic agents and embolic agents has long been performed. However, the ability to deliver radiation selectively to numerous tumor deposits and to spare the normal parenchyma is only now being realized. Only in the past 6 years have US investigators had sustained access to radioactive microspheres, although there is an extensive history of their use in Asia, particularly in Australia [20, 21, 22, 23]. In August 2000, using glass microspheres, the gastrointestinal (GI) oncology team at the University of Maryland School of Medicine was the first to reintroduce this procedure in the United States [24, 25, 26, 27]. Important phase I clinical data had previously been developed by Andrews [28] in 1994, shortly thereafter it was unavailable in the United States, although the product continued to be used in Canada for hepatocellular carcinoma [29]. When a second microsphere product (resin based spheres) became available in the United States in March 2002, they were utilized in a manner similar to that of glass microspheres [30, 31, 32] (see Fig. 10.1).

D.M. Coldwell (✉)
Interventional Radiologist, Department of Radiology, Jane Phillips Medical Center, Bartlesville, OK, USA

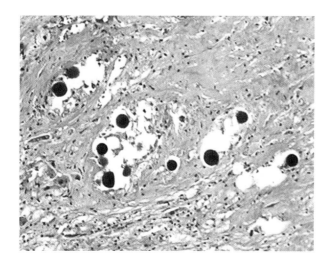

Fig. 10.1 H&E stained slide of ^{90}Y-microspheres in the liver of a patient who received treatment for chemo-insensitive metastatic colon cancer. The microspheres (*dark spheres*) are composed of resin material and take up the tissue stain. Original magnification 100×

Radioactive Material

Yttrium-90 (^{90}Y) is a pure beta emitter, which decays to stable zirconium-90 with an average energy of 0.94 MeV via a half-life of 2.67 days (64.2 hours). It is produced by neutron bombardment of ^{89}Y in a commercial reactor, yielding ^{90}Y beta radiation with a tissue penetration of 2.5 mm, and a maximum range of 1.1 cm. One GBq (27 mCi) of ^{90}Y delivers a total dose of 50 Gy/Kg in tissue. Commercially available radioactive microspheres in North America include a glass (TheraSphere$^{®}$—MDS Nordion, Inc., Ontario, Canada) and a resin (SIR-Spheres$^{®}$—SIR-Tex Medical Limited, Sydney, Australia) product using ^{90}Y that is permanently embedded within the glass or resin structure. Each glass sphere has a diameter of 25 ± 10 μm, and each resin sphere of 32 + 10 μm, causing them to be permanently embolized in terminal arterioles, i.e., within the tumor. No significant amount of ^{90}Y leaches in the patient from the resin spheres, and none escapes the glass spheres. A standard dose of 5 GBq glass microspheres contains approximately 4 million spheres; these numbers increase if the average sphere size is smaller than 25 μm and decrease as the average sphere size approaches 35 μm. A standard dose of resin microspheres is 2 GBq containing approximately 50 million microspheres (range 40–80 million). The difference in dose per microsphere is estimated to be 2500 Bq (glass) versus 50 Bq (resin) [33].

Radiation Treatment Planning

All patients should undergo CT treatment planning with reconstruction of the liver volumes (whole liver, right, and left lobes) (see Fig. 10.2). The required activity for the

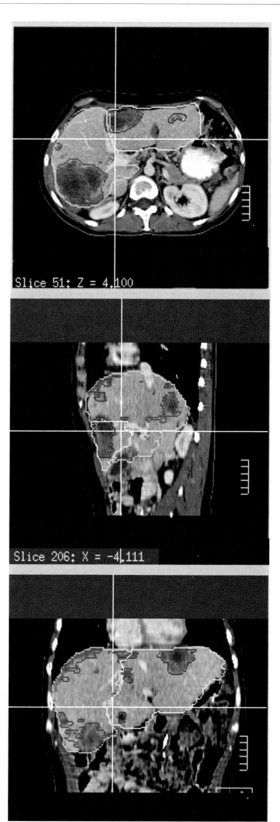

Fig. 10.2 Axial, sagittal, and coronal views of a treatment planning CT scan used to calculate the proper activity of ^{90}Y-microspheres for a delivery. Note the color outlines demarcating right and left lobes, and tumor that is encompassed in each lobe

treatment of each patient is calculated differently based on microsphere type. For glass microspheres a medical internal radiation dose (MIRD) calculation similar to most nuclear medicine therapies is recommended. The target dose is 100–120 Gy but assumes uniform distribution of radiation throughout the liver, which is known not to be true. However, clinical experience with thousands of patients has determined that this approach is safe and effective. Once the treatment plan has been defined, the appropriate volume and mass (whole liver or single lobe) are determined using the CT or MR images, assuming a conversion factor of 1.03 g/cm³.

The amount of radioactivity of glass microspheres required to deliver the dose to the selected liver target (whole liver or single lobe) is calculated using the following formula:

Activity Required (GBq)

$$= \frac{[\text{Desired dose (Gy)}][\text{Mass of selected liver target (kg)}]}{50[1 - F]}$$

Calculation of the liver dose (Gy) delivered after injection is provided by the following formula:

$$\textbf{Dose(Gy)} = \frac{50 \,[\text{Injected activity (GBq)}][1 - F]}{\text{Mass of selected liver target (kg)}}$$

where F is the fraction of injected activity deposited into the lungs as measured by Tc-99 macro-aggregated albumin (MAA). If F is unknown, the value, $F = 0.61$ GBq is used (representing the upper limit of activity that can safely be delivered to the lungs in a single administration) to estimate the fraction of dose that could be deposited into the lungs.

Resin microsphere radioactivity is calculated by either one of three methods as suggested by the manufacturer: body surface area (BSA) method, partition theory, or empiric. The methods were described in the product package insert, and from the equations below:

$$A(\text{GBq})_{\text{resin}} = \frac{[D\text{liver}((T : N \times M\text{tumor}) + M\text{liver})]}{[49,670 \,(1 - L/100)]}$$

D_{liver} = nominal dose (Gy) to the liver
$T{:}N$ = tumor to normal ratio as calculated below
L = shunt fraction (%) of microspheres from liver to lung based on macro-aggregated albumin (MAA) nuclear medicine scan (see below)
M_{liver} = total mass of liver (kg) from CT volume
$T{:}N$ = tumor to normal ratio for an individual patient (Equation 3)
$T{:}N$ ratio = $(A_{\text{tumor}}/M_{\text{tumor}})/(A_{\text{liver}}/M_{\text{liver}})$
A_{tumor} = activity in tumor from MAA scan
A_{liver} = activity in liver from MAA scan

M_{liver} = mass of normal liver (excluding tumor) (kg) from CT scan
M_{tumor} = mass of tumor in liver (excluding normal liver tissue) (kg) from CT scan

Empiric Method

The dose calculated from the empiric method is determined by the amount of tumor present in the liver:

Tumor <25% of the total mass of the liver by CT scan = 2 GBq whole liver delivery
Tumor >25% but <50% of liver mass by CT scan = 2.5 GBq whole liver delivery
Tumor >50% of liver mass by CT scan = 3 GBq for whole liver delivery

The partition method utilizes the equations listed above and determines the dose by utilizing the relative uptake of the MAA in the screening arteriogram versus the uptake in the normal liver.

Experience has shown that the partition method using the activity of the MAA scan to determine the activity is far too complex for most centers to utilize effectively. Additionally, the empiric method, while attractive in its simplicity, generally recommends activity that is too high and that can cause irreversible liver damage. From personal observation, the authors have noted that the only cases of radiation-induced liver disease (RILD) seen were in patients in whom the activity was determined by the empiric method. Consequently, the only method that is utilized routinely in most centers is the BSA method.

This calculation originated in Australia when the resin spheres were developed. It is important to note that the patients in whom this formula was applied were treatment-naïve patients with intact liver function who received a vasoactive agent to further protect the normal liver. These are not the patients that are currently being treated in the United States and Europe. Patients now seen are those in whom significant prior chemotherapy has been given and their liver functions are usually impaired. We feel that even the BSA formula overdoses most of the patients having colon cancer and it is now being routinely discounted by 20% in the face of data demonstrating that the tumors receive up to 30 times the tumoricidal dose of radiation.

Dosimetry is the most difficult aspect of this therapy and there is not a proven objective means to preplan an activity. However, the estimate for preplanned activity is placed in an acceptable range using a combination of tumor and liver volumes, clinical liver function parameters, and clinical experience. The actual activity implanted in each lobe or segment, or in the entire liver, is dependent upon the tumor vasculature capacity. Fortunately, there have been few patients in whom late radiation damage is seen. Current research is focusing on new methods to plan the delivered activity.

Dose Delivery

Each patient is screened and preplanned via CT, hepatic angiogram, and macro-aggregated albumin (^{99m}Tc) with single photon emission computed tomography (SPECT) imaging [24, 25, 29, 30, 34, 35 ,36, 37, 38]. The CT is used for dose planning and identifying tumor distribution by segment for targeting. The hepatic angiogram confirms the capability of microsphere release into the correct hepatic artery branch, and provides an opportunity to embolize arteries if necessary to spare the gastric and duodenal arterial flow from being exposed to radioactive spheres. The MAA SPECT images provide a measure of the amount of activity injected into the liver that may abnormally deposit in the lungs via tumoral arteriovenous (AV) shunts. These AV shunts are too small to be visualized, but the resultant activity identified in the lung can be measured. Each manufacturer recommends a different way to calculate the appropriate amount of ^{90}Y microspheres to deliver. A standard dose of resin microspheres (specific gravity, 1.6 g/mL) is 2 GBq and contains approximately 50 million microspheres. From the discussion above, we see that the activity at the typical time of infusion is 50 Bq/resin sphere. Moreover, for a standard 2 GBq dose of resin spheres at calibration time, 50 million spheres would be infused. If the infusion took place 8 hours prior to the calibration time, only 46.3 million spheres would be used. Similarly, if the infusion took place 16 hours post-calibration time—i.e., the day after receiving them, 59.5 million spheres would be used. A variety of different scenarios occurred in clinical practice. It is critical to the success of the microsphere therapy program to have this dose delivery occur at a particular time. The amount to be administered must be determined in advance and pegged to a particular time, the dose drawn in the nuclear pharmacy and delivered to the interventional radiology suite in a timely manner so that the actual amount delivered is the calculated one, not a decayed and lesser dose.

Laboratory Studies

Pre- and post-treatment laboratory tests include liver function tests (alkaline phosphatase, alanine aminotransferase (ALT), aspartate aminotransferase (AST), and total bilirubin); also electrolytes, complete blood count with differential, prothrombin time (PT), partial thromboplastin time (PTT), international normalized ratio (INR), and tumor markers specific for the tumor being treated. Laboratory tests should be conducted every 2 weeks post-treatment for

6 weeks, then monthly for 3 months to monitor both acute and late toxicities. If toxicity is noted to be grade 3, it should be followed until resolved.

Imaging Studies

All patients are evaluated via chest, abdomen, and pelvic CT or MRI to detect extrahepatic metastases and determine liver tumor location, size, and number. All scans of the abdomen should be three phase, performed with oral and IV contrast, with slice thickness less than or equal to 7 mm through the abdomen. Standard response evaluation criteria in solid tumors (RECIST) should be utilized to determine CT response as:

- Complete response (CR): All lesions from the pre-treatment CT or MRI were not seen on the 12 week follow-up CT/MRI.
- Partial response (PR): A 50% decrease in tumor number or size by one measurement or necrosis of most lesions as determined by water-equivalent Hounsfield unit values in the center of a lesion.
- Stable disease (SD): Less than 50% response of lesions or less than 25% growth in number or size of lesions.
- Progressive disease (PD): Growth of more than 25% in number or size of any lesion without necrosis at the 12-week post-treatment follow-up scan.

However, the RECIST criteria routinely underestimates the response of the tumor when compared with that seen on PET scans. Positron emission tomography (PET) scan response criteria are currently being developed but a decrease in the standard uptake value of the most intense lesion by 25% is judged to be a response. Disappearance of the 2-fluoro-2-deoxy-D-glucose (FDG) uptake is evidence of a complete response in the tumor deposit. A novel development using the functional volume of the tumor, as determined by PET/CT, multiplied by the most intense uptake value is the total glyclolytic index. This is quite sensitive to the application of the microspheres with the value decreasing in response to treatment [39] These values and PET or PET/CT are used to evaluate response at 12 weeks post-treatment, compared to a pre-treatment study performed within 4 weeks prior to the treatment.

Hepatic Angiography

All patients undergo mapping of the superior mesenteric, celiac, and hepatic vasculature via femoral catheter approach. Treatment routes as well as determination of the hepatic volumes supplied by the right or left hepatic arteries are reviewed by the treatment team. This is essential in aiding pre-treatment planning and dosimetry calculations. Typically the angiogram is performed the week before treatment, but on occasion, it can be up to 3 weeks prior to the actual delivery of microsphere therapy. If it is determined during the angiogram that the gastroduodenal or right gastric artery would pose a significant opportunity for microspheres to escape into the GI tract, coil embolization or gel-foam blockade is performed. Tumors may parasitize other arteries, e.g., the subphrenic or lumbars; if so, these should also be embolized with particles to minimize the amount of untreated tumor which is fed from arteries that will not have microspheres injected into them [40, 41].

Nuclear Medicine Studies

All patients are tested for an occult AV shunt from the hepatic arterial system to the pulmonary or GI venous systems via planar and SPECT imaging of 4.0–6.0 mCi ^{99m}Tc MAA. The MAA particles approximate the size of the microspheres but can be imaged and quantified easily via a gamma camera. Each ^{99m}Tc MAA infusion contains 3.6–6.5 million particles, with >85% between 20 μm and 40 μm [42]. Planar and SPECT imaging were performed on all patients to better determine if a shunt is present. The treatment protocol outlines an upper limit of 30 Gy or 16.5 mCi for cumulative total dose to the lungs. A shunt value of 20% of the infused ^{99m}Tc MAA activity on any screening study detected in the lungs would require at least a 20% dose reduction. Alternatively, an incomplete bland particulate embolization can be performed, and then the patient re-evaluated with MAA a week later. This can be difficult to perform since the amount of embolic agent to use is less than the amount to cause complete stasis but only enough to close the AV shunts. Also, to prevent GI toxicity, if any uncorrectable anatomic shunting is detected in the GI tract, the patient would be disqualified from microsphere treatment. Because the shunt fraction estimate is significantly affected by the estimation procedure used, a geometric mean analysis with a liberal hepatic region of interest (ROI) is chosen. The liberal hepatic ROI is obtained by increasing the image intensity to include most of the scatter originating from the liver. All ROI counts are corrected for background obtained from the abdominal region that is well below the liver and avoiding the urinary tract. Regions of interest are drawn around the liver and lungs in both anterior and posterior whole body planar images, and the shunt calculated using:

$$\text{Shunt fraction} = \frac{\text{ROI lung counts}}{\text{ROI lung counts} + \text{ROI liver counts}}$$

SPECT imaging is performed to better determine if a GI shunt is present and to provide three-dimensional data to view the tissues behind the often very intense uptake in the left and anterior right lobes.

Within 1–24 hours after microsphere therapy, patients return to the nuclear medicine department for acquisition of planar torso and SPECT images that the microspheres produce by releasing Bremsstrahlung (gamma) radiation. This quality assurance test confirms that the radiation dose is deposited only in the liver. It is compared to the distribution of activity present on the pre-treatment ^{99m}Tc MAA scans. This reflects the common practice in all types of brachytherapy in attempting to verify the final position of radioactive sources within the body.

If patients are able to undergo an initial PET scan prior to therapy, a follow-up PET is performed at 6 and 12 weeks. Review is not only for liver response but also to detect any extrahepatic disease, since patients are not usually placed on maintenance chemotherapy.

Toxicity

Patients are followed closely until all acute toxicities are resolved, or at least every 2 weeks for 6 weeks, then monthly for 3 months to observe for possible RILD or other late toxicities. RILD is typically defined as a transient condition of variable severity characterized by jaundice, weight gain, and painful hepatomegaly with elevation of liver enzymes. Rarely thrombocytopenia and encephalopathy are seen. Clinical findings include a rise in the liver function tests, especially bilirubin, 30–120 days from the date of therapy, large volume ascites, and hypoalbuminemia. Perihepatic ascites may develop that is detectable on CT but usually not frank liver failure and is not considered RILD. Acute events are those that occurred within 30 days of treatment and late effects are defined as occurring on 31–90 days post-treatment. Acute events include the development of gastritis, ulceration, or pancreatitis due to the deposition of the microspheres in vessels that serve these organs. The National Cancer Institute's Common Terminology Criteria for Adverse Events v3.0 (CTCAE) [43] is used as appropriate [41].

Patient Selection

All patients are selected according to strict inclusion/ exclusion criteria. Eligible patients are >18 years of age; of any race and either gender; who had a confirmed diagnosis of cancer; with measurable unresectable disease predominately involving the liver; who are able to give informed consent; with an Eastern Cooperative Oncology Group (ECOG) Performance Status score of less than or equal to 2; adequate bone marrow (granulocytes >1500/μl, platelets >60,000/μl); hepatic (total bilirubin <2.0 mg/dl) serum glutamic-oxalocetic transaminase/serum glutamic-pyruvic transaminase (SGOT/SGPT) or alkaline phosphatase <5 times the upper limit of normal; and pulmonary function (FEV$_1$ >1 L) and no contraindications for angiography and selective visceral catheterization. In addition, absolute contraindications include pulmonary shunt >20% of technetium-labeled MAA (^{99m}Tc MAA) or any uncorrectable delivery to the GI tract; hepatofugal flow in the portal vein, complete portal vein thrombosis or planned need for systemic chemotherapy within 4 weeks of treatment or chemotherapy in the immediate past 4 weeks prior to proposed treatment.

Colorectal Cancer Metastases

Several reports in abstract form have been published regarding delivery of microspheres for colorectal hepatic metastases [24, 25, 26, 27, 30, 31, 32]. Resin microspheres are fully Food and DrugAdministration (FDA)-approved and indicated for colorectal cancer with a similar delivery method as for glass spheres. Therefore, enrollment on an Institutional

Review Board (IRB)-approved protocol is not required, but informed consent must be obtained for all patients prior to treatment. Since this therapy has not been proven to be as effective as current chemotherapeutic regimens, patients are accepted for therapy who had already received and failed standard first-line and often second- and third-line therapies for their primary tumor. Documentation in their chart of either progression on, or inability to receive: oxaliplatin, irinotecan, capecitabine, and various 5FU/leucovorin schedules with Avastin and Erbitux should be obtained before enrollment into a microsphere therapeutic program. Evaluation of patients by medical oncology, radiation oncology, hepatobiliary surgery, and interventional radiology also should be completed prior to acceptance for microsphere treatment. These patients should not be candidates for RFA, transarterial chemoembolization (TACE), resection, intensity modulated radiation therapy (IMRT) or stereotactic radiotherapy by consensus. In addition, careful review of screening tests – in particular nuclear medicine and body CT or MRI – requires significant consultations with subspecialist physicians in those disciplines.

Current publications demonstrate the efficacy of this therapy in a previously rigorously treated group of patients with excellent results [44, 45]. A mean dose of 1.75 GBq of microspheres has been used usually as whole liver therapy. The response rate to this treatment is 35% on CT but an impressive 85% on PET scan. Those patients that responded lived an average of 10.5 months

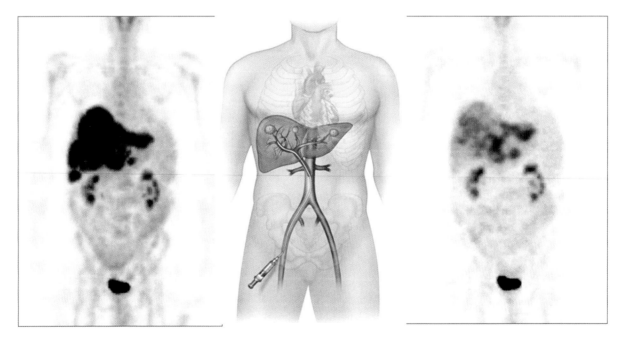

Fig. 10.3 Chemorefractory metastatic colon cancer in a 56-year-old man. *The first panel* shows near complete replacement of the liver on a coronal image of a pre-^{90}Y-microspheres FDG PET scan. *The second panel* is an illustration of the treatment given to the right

hepatic lobe with ^{90}Y-microspheres via a microcatheter placed into the right hepatic artery. *The third panel* is the same patient imaged via PET at 6 weeks post-microsphere treatment showing near complete clearing of active tumor in the treated right lobe and those not responding 4.5 months. The differing response rate of CT versus PET is thought to be due to the highly restrictive criteria for response. The tumors will die more quickly than the response is demonstrated on CT. Due to the more sensitive nature of PET scanning, the response is more readily discerned (see Fig. 10.3).

Breast Cancer Metastases

Recent papers outline the use of this therapy in women with breast cancer metastases [46, 47]. The mean survival of breast cancer patients after developing liver metastases is 14 months. Serendipitously, the mean follow-up of patients in one of these series was 14 months. Survival after having been treated with ^{90}Y SIR-Spheres at 14 months was 86% while expected survival with chemotherapy at that time was 50%. The response of these tumors to microsphere therapy is due to their extraordinary hypervascularity and reasonably slow growth rate. It was seen in these papers that complete PET response in the liver was not an unusual event; however, the development of extrahepatic disease was common.

Neuroendocrine Tumor Metastases

A number of abstracts have been presented on the use of yttrium microspheres in the treatment of neuroendocrine metastases [48, 49]. Not surprisingly, the response of these patients has been excellent. The most commonly utilized therapy for liver metastases from these tumors

has been hepatic arterial embolization, either bland or combined with chemotherapy. Control of disease has been shown to be effective for as long as 1 year per embolization. However, over time, the tumors re-grow and parasitize their blood supply from successively smaller vessels. Eventually, after several treatments, the patient's hepatic arterial supply has the "pruned tree" appearance without the presence of tumor vessels. At this point the patient becomes untreatable by directed therapy. The yttrium microspheres change this paradigm. The re-appearance of the metastases is due to islets of viable tumor that is left behind after the embolization is complete. These islets grow into new tumors over time. Because the zone of effect is increased for the microspheres due to their radioactivity, more of these islets of tumor receive therapeutic doses of radiation causing fewer of them to re-grow. Again, the slow growth and hypervascularity of these tumors is an asset when utilizing microsphere therapy (see Fig. 10.4).

Discussion

The use of brachytherapy in treating primary and secondary liver tumors has a long history. Müller and Rossier first reported the use of radiolabeled particles for therapeutic use in 1951 when they injected ^{65}Zn and ^{98}Au tagged to carbon particles to treat primary lung tumors and metastases [50]. The first use of yttrium-90 attached to microspheres was in 1961 [51]. Kim et al, in 1962, reported using this isotope with ceramic microspheres to treat both animals and 17 patients, 7 of whom (41%) showed tumor size reduction or amelioration of clinical

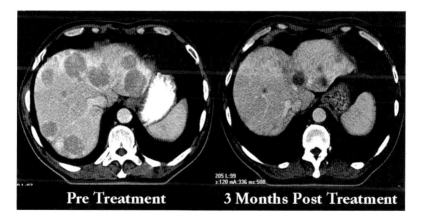

Fig. 10.4 Axial CT scans before (*left*) and after (*right*) a single treatment of 2.25 GBq of ^{90}Y-microspheres in a patient with symptomatic carcinoid tumor metastatic to the liver from an ileum primary site. Chromogranin A serum marker decreased to normal by 6 weeks with the CT scan findings eventually confirming a complete response

symptoms [52]. In the subsequent decades a number of investigators in a handful of countries advanced their protocol techniques using a variety of radiolabels, either glass or resin microspheres, and to some extent, adjunctive agents [53, 54, 55, 56, 57, 58, 59, 60, 61, 62, 63, 64, 65, 66, 67, 68]. However, in the early 1970s, though a few groups continued to gather relatively successful and illuminating results, a number of obstacles to the use of microspheres – particularly that of radiation leaching to extrahepatic sites – led to its discontinuation. For this reason, and because the concept of multidisciplinary or combined oncologic modalities was yet to become well recognized, this once promising line of treatment became virtually relegated to dormancy in most centers around the world. With the development of non-leaching yttrium TheraSpheres™ (glass) and SIR-Spheres® (resin) in the late 1980s, and the independent ongoing work of two groups in Australia and the United States, plus the advent of widely used computerized technology to assist in much-needed dosimetry and evaluation methods, a resurgence of interest for this intervention occurred in the 1990s and continues to date.

The earliest exclusively clinical evaluations of hepatic metastases using yttrium-90 microspheres alone in at least one study arm led to an average survival of 6 months post-treatment [60]. Blanchard's work, more than a decade later, resulted in a post-operative survival average of 62.6 weeks with a radiation dose range of 1.85–2.7 GBq [66]. Although more sensitive data were being increasingly defined over time, response rates, end points, and follow-up in subsequent reports [67, 68, 69] were poorly recorded until a series conducted by Anderson et al. (with glass spheres) in 1992 [70]. At this point, new microspheres – both glass and resin – were being manufactured and the fundamental problem of leaching to extra-tumor sites, especially bone marrow, was remedied. This resulted in a documented median survival of 11 months post-treatment in 7 patients, an increase of 4 months over the acknowledged survival estimate without treatment [64, 71]. A number of other developments in the 1990s led to better outcomes and therefore increased use of both resin and glass spheres. These developments included use of angiography and other advanced imaging techniques [58, 61, 64, 72], use of simulated infusion of ^{99m}Tc MAA to better assess pre-treatment sphere distribution [73], more discrete determination of histology and vascularity of tumors [67, 74], a refinement of dosimetry [69, 75, 76, 77], use of angiotensin II to confine blood flow to tumorous tissue [68, 78], methodology control of potential toxicities [7, 20, 28, 58, 70, 79, 80, 81, 82], and clear indications and contraindications for patient selection [83].

The earliest recorded radiation-induced toxicities were a transient elevation of serum transaminase [62]. Later more serious problems included radiation pneumonitis [83], veno-occlusive disease [84], gastroduodenal ulceration [79] and gastritis, and radiation hepatitis, which was subsequently declared a misnomer and renamed RILD since no true inflammation was apparent [7]. Although records are imprecise over these years and a clear assessment of success rates was compromised due to concomitant use of chemotherapeutic agents, prior to 2000 a partial response can be said to have been achieved in over 50% of patients (approximately 225 patients), stable disease or time to progressive disease was noted for longer durations, and survival rates exceeded previous peaks [85].

Despite the difficulty in imaging a beta emitter, and the minute size of each sphere, extensive animal studies of microsphere implantation within liver tumors have been published confirming preferential accumulation within tumors versus normal liver [77, 86]. In summary, clusters of microspheres non-randomly but heterogeneously embed in the outer 6 mm of tumor–normal liver interface. Kennedy and colleagues recently completed a detailed report on animal and human microsphere location within liver tumors confirming prior investigator's conclusions that the majority of radioactive spheres embed within the periphery of tumor nodules, delivering doses as high as 3000 Gy to the tumor [33]. Microsphere implantation within the tumor spares adjacent normal liver allowing the liver to tolerate this therapy well while destroying tumors, even large ones [76, 87, 88, 89].

The toxicities from radiation alone given as salvage treatment are generally mild and self-limiting in 3–5 days. In decreasing order and severity, the toxicities included fatigue, nausea, abdominal pain, and emesis. Many patients benefit from a methylprednisolone dose pack (24 mg/on day 1 to 0 mg on day 7) for nausea and fatigue in the first 6 days after sphere treatment, particularly if the whole liver was treated. It is our opinion that both the embolic- and radiation-related edema effects in the liver, and the intensity of liver radiation during this time, are stressful on the body and counteracted by a short burst of steroid therapy, which acts in concert with anti-emetics to relieve nausea. Some patients only require anti-emetic therapy in the first 24 hours; others need mild pain relief only during the first week.

Whereas brachytherapy for GI cancers of the anus, rectum, stomach, and esophagus uses a standard approach of concurrent chemotherapy and spheres delivery, the same is needed to improve this approach for metastatic colorectal cancer. Clinical trials of resin spheres for colorectal cancer have been conducted in Australia in chemotherapy-naïve patients, but as reflected in this report, United States' experience is only in salvage patients. The pivotal resin sphere trial accepted by the

FDA was interesting but not applicable to current accepted practice with modern chemotherapy. Gray [35] randomized 74 patients with liver-only colon cancer metastases to hepatic artery infusion of FUDR versus FUDR plus one treatment of resin microspheres, termed *selective internal radiation therapy* (SIRT). The partial and complete response rate by CT and carcinoembryonic antigen (CEA) was improved for patients receiving SIRT. The median time to disease progression in the liver was significantly longer for patients receiving SIRT in comparison to patients receiving HAC alone. The one, two, three and five-year survival for patients receiving SIRT was 72%, 39%, 17% and 3.5%, compared to 68%, 29%, 6.5% and 0% for hepatic artery catheter (HAC) alone. Cox regression analysis suggested an improvement in survival for patients treated with SIR-Spheres who survive more than 15 months ($P = 0.06$). There was no increase in grade 3–4 treatment related toxicity for patients receiving SIRT in comparison to patients receiving HAC alone.

Resin microspheres in the United States are used in patients with chemorefractory liver metastases but minimal extrahepatic disease, treated with one, two, and sometimes three courses of SIRT without concurrent chemotherapy. The ECOG (ECOG #3202) plans to open enrollment in 2005 of a phase II study of resin spheres in combination with bolus 5FU/LV. Combining the newest and most effective chemotherapy agents for colorectal cancer with microspheres is the logical next step now that the effectiveness and safety have been established in microsphere-alone treated patients. Two important phase I studies have been reported in abstract form in patients with liver metastases from colon cancer. Van Hazel [90] treated newly diagnosed patients with oxaliplatin, 5-FU, and leucovorin concurrent with one application of microspheres during the first week of chemotherapy. The dose escalation involved oxaliplatin, which was found to be well-tolerated at full dose (85 mg/m^2) for that regimen with concurrent resin microspheres. Response (RECIST) by CT scan was significant in 10 of 11 evaluable patients. Van Hazel [91] also tested chemotherapy and microspheres in 23 patients that had failed 5-FU, but were irinotecan naïve. The median time to liver progression was 6.3 months, and median survival was 12.0 months (2–25+ months).

All patients are evaluated for existing therapies, including RFA, conformal radiotherapy, surgery, and TACE, but their disease is usually too large, too widely distributed, or too close to critical structures for these approaches. We conclude from our experience that ^{90}Y-microsphere therapy can provide significant benefit for heavily pretreated heterogeneous group of good-performance patients with liver-predominant metastases.

References

1. Ellis LM, Curley SA, Tanabe KK. Radiofrequency Ablation for Cancer: Current Indications, Techniques and Outcomes. New York: Springer-Verlag; 2004.
2. Vogl TJ, Straub R, Eichler K, et al. Colorectal carcinoma metastases in liver: laser-induced interstitial thermotherapy—local tumor control rate and survival data. Radiology. 2004; 230: 450–458.
3. Ricke J, Wust P, Stohlmann A, et al. CT-guided interstitial brachytherapy of liver malignancies alone or in combination with thermal ablation: phase I-II results of a novel technique. Int J Radiat Oncol Biol Phys. 2004; 58: 1496–1505.
4. Martinez-Monge R, Nag S, Nieroda CA, et al. Iodine-125 brachytherapy in the treatment of colorectal adenocarcinoma metastatic to the liver. Cancer. 1999; 85: 1218–1225.
5. Dritschilo A, Grant EG, Harter KW, et al. Interstitial radiation therapy for hepatic metastases: sonographic guidance for applicator placement. AJR Am J Roentgenol. 1986; 147: 275–278.
6. Lawrence TS, Ten Haken RK, Kessler ML, et al. The use of 3-D dose volume analysis to predict radiation hepatitis. Int J Radiat Oncol Biol Phys. 1992; 23: 781–788.
7. Lawrence TS, Robertson JM, Anscher MS, et al. Hepatic toxicity resulting from cancer treatment. Int J Radiat Oncol Biol Phys. 1995; 31: 1237–1248.
8. Lawrence TS, Kessler ML, Robertson JM. 3-D conformal radiation therapy in upper gastrointestinal cancer. The University of Michigan experience. Front Radiat Ther Oncol. 1996; 29: 221–228.
9. Lawrence TS, Kessler ML, Robertson JM. Conformal high-dose radiation plus intraarterial floxuridine for hepatic cancer. Oncology (Williston Park). 1993; 7(10): 51–57; discussion 57–58, 63. (from Pub Med)
10. Lawrence TS, Dworzanin LM, Walker-Andrews SC, et al. Treatment of cancers involving the liver and porta hepatis with external beam irradiation and intraarterial hepatic fluorodeoxyuridine. Int J Radiat Oncol Biol Phys. 1991; 20: 555–561.
11. Lawrence TS, Davis MA, Maybaum J, et al. The potential superiority of bromodeoxyuridine to iododeoxyuridine as a radiation sensitizer in the treatment of colorectal cancer. Cancer Res. 1992; 52: 3698–3704.
12. Lawrence TS, Tesser RJ, Ten Haken RK. An application of dose volume histograms to the treatment of intrahepatic malignancies with radiation therapy. Int J Radiat Oncol Biol Phys. 1990; 19: 1041–1047.
13. Sailer SL. Three dimensional conformal radiotherapy. In: Gunderson L, Tepper J, editors. Clinical Radiation Oncology. Philadelphia: Churchill Livingstone; 2000: 236–255.
14. Fuss M, Thomas CR Jr. Stereotactic body radiation therapy: an ablative treatment option for primary and secondary liver tumors. Ann Surg Oncol. 2004; 11: 130–138.
15. Gunven P, Blomgren H, Lax I. Radiosurgery for recurring liver metastases after hepatectomy. Hepatogastroenterology. 2003; 50: 1201–1204.
16. Herfarth KK, Debus J, Lohr F, et al. Stereotactic single-dose radiation therapy of liver tumors: results of a phase I/II trial. J Clin Oncol. 2001; 19: 164–170.
17. Herfarth KK, Debus J, Lohr F, et al. Extracranial stereotactic radiation therapy: set-up accuracy of patients treated for liver metastases. Int J Radiat Oncol Biol Phys. 2000; 46: 329–335.
18. Lax I, Blomgren H, Naslund I, et al. Stereotactic radiotherapy of malignancies in the abdomen. Methodological aspects. Acta Oncol. 1994; 33: 677–683.
19. Fuss M, Salter BJ, Cavanaugh SX, et al. Daily ultrasound-based image-guided targeting for radiotherapy of upper abdominal malignancies. Int J Radiat Oncol Biol Phys. 2004; 59: 1245–1256.

20. Gray BN, Anderson JE, Burton MA, et al. Regression of liver metastases following treatment with yttrium-90 microspheres. Aust N Z J Surg. 1992; 62: 105–110.

21. Stubbs RS, Cannan RJ, Mitchell AW. Selective internal radiation therapy (SIRT) with 90Yttrium microspheres for extensive colorectal liver metastases. Hepato-Gastroenterology. 2001; 48: 333–337.

22. Lau WY, Leung WT, Ho S, et al. Treatment of inoperable hepatocellular carcinoma with intrahepatic arterial yttrium-90 microspheres: a phase I and II study. Br J Cancer. 1994; 70: 994–999.

23. Lau WY, Ho S, Leung TW, et al. Selective internal radiation therapy for nonresectable hepatocellular carcinoma with intraarterial infusion of 90yttrium microspheres. Int J Radiat Oncol Biol Phys. 1998; 40: 583–592.

24. Kennedy AS, Murthy R, Sarfaraz M, et al. Outpatient hepatic artery brachytherapy for primary and secondary hepatic malignancies. Radiology. 2001; 221P: 468.

25. Kennedy AS, Murthy R, Van Echo DA. Preliminary results of outpatient hepatic artery brachytherapy for colorectal hepatic metastases. Eur J Cancer. 2001; 37: 289.

26. Van Echo DA, Kennedy AS, Coldwell D. TheraSphere (TS) at 143 Gy median dose for mixed hepatic cancers; feasibility and toxicities. Amer Soc Clin Oncol. 2001; 260a: 1038.

27. Coldwell D, Kennedy AS, Van Echo DA, et al. Feasibility of treatment of hepatic tumors utilizing embolization with yttrium-90 glass microspheres. J Vasc Interv Radiol. 2001; 12: S113.

28. Andrews JC, Walker SC, Ackermann RJ, et al. Hepatic radioembolization with yttrium-90 containing glass microspheres: preliminary results and clinical follow-up. J Nucl Med. 1994; 35: 1637–1644.

29. Dancey JE, Shepherd FA, Paul K, et al. Treatment of nonresectable hepatocellular carcinoma with intrahepatic 90Y-microspheres [In Process Citation]. J Nucl Med. 2000; 41: 1673–1681.

30. Murthy R, Kennedy AS, Coldwell D, et al. Technical aspects of TheraSphere (TS) infusion. J Vasc Interv Radiol. 2002; 13: S2.

31. Murthy R, Kennedy AS, Tucker G, et al. Outpatient trans arterial hepatic 'low dose rate' (TAH-LDR) brachytherapy for unresectable hepatocellular carcinoma. Proc Amer Assoc Cancer Res. 2002; 43: 485.

32. Murthy R, Line BR, Kennedy AS, et al. Clinical utility of Brehmstralung scan (BRM-Scan) after TheraSphere (TS). J Vasc Interv Radiol. 2002; 13: S2.

33. Kennedy AS, Nutting C, Coldwell D, et al. Pathologic response and microdosimetry of 90Y microspheres in man: review of four explanted whole livers. Int J Radiat Oncol Biol Phys. 2004; 60: 1552–1563.

34. Kennedy AS, Murthy R, Kwok Y, et al. Hepatic artery brachytherapy for unresectable hepatocellular carcinoma: an outpatient treatment approach. Proceedings of the 12th International Congress on Anti-Cancer Treatment 2002; 1: 198–199.

35. Gray B, Van Hazel G, Hope M, et al. Randomised trial of SIR-Spheres plus chemotherapy vs. chemotherapy alone for treating patients with liver metastases from primary large bowel cancer. Ann Oncol. 2001; 12: 1711–1720.

36. Sarfaraz M, Kennedy AS, Cao ZJ, et al. Radiation dose distribution in patients treated with Y-90 microspheres for nonresectable hepatic tumors. Int J Rad Biol Phys. 2001; 51: 32–33.

37. Salem R, Thurston KG, Carr B, et al. Yttrium-90 microspheres: Radiation therapy for unresectable liver cancer. J Vasc Interv Radiol. 2002; 13: S223–229.

38. Murthy R, Xiong H, Nunez R, et al. Yttrium 90 resin microspheres for the treatment of unresectable colorectal hepatic metastases after failure of multiple chemotherapy regimens: preliminary results. J Vasc Interv Radiol. 2005; 16: 937–945.

39. Gulec, SA, Mesoloras G, Bruetman D, Pennington K. Effectiveness of yttrium-90 microspheres selective internal radiation treatment with concomitant chemotherapy as a front-line treatment in patients with colorectal cancer liver metastases. Poster presentation, Soc Nuc Med Annual Meeting, 2007.

40. Liu DM, Salem R, Bui JT, et al. Angiographic considerations in patients undergoing liver-directed therapy. JVIR. 2005; 16: 911.

41. Murthy R, Brown DB, Salem R, et al. Gastrointestinal complications associated with hepatic arterial yttrium-90 microsphere therapy. JVIR. 2007; 18: 553–562.

42. Pulmolite [package insert]. Bedford, MA: CIS-US, Inc.

43. Cancer Therapy Evaluation Program, Published 12 December 2003; http://ctep.cancer.gov Accessed 9 August 2007.

44. Kennedy AS, Nutting C, Coldwell DM, et al. Resin 90Y-microsphere brachytherapy for unresectable colorectal liver metastases: Modern USA experience. Int J Radiat Oncol Biol Phys. 2006; 65: 412.

45. Lewandowski RJ, Thurston KG, Goin JE, et al. 90Y microsphere (TheraSphere) treatment for unresectable colorectal cancer metastases of the liver: response to treatment at targeted doses of 135–150 Gy as measured by [18F]fluorodeoxyglucose positron emission tomography and computed tomographic imaging. JVIR. 2005; 16: 1641.

46. Coldwell DM, Kennedy AS, Nutting CW. The use of resin Y90 microsphere brachytherapy for unresectable hepatic metastases from breast cancer. Int J Radiat Oncol Biol Phys. 2007; 69(3): 800–804.

47. Bangash AK, Atassi B, Kaklamani V, et al. 90Y radioembolization of metastatic breast cancer to the liver: toxicity, imaging response, survival. JVIR. 2007; 18: 621.

48. Coldwell DM, Kennedy AS, et al. Treatment of unresectable metastatic neuroendocrine tumors in the liver with intra-arterial brachytherapy using yttrium-90 microspheres. World Congress of Gastrointestinal Cancer, Barcelona, 2005.

49. Kennedy A, Coldwell D, Nutting C, et al. Hepatic brachytherapy for GI neuroendocrine tumors with 90-Y microspheres: Long term US experience. ICACT Annual Meeting, Paris, France, February, 2005.

50. Muller JH, Rossier PH. A new method for the treatment of cancer of the lungs by means of artificial radioactivity (Zn63 and Au198). Acta Radiol. 1951; 35: 449–468.

51. Ya PM, Guzman T, Loken MK, et al. Isotope localization with tagged microspheres. Surgery. 1961; 49: 644–650.

52. Kim YS, LaFave JW, MacLean LD. The Use of radiating microspheres in the treatment of experimental and human malignancy. Surgery. 1962; 52: 220.

53. Grady ED, Sale WT, Rollins LC. Localization of radioactivity by intravascular injection of large radioactive particles. Ann Surg. 1963; 157: 97–114.

54. Ariel IM. Radioactive isotopes for adjuvant cancer therapy. Arch Surg. 1964; 89: 244–249.

55. Nolan T, Grady ED, Crumbley AJ. Regional internal radiation for hepatic cancer. Minerva Oncol. 1973; 1: 104–106.

56. Nolan T, Grady ED, Crumbley AJ, et al. Internal hepatic radiotherapy: I. Organ distribution of colloidal Cr32 P04 injected into a peripheral vein, the portal vein, or the arterial supply of the gastrointestinal tract in the rat. Am J Roentgenol Radium Ther Nucl Med. 1975; 124: 590–595.

57. Grady ED, Nolan T, Larose JH, et al. Internal hepatic radiotherapy: II. Intra-arterial radiocolloid therapy for hepatic tumors. Am J Roentgenol Ther Nucl Med. 1975; 124: 596–599.

58. Grady ED. Internal radiation therapy of hepatic cancer. Dis Colon Rectum. 1979; 22: 371–375.

59. Ariel IM. Treatment of inoperable primary pancreatic and liver cancer by the intra-arterial administration of radioactive

isotopes (Y90 radiating microspheres). Ann Surg. 1965; 162: 267–278.

60. Ariel IM, Pack GT. Treatment of inoperable cancer of the liver by intra-arterial radioactive isotopes and chemotherapy. Cancer. 1967; 20: 793–804.

61. Mantravadi RV, Spigos DG, Tan WS, et al. Intraarterial yttrium 90 in the treatment of hepatic malignancy. Radiology. 1982; 142: 783–786.

62. Ariel IM, Padula G. Treatment of asymptomatic metastatic cancer to the liver from primary colon and rectal cancer by the intraarterial administration of chemotherapy and radioactive isotopes. J Surg Oncol. 1982; 20: 151–156.

63. Blanchard RJW. Treatment of liver tumours with yttrium-90 microspheres. Can J Surg. 1983; 26: 442–443.

64. Gyves JW, Ziessman HA, Ensminger WD, et al. Definition of hepatic tumor microcirculation by single photon emission computerized tomography (SPECT). J Nuclear Med. 1984; 25: 972–977.

65. Gray BN. Colorectal cancer: the modern treatment of disseminated disease—a review. Aust N Z J Surg. 1980; 50: 647 658.

66. Blanchard RJ, Morrow IM, Sutherland JB. Treatment of liver tumors with yttrium-90 microspheres alone. Can Assoc Radiol J. 1989; 40: 206–210.

67. Burton MA, Gray BN, Klemp PF, et al. Selective internal radiation therapy: distribution of radiation in the liver. Eur J Cancer Clin Oncol. 1989; 25: 1487–1491.

68. Gray BN, Burton MA, Kelleher DK, et al. Selective internal radiation (SIR) therapy for treatment of liver metastases: measurement of response rate. J Surg Oncol. 1989; 42: 192–196.

69. Gray BN, Burton MA, Kelleher D, et al. Tolerance of the liver to the effects of yttrium-90 radiation. Int J Radiat Oncol Biol Phys. 1990; 18: 619–623.

70. Anderson JH, Goldberg JA, Bessent RG, et al. Glass yttrium-90 microspheres for patients with colorectal liver metastases. Radiother Oncol. 1992; 25: 137–139.

71. Gray BN. Colorectal cancer: the natural history of disseminated disease—a review. Aust N Z J Surg. 1980; 50: 643–646.

72. Marn CS, Andrews JC, Francis IR, et al. Hepatic parenchymal changes after intraarterial Y-90 therapy: CT findings. Radiology. 1993; 187: 125–128.

73. Stribley KV, Gray BN, Chmiel RL, et al. Internal radiotherapy for hepatic metastases I: The homogeneity of hepatic arterial blood flow. J Surg Res. 1983; 34: 17–24.

74. Stribley KV, Gray BN, Chmiel RL, et al. Internal radiotherapy for hepatic metastases II: The blood supply to hepatic metastases. J Surg Res. 1983; 34: 25–32.

75. Burton MA, Gray BN, Jones C, et al. Intraoperative dosimetry of 90Y in liver tissue. Int J Rad Appl Instrum B. 1989; 16: 495–498.

76. Fox RA, Klemp PF, Egan G, et al. Dose distribution following selective internal radiation therapy. Int J Radiat Oncol Biol Phys. 1991; 21: 463–467.

77. Roberson PL, Ten Haken R, McShan DL, et al. Three-dimensional tumor dosimetry for hepatic Yttrium-90 microsphere therapy. J Nuclear Med. 1992; 33: 735–738.

78. Burton MA, Gray BN, Coletti A. Effect of angiotensin II on blood flow in the transplanted sheep squamous cell carcinoma. Eur J Cancer Clin Oncol. 1988; 24: 1373–1376.

79. Herba MJ, Illescas FF, Thirlwell MP, et al. Hepatic malignancies: improved treatment with intraarterial Y-90. Radiology. 1988; 169: 311–314.

80. Ehrhardt G, Day DE. Therapeutic use of 90Y microspheres. Int J Rad Appl Instrum B. 1987; 14: 233–242.

81. Russell JL Jr, Carden JL, Herron HL. Dosimetry calculations for yttrium-90 used in the treatment of liver cancer. Endocurietherapy/Hyperthermia Oncology. 1988; 4: 171–186.

82. Leung TW, Lau WY, Ho SK, et al. Radiation pneumonitis after selective internal radiation treatment with intraarterial 90yttrium-microspheres for inoperable hepatic tumors. Int J Radiat Oncol Biol Phys. 1995; 33: 919–924.

83. Harbert JC, Ziessman HA. Therapy with intraarterial microspheres. Nucl Med Annu. 1987; 295–319.

84. Fajardo LF, Colby TV. Pathogenesis of veno-occlusive liver disease after radiation. Arch Pathol Lab Med. 1980; 104: 584–588.

85. Ho S, Lau WY, Leung TW, et al. Internal radiation therapy for patients with primary or metastatic hepatic cancer: a review. Cancer. 1998; 83: 1894–1907.

86. Pillai KM, McKeever PE, Knutsen CA, et al. Microscopic analysis of arterial microsphere distribution in rabbit liver and hepatic VX2 tumor. Selective Cancer Therapeutics. 1991; 7: 39–48.

87. Campbell AM, Bailey IH, Burton MA. Analysis of the distribution of intra-arterial microspheres in human liver following hepatic yttrium-90 microsphere therapy. Phys Med Biol. 2000; 45: 1023–1033.

88. Campbell AM, Bailey IH, Burton MA. Tumor dosimetry in human liver following hepatic yttrium-90 microsphere therapy. Phys Med Biol. 2001; 46: 487–498.

89. Coldwell D, Kennedy AS, Van Echo DA. Comparative side effects of yttrium-90 based intra-arterial brachytherapy. J Clin Oncol. 2004; 22: 3760.

90. Van Hazel G, Price D, Bower G, et al. Selective internal radiation therapy (SIRT) plus systemic chemotherapy with Oxaliplatin, 5-Fluorouracil and Leucovorin: A phase I dose escalation study. Proceedings of the ASCO GI Cancers Symposium 2005: 133.

91. Van Hazel G, Pavlakis N, Goldstein D, et al. Selective internal radiation therapy (SIRT) plus systemic chemotherapy with irinotecan. A phase I dose escalation study. Proceedings of the ASCO GI Cancers Symposium 2005: 223.

Barbara L. van Leeuwen, N. de Liguori Carino, G.J. Poston, and R.A. Audisio

Epidemiology Of Aging And Colorectal Cancer In The Western World

Life expectancy has increased dramatically in the past century and is now 75–77 years for men and 80–81 years for women in the western world [1]. The demographics of the changing world have important consequences for health care professionals dealing with cancer patients. Cancer is a disease mainly of the elderly, due to a combination of lifetime exposure to carcinogens and lifestyle-related risks [2]. It is predicted that due to the overall increase in life expectancy in 2030, when the baby boomers born in the 1950–1960s will reach the age of 65, cancer will be the leading cause of death worldwide [1]. Currently, over half of all cancer types are diagnosed among the elderly, and 76% of all patients with a newly diagnosed colorectal tumour are between 65 and 85 years old [3, 4].

In most developed countries, colorectal cancer is among the top three most prevalent cancers in both men and women over the age of 65 [2]. Although the prevalence of elderly colorectal cancer patients is increasing, survival in this patient category has not improved accordingly. Postoperative mortality has decreased over the past decades, but there has been no improvement in stage specific survival in the elderly [5]. Data suggest that this age difference in outcome is less pronounced in the USA than in Europe [6], but US patients over the age of 75 with colorectal cancer are equally less likely to undergo operative surgery [7]. Age standardised survival rates are lower for elderly patients with colorectal cancer, especially in the first year after diagnosis [3], and there is also debate as to whether survival in elderly women is better when compared to men [8, 9]. Certainly, socio-economic factors are partly responsible for these unacceptable differences in treatment outcome. The elderly, especially those widowed or socially isolated, do not seek medical help in the early stages of disease and are often not involved in screening programs. They are, therefore, more likely to present with stage IV disease and liver metastases.

Sadly, population-based studies have shown that younger age is an independent factor associated with a curative resection for colorectal liver metastases [10, 11]. It was demonstrated in a large French series of more than 13,000 patients with colorectal liver metastases that patients older than 75 years were 2–5 times less likely to be offered resection of their liver metastases than younger patients. Not surprisingly, cancer specific survival was worse in the senior group [10]. The elderly are less likely to undergo curative surgery and even less likely to be offered the option of metastasectomy when liver metastases are present [7]. Although such a minimalist approach would seem unacceptable as resection of liver metastases is still the only way to cure these patients, it is likely that the risk of postoperative morbidity and mortality might have been a reason not to treat metastatic cancer for the past decades.

Nowadays, perioperative care has improved dramatically, and mortality rates vary between 0% and 11%, even for procedures combining colon resection with metastasectomy [12]. When patients with stage IV colorectal cancer and liver metastases receive palliative care only, 5-year survival is 0–14% depending on the grade of the liver involvement [9, 13], even with the recent advances made in chemotherapeutic treatment. Oxaliplatin- and irinotecan-based regimens lead to a progression-free survival of 7–10 months and median survival of 9–22 months only [14, 15, 16]. An extensive review of 30 independent studies investigating the efficacy and safety of surgical resection of colorectal liver metastases reported that approximately 30% of patients remain alive 5 years after resection and around two-thirds of these are disease free [17]. A recently published series of 13,599 patients over the age of 65 diagnosed with incident colorectal and liver metastases from 1991 to 2001 from the Surveillance,

B.L. van Leeuwen (✉)
Department of Surgery, University Medical Center Groningen, Groningen, The Netherlands

J.-N. Vauthey et al. (eds.), *Liver Metastases*, DOI 10.1007/978-1-84628-947-7_11,
© Springer-Verlag London Limited 2009

Epidemiology and End Results (SEER)-Medicare database showed that hepatectomy was associated with improved survival [18]. Median survival was 17 months without resection and 46 months if liver resection was performed.

Yet, when balancing the benefits of surgical resection of liver metastases against the potential risks of surgery (i.e. complications, decreased quality of life and even death), many clinicians are still reluctant to advise in favour of surgical treatment in the elderly. There is an increasing need to educate and inform physicians treating elderly patients with colorectal liver metastases. Awareness should be raised regarding life expectancy: at present, 65-year-old men and women have a life expectancy of 82.1 years and 85.0 years, respectively [19]. Once a patient has reached the age of 75 years, life expectancy is 85.7 years for men and 87.8 years for women. This entails that physicians have an obligation to allow patients to enjoy the remaining years of their life in the best possible way. Offering only palliative care for liver metastases with a 0% chance of survival in an era when safe liver resection is technically feasible is unacceptable. There are, however, several factors to consider when selecting elderly patients for hepatic resection.

Physiological Changes In The Aging Liver

A worrying postoperative complication with significant mortality is postoperative liver failure [20, 21]. Reported rates vary between 0% and 48% in mixed case groups of elderly undergoing liver resections [21, 22, 23, 24, 25, 26, 27]. Elderly patients may be prone to liver failure for several reasons. With increasing age, hepatic blood flow decreases and from the age of 50 years, the size of the liver starts to decrease from 2.5% of total body mass to roughly 1.5% in the octogenarian [28]. The total number of hepatocytes is reduced, but the individual size of the cells may be increased due to an increased biological demand. Hepatic synthesis of clotting factors may be reduced, but liver function itself is not usually impaired in the elderly. Hepatic filtration, detoxification, ethanol elimination and conjugation are not impaired under normal circumstances in the elderly person. However, when challenged, because of the decreased number of hepatocytes, hepatic synthesis of several proteins may be impaired [28].

In a small study comparing 12 patients over the age of 70 years versus 29 younger patients undergoing partial hepatectomy for several different diagnoses, a reduction of the hepatic acute phase response was noticed in the elderly group [29]. In the younger patients mean levels of

serum α_1-antitrypsin and plasma fibrinogen levels (acute phase proteins, APPs) increased 30% compared to the preoperative levels, whereas in the older patients, no such change was observed. APPs play an important role in the body's defence against bacterial invasion and the control of leukocyte generated mechanisms necessary for the removal of bacteria and dead cells. The increased rate of postoperative infection found in the elderly patients was thought to be caused by the impaired acute phase response. Postoperative albumin levels and hepaplastin test values were also significantly lower in the elderly postoperatively, and prothrombin time was increased. It takes 3 months in the elderly for these values to return to their normal preoperative level. This observation conflicts with Ettore's findings which showed no difference in postoperative liver function after right hepatectomy when comparing 24 patients aged 65 years or more to 22 patients aged younger than 40 [30]. Postoperative serum levels of bilirubin, aminotranferases, γ-glutamyl transpeptidase, alkaline phosphatase and prothrombin time were similar in both age groups. There were no significant differences in postoperative mortality and morbidity. This is in accordance with reports that showed that using donor livers from elderly patients resulted in comparable outcomes in orthotopic liver transplantation [31, 32].

Therefore, the healthy aging liver is very well able to withstand the test of surgical resection. Conversely, cirrhotic livers are less able to cope with the stress of hepatic resection, and the consensus holds that the presence of Child-Pugh stages B and C cirrhosis, especially in octogenarians, is a contraindication for hepatic resection [21, 26]. With careful patient selection postoperative liver failure in the elderly can be minimised and even completely avoided [25].

Comorbidity

With increasing age patients are more likely to present with increasing comorbidity. Associated illnesses may be the main reason why elderly patients with well functioning livers are not able to withstand the cardiovascular or pulmonary stress of major surgery. It is clear that the presence of comorbid conditions in itself is not a contraindication for major surgery. However, it is important to identify those patients that are too frail to undergo major surgery. American Society of Anesthesiology (ASA) scores can be utilised but are highly user dependent and not specific enough to predict outcome in individual elderly patients. The comprehensive geriatric assessment scale (CGA) is an instrument used by geriatricians to evaluate the condition of elderly patients and entails activities of daily living (ADL), instrumental activities of daily living (IADL), comorbidity, social support, cognitive status and the presence of geriatric syndromes. This tool has been adapted by several investigators to predict short- and long-term mortalities [33]. There are, however, very few tools that have been tested in the surgical setting. One CGA instrument that shows great promise in this respect is the Preoperative Assessment of Cancer in the Elderly (PACE). It has been proven to be a valuable tool in describing the functional capacity and preoperative health status in an international cohort of elderly cancer patients [34]. Preliminary data suggest that 30-day morbidity is related to IADL and the brief fatigue inventory [35].

Techniques In Hepatic Resection

In recent years techniques in hepatic resection have improved, surgical instruments have evolved dramatically and anesthetic interventions have been optimised. With the introduction of new tools such as ultrasonic dissection devices, argon lasers and tissue glue, parenchymal transection is now possible and safe [36]. These techniques enable the surgeon to minimise blood loss and preserve as much healthy liver tissue as possible. Still, some authors advocate anatomical resections to prevent bile leakage and the risk of infection, sepsis and liver failure [37]. An unnecessarily long Pringle manoeuvre (portal pedicle inflow occlusion) should be avoided at all costs. As the older liver tissue may be less resistant to normothermic ischaemia, it is advised to use this manoeuvre selectively, and when indicated, limiting the time to 15 minutes with intervals of at least 5 minutes [37].

Outcome

Most studies reporting outcome after hepatic resection in the elderly deal with mixed caseloads and different types of resection, making uniform conclusions difficult. Many series include a substantial number of patients with hepatocellular carcinoma (HCC), a disease completely different from colorectal liver metastases. HCC most often occurs in patients with cirrhotic livers with impaired functional reserve and an increased risk of postoperative complications, liver failure and death. However, even with these mixed caseloads, early outcomes after hepatic resection in the elderly seem promising, with mortality rates varying between 0 and 11.1% and morbidity between 3.1 and 43% [20, 21, 23, 24, 25, 26, 27, 38, 39]. Results of studies focusing only on patients with colorectal liver metastases are of more importance when deciding whether or not resectional surgery for colorectal liver metastases is appropriate in the elderly. One early study reported on age as a poor prognostic factor for outcome after liver resection [40]. However, several studies have since reported the effect of age on outcome after hepatectomy for liver metastases, all showing favourable results. All these findings should be interpreted with great caution, as a selection bias is suspected in these single centre reports. In a recent study by Menon et al. [22], a subgroup analysis on 126 elderly patients undergoing a major hepatectomy for colorectal liver metastases showed 3-year overall and disease-free survival to not be different from the younger group (61% vs. 55% and 60% vs. 47%, respectively).

A summary of studies reporting on series of elderly patients undergoing resection for colorectal liver metastases is given in Table 11.1. Early results of liver resection in patients with colorectal liver metastases over the age of 70 years were published by Zieren [41, 42]. He compared a small group of 18 patients to the overall series (90 patients) and found comparable postoperative morbidity (28% vs. 26%), mortality (6% vs. 3%) and 1-, 3- and 5-year survival (69% vs. 78%, 38 vs. 45% and 25 vs. 32%, respectively).

A large series reported by Fong [43] comparing patients aged 70 years and older to younger ones also showed no differences in outcome, except for a shorter hospital stay for the younger patients (12 vs. 13 days). As can be expected, comorbidities were common in this group, with 55% of the elderly patients suffering from cardiopulmonary disease and 11% presenting with a history of diabetes. Postoperative complications occurred in 42%, and the majority of these were cardiopulmonary. Liver failure occurred in only 2%, even though cirrhosis was preoperatively detected in 6% of the cases. Men had a 2.6 times greater risk of developing postoperative complications than women. Abnormal preoperative ECGs and operative time >240 minutes were predictors of postoperative complications. Postoperative mortality, ICU admission and long-term survival were not different between younger and senior patients. Interestingly, a comparison of patients >80 years versus those aged 70–74 years showed comparable mortality (8% vs. 5%) but a lower complication rate in the older group (probably indicative of patient selection).

Brunken found that in a group of patients with liver metastases a hepatic resection was performed in 56% of those 70 years and older versus 68% in the younger age group [44]. Surprisingly, 5-year survival after resection was better in the elderly, but this observation was explained by the greater rate of R0 resections. Even though the incidence of preoperative cardiac comorbidities was significantly higher among older patients (43%

Table 11.1 Published articles on series of elderly patients undergoing resection for colorectal liver metastasis

Author	Period	N	Age (years)	Postoperative morbidity	Postoperative mortality	Overall 5-yr survival	Disease-free survival (months)	Median survival (months)	Type of resection
Zieren [41, 42]		18	>70	28%	6%	25%	n.a.	18	First
		90	27–78	26%	3%	32%		27	
Fong [43]	1985–1994	128	≥70	42%	4%	35%	n.a.	40	First
		449	<70	40%	4%	39%		44	
Brunken [44]	1987–1996	25	≥70	28%	4%	44%	n.a.	49	First
		141	<70	26%	3.5%	33%		28	
Brand [45]	1971–1995	41	≥70	29%	7.3%	16%	10.1	22.9	First
		126	<70	17.5%	2.4%	21%	9.5	33.5	
Zacharias [46]	1990–2000	56	>70	41%	0%	22%	12	33	First
		16	>70	38%	7%	0%		17	repeat resection
Cummings [18]	1991–2001	833	≥65	31.9%	4.3%	32.8%	n.a.	45	Mixed
Mazzoni [37]	1987–2002	53	≥70	20.7%	5.7%	30%	25	28	First
		144	<70	14.6%	2.1%	38%	25	31	
Adam [47]	Jan—July	735	≥70	32%	4.3%	35%	n.a.	41.8	Mixed
	2006	3698	<70	30%	1.6%	43%		46.8	

n.a.: Not applicable.

vs. 2%), overall postoperative morbidity was comparable in both groups (28 vs. 26%), as well as duration of hospital stay (14 vs. 15 days). Brand found similar results when comparing outcomes in elderly patients treated surgically in his centre over a 25-year period [45]. There were no differences between the older and younger patients regarding ICU stay (3.9 vs. 2.0 days, respectively), length of hospital stay (13 vs. 16 days), major morbidity (29% vs. 17.5%) or mortality (7.3% vs. 2.4%). Elderly patients tended to require more blood transfusion (46% vs. 29%), but again, this difference did not reach statistical significance. A higher frequency of anatomic resections in the younger group was detected (68% vs. 49%). With respect to long-term outcome, recurrence rate (56% in the senior group vs. 66% in the younger group), disease-free interval and 5-year overall survival were comparable in both groups.

Zacharias [46] evaluated short- and long-term outcomes after first and repeat hepatic resections in patients older than 70 years. Results were promising but not as good as the outcomes seen in younger patients. Morbidity and mortality rates were comparable to previous series. The presence of extrahepatic disease, three or more liver metastases and high preoperative carcinoembryonic antigen (CEA) level over 200 ng/ml were independent risk factors for recurrence and poor disease-free survival. The latter two factors were also risk factors for poor overall survival. When these factors were not present, 5-year survival was 36%, median overall survival was 42 months and 5-year disease-free survival was 33%. With one or two risk factors present, 3-year overall survival rates were

47% and 20%, respectively. Resection of recurrent metastatic disease proved technically feasible with low morbidity and mortality rates. Rates of 1-, 2- and 3-year survival were 61%, 37% and 25%, respectively, but there were no 5-year survivors after repeat resection, as disease recurred in all of them. It was concluded that repeat resection of liver metastases remains controversial.

Cummings studied 13,599 patients aged 65 years and over with incident colorectal cancer and liver metastases [18]. A subgroup of 833 patients underwent hepatic resection with acceptable morbidity and mortality results (31.9 and 4.3%, respectively). Lack of hepatic resection was associated with a 2.78-fold increased risk of death. In the most recent series to date, Adam found 35% 5-year survival rates for patients aged ≥70 years [47]. Synchronous metastases, bilateral distribution and concomitant extrahepatic disease were associated with poor survival in this group.

A clinical score for predicting recurrence after hepatic resection for metastatic colorectal cancer was designed by Fong et al. in 1999 [48]. Seven factors were found to be predictors of poor long-term outcome: positive resection margins, extrahepatic disease, node positive primary, disease-free interval from primary to metastases <12 months, largest hepatic tumour >5 cm, number of hepatic tumours >1 and CEA level >200 ng/ml. A total of 1001 cases were evaluated to design this score, and 199 patients were aged 70 years or over. Age was not found to be a factor influencing long-term outcome. Recently, Mazzoni adapted this scoring system for use in the elderly population [37]. He constructed a modified clinical risk score of five factors:

node positive primary, disease-free interval >12 months, number of metastases >1, preoperative CEA level >100 ng/ml and size of tumours >5 cm. The presence of one of these factors added one point to the total modified clinical risk score. Patients with a score of 3 or more had a median survival of 20 months or less, compared to 30.5–46.0 months in the patients with a score of 0–2. The authors concluded that patients with a clinical risk score of 3 or more should be excluded from liver resection. Also, they denied surgery to patients with an ASA score of III or greater: in these cases radiofrequency ablation or transarterial chemoembolization was advised.

Summary

Hepatic resection of liver metastases in the elderly is feasible, safe and may offer long-term survival to a substantial percentage of patients. Several selection criteria are of importance in this subgroup of patients. The presence of liver cirrhosis (Child-Pugh stages B and C), particularly in patients >80 yrs, is a contraindication for resectional surgery. Comorbidities are not a contraindication for hepatic resection. Although not evidence based, ASA grade III or more is considered a contraindication. In the presence of extrahepatic disease and 3 or more factors of the modified clinical risk score by Mazzoni et al., the benefit of hepatic resection is also doubtful. After careful assessment of these risk factors, we strongly recommend considering senior patients for surgical treatment whenever possible.

References

1. World Health Organisation. World Health statistics. Anonymous. WHO Library Cataloguing-in-Publication Data, 2007.

2. Franceschi S, La Vecchia C. Cancer epidemiology in the elderly. Crit Rev Oncol Hematol. 2001; 39(3): 219–226.

3. Quaglia R, Capocaccia A, Micheli E, et al. A wide difference in cancer survival between middle aged and elderly patients in Europe. Int J Cancer. 2007; 120(10): 2196–2201.

4. Petrowsky H, Clavien PA. Should we deny surgery for malignant hepato- pancreatico-biliary tumors to elderly patients? World J Surg. 2005; 29(9): 1093–1100.

5. Mitry E, Bouvier AM, Esteve J, Faivre J. Improvement in colorectal cancer survival: a population-based study. Eur J Cancer. 2005; 41(15): 2297–2303.

6. Gatta G, Capocaccia R, Coleman MP, et al. Toward a comparison of survival in American and European cancer patients. Cancer. 2000; 89(4): 893–900.

7. Temple LK, Hsieh L, Wong WD, et al. Use of surgery among elderly patients with stage IV colorectal cancer. J Clin Oncol. 2004; 22(17): 3475–3484.

8. Vercelli M, Lillini R, Capocaccia R, et al. Cancer survival in the elderly: effects of socio-economic factors and health care system features (ELDCARE project). Eur J Cancer. 2006; 42(2): 234–242.

9. Yun HR, Lee WY, Lee OS, et al. The prognostic factors of stage IV colorectal cancer and assessment of proper treatment according to the patient's status. Int J Colorectal Dis. 2007; 22(11): 1301–10.

10. Manfredi S, Lepage C, Hatem C, O. et al. Epidemiology and management of liver metastases from colorectal cancer. Ann Surg. 2006; 244(2): 254–259.

11. Leporrier J, Maurel L, Chiche S, et al. A population-based study of the incidence, management and prognosis of hepatic metastases from colorectal cancer. Ann Surg. 2006; 93(4): 465–474.

12. Tocchi A, Mazzoni G, Brozzetti S, et al. Hepatic resection in stage IV colorectal cancer: prognostic predictors of outcome. Int J Colorectal Dis. 2004; 19(6): 580–585.

13. Okuno K. Surgical treatment for digestive cancer. Current issues—colon cancer. Dig Surg. 2006; 24(2): 108–114.

14. Cunningham S, Pyrhonen R D, James C J, et al. Randomised trial of irinotecan plus supportive care versus supportive care alone after fluorouracil failure for patients with metastatic colorectal cancer. Lancet. 1998; 352(9138): 1413–1418.

15. Scheithauer W, Kornek GV, Raderer M, et al. Randomized multicenter phase II trial of oxaliplatin plus irinotecan versus raltitrexed as first-line treatment in advanced colorectal cancer. J Clin Oncol. 2002; 20(1): 165–172.

16. Falcone S, Ricci S, Brunetti I, et al. Phase III trial of infusional fluorouracil, leucovorin, oxaliplatin, and irinotecan (FOLFOXIRI) compared with infusional fluorouracil, leucovorin, and irinotecan (FOLFIRI) as first-line treatment for metastatic colorectal cancer: the Gruppo Oncologico Nord Ovest. J Clin Oncol. 2007; 25(13): 1670–1676.

17. Simmonds PC, Primrose JN, Colquitt JL, et al. Surgical resection of hepatic metastases from colorectal cancer: a systematic review of published studies. Br J Cancer. 2006; 94(7) 982–999.

18. Cummings LC, Payes JD, Cooper GS. Survival after hepatic resection in metastatic colorectal cancer: a population-based study. Cancer. 2007; 109(4): 718–726.

19. US Department of Health and Human Services. Health, United States, 2006. Centers for Disease Control and Prevention and National Center for Health Statistics. 2006.

20. Fortner JG, Lincer RM. Hepatic resection in the elderly. Ann Surg. 1990; 211(2): 141–145.

21. Koperna T, Kisser M, Schulz F. Hepatic resection in the elderly. World J Surg. 1998; 22(4): 406–412.

22. Menon KV, Al Mukhtar A, Aldouri A, et al. Outcomes after major hepatectomy in elderly patients. J Am Coll Surg. 2006; 203(5): 677–683.

23. Ferrero A, Vigano L, Polastri R, et al. Hepatectomy as treatment of choice for hepatocellular carcinoma in elderly cirrhotic patients. World J Surg. 2005; 29(9): 1101–1105.

24. Aldrighetti L, Arru M, Caterini R, et al. Impact of advanced age on the outcome of liver resection. World J Surg. 2003; 27(10): 1149–1154.

25. Aldrighetti L, Arru M, Catena M, et al. Liver resections in over-75-year-old patients: surgical hazard or current practice? J Surg Oncol. 2006; 93(3): 186–193.

26. Cescon M, Grazi GL, Del Gaudio M, et al. Outcome of right hepatectomies in patients older than 70 years. 2003; 138(5): 547–552.

27. Cosenza CA, Hoffman AL, Podesta LG, et al. Hepatic resection for malignancy in the elderly. Am Surg 1995; 61(10): 889–895.

28. Aalami OO, Fang TD, Song HM, Nacamuli RP. Physiological features of aging persons. Arch Surg. 2003; 138(10): 1068–1076.

29. Kimura F, Miyazaki M, Suwa T, Kakizaki S. Reduction of hepatic acute phase response after partial hepatectomy in elderly patients. Res Exp Med (Berl). 1996; 196(5): 281–290.

30. Ettorre GM, Sommacale D, Farges O, et al. Postoperative liver function after elective right hepatectomy in elderly patients. Br J Surg. 2001; 88(1): 73–76.

31. Grande L, Rull A, Rimola A, et al. Outcome of patients undergoing orthotopic liver transplantation with elderly donors (over 60 years). Transplant Proc. 1997; 29(8): 3289–3290.

32. Tisone G, Manzia TM, Zazza S, et al. Marginal donors in liver transplantation. Transplant Proc. 2004; 36(3): 525–526.

33. Balducci L. Aging, frailty, and chemotherapy. Cancer Control. 2006; 14(1): 7–12.

34. Pope D, Ramesh H, Gennari R, et al. Pre-operative assessment of cancer in the elderly (PACE): A comprehensive assessment of underlying characteristics of elderly cancer patients prior to elective surgery. Surg Oncol. 2006; 15(4): 189–197.

35. Audisio RA, Zbar AP, Jaklitsch MT. Surgical management of oncogeriatric patients. J Clin Oncol. 2007; 25(14): 1924–1929.

36. Gruttadauria Doria C, Vitale CH, et al. Preliminary report on surgical technique in hepatic parenchymal transection for liver tumors in the elderly: a lesson learned from living-related liver transplantation. J Surg Oncol. 2004; 88(4): 229–233.

37. Mazzoni G, Tocchi A, Miccini M, et al. Surgical treatment of liver metastases from colorectal cancer in elderly patients. Int J Colorectal Dis. 2007; 22(1): 77–83.

38. Zhou L, Rui JA, Wang SB, et al. Clinicopathological features, post-surgical survival and prognostic indicators of elderly patients with hepatocellular carcinoma. Eur J Surg Oncol. 2006;32(7): 767–772.

39. Audisio RA, Veronesi P, Ferrario L, et al. Elective surgery for gastrointestinal tumours in the elderly. Ann Oncol. 1997; 8(4): 317–326.

40. Gayowski TJ, Iwatsuki S, Madariaga JR, et al. Experience in hepatic resection for metastatic colorectal cancer: analysis of clinical and pathologic risk factors. Surgery. 1994; 116(4): 703–710.

41. Zieren HU, Muller JM, Zieren J. Resection of colorectal liver metastases in old patients. Hepatogastroenterology. 1994; 41(1): 34–37.

42. Zieren HU, Muller JM, Zieren J, Pichlmaier H. The impact of patient's age on surgical therapy of colorectal liver metastases. Int Surg. 1993; 78(4): 288–291.

43. Fong Y, Blumgart LH, Fortner JG, Brennan MF. Pancreatic or liver resection for malignancy is safe and effective for the elderly. Ann Surg. 1995; 222(4): 426–434.

44. Brunken C, Rogiers X, Malago M, et al. [Is resection of colorectal liver metastases still justified in very elderly patients?]. Chirurg. 1998; 69(12): 1334–1339.

45. Brand MI, Saclarides TJ, Dobson HD, Millikan KW. Liver resection for colorectal cancer: liver metastases in the aged. Am Surg. 2000; 66(4): 412–415.

46. Zacharias T, Jaeck D, Oussoultzoglou E, et al. First and repeat resection of colorectal liver metastases in elderly patients. Ann Surg. 2004; 240(5): 858–865.

47. Adam R, Laurent C, Poston G, et al. Liver resection of colorectal metastases in elderly patients: is it worthwhile and is there an age limit? Annual Meeting European Surgical Association, 2007.

48. Fong Y, Fortner J, Sun RL, et al. Clinical score for predicting recurrence after hepatic resection for metastatic colorectal cancer: analysis of 1001 consecutive cases. Ann Surg. 1999; 230(3): 309–318.

Health-Related Quality of Life and Palliative Care in Colorectal Liver Metastases

12

Clare Byrne and Mari Lloyd-Williams

Background

The liver is the most frequent site of metastatic spread from colorectal cancer, with more than half of colorectal cancer patients (492,000) dying from their metastases [1]. Until recently the presence of untreated liver metastases in advanced colorectal cancers resulted in a mean survival of only 8 months [2, 3], but with new therapeutic agents the mean life expectancy has now increased to 21 months [4]. Access to multi-modal therapy (e.g., ablative techniques) may also contribute to increased length of life, although the impact of such treatments on survival remains uncertain in the lack of prospective randomised trials demonstrating any advantage over palliative chemotherapy [5].

The recent trend of longer survival rates has prompted a marked interest in reviewing and refining the contribution of health-related quality of life (HRQoL) outcome measures of palliative treatment in advanced colorectal cancer. This seems to have been strengthened following a systematic review and meta-analysis of trials comparing palliative chemotherapy and supportive care undertaken by the Colorectal Cancer Collaborative [6]. HRQoL data in relation to palliative chemotherapy trials were considered to be inadequate for a number of reasons including:

- poor consensus over the use of a wide range of different instruments,
- use of tools that were not always validated,
- missing data, and
- lack of clinical interpretation of HRQoL data.

Such major methodological flaws made it impossible to draw any useful conclusions.

Concern has also been expressed that "there are relatively few examples of formal quality-of-life measurement that have influenced individual patient decision making or treatment policies [7]."

In a very proactive response, a number of valuable reviews of HRQoL in colorectal cancer have emerged [8, 9] as well as a prognostic factor analysis of HRQoL data [10]. The synthesis of these suggests that if HRQoL data are to be of clinical value and are going to help both physicians and patients make decisions, there is a need for a consensus on both the design and methods of measurement of HRQoL, and an acknowledgement and application of the important HRQoL methodological issues, including limitations, when planning clinical trials, interpreting outcomes, and presenting results.

Furthermore, the context of the cultural shift in healthcare where patients are becoming increasingly better-informed than their predecessors must also be considered. A recent study concluded that different ways of describing the outcome of treatments for colorectal liver metastases can have a dramatic impact on patient treatment decisions [11]. This observation has implications not only for what is said, but how it is said, and by whom; it emphasises the complexity of information giving and decision making in present-day multi-modal therapy for advanced colorectal cancer. Recent studies in newly diagnosed colorectal cancer patients, though small in sample size, show that only a minority of individuals with advanced colorectal cancer want to be involved in decisions about their care [12, 13, 14]. Patients with colorectal liver metastases present for treatment with the double blow of either synchronous disease or the discovery of recurrence following seemingly curative resection of their primary tumour. In the context of multi-modal therapy for advanced colorectal cancer (where there are difficulties in translating scientific data from clinical trials into layman's language), patient involvement in treatment decisions might be assisted by the inclusion of HRQoL outcome data. One of the challenges is how we inform

C. Byrne (✉)
Advanced Nurse Practitioner, Liverpool Supra-Regional
Hepatobiliary Unit, University Hospital Aintree, Liverpool, UK

cancer patients of the interpretation of HRQoL outcome data, recognising that such data have the potential to provide individualised information strategies.

Another key dimension of cancer care that has influenced HRQoL has been the development of supportive and palliative care services. This multidisciplinary approach refers to a culture of care that has evolved from the hospice movement to help patient and their caregivers cope with life threatening illness through the prevention and relief of suffering by assessment and treatment of their physical, psychological, social, and spiritual needs. This philosophy is summarised in the World Health Organisation definition [15]. Palliative care:

- provides relief from pain and other distressing symptoms;
- affirms life and regards dying as a normal process;
- intends neither to hasten nor postpone death;
- integrates the psychological and spiritual aspects of patient care;
- offers a support system to help patients live as actively as possible until death;
- offers a support system to help the family cope during the patient's illness and in their own bereavement;
- uses a team approach to address the needs of patients and their families, including bereavement counselling, if indicated;
- will enhance quality of life, and may also positively influence the course of illness;
- is applicable early in the course of illness, in conjunction with other therapies that are intended to prolong life, such as chemotherapy or radiation therapy, and includes those investigations needed to better understand and manage distressing clinical complications.

What Is Health-Related Quality of Life?

Our quality of life is as unique as every one of us. Our quality of life is defined by the meaning of events, how we make sense of them and how they all add up to the whole. I well remember a patient who in addition to advanced cancer had advanced neurological disease and could only communicate by blinking—for many professionals and lay people, his quality of life would have been defined at the very least as poor. When asked, this patient responded by blinking to the letters on his communication device that his quality of life was "great". It is very hard to measure and indeed some would argue whether it is something that can be measured at all.

However, measurement of quality life is now a standard part of the majority of clinical trials and increasingly used in clinical practice.

Measurements of Health-Related Quality of Life

All tools used for measuring HRQoL must be multidimensional—they must measure all aspects of HRQoL that may be affected by life limiting illness including the physical, psychological, social, spiritual, and financial domains.

Several one dimensional tools can be used but there is a danger that these may be burdensome to the patients [16]. Such tools may include measures of physical health, socioeconomic status, affect, social support, family, achievement of life goals, etc. All instruments must be useful in the setting in which they are used (e.g. their readability and length are very important) and lastly all instruments must be valid (i.e. the measure what they are purported to measure) and reliable—repeated measures give consistent results. There are many quality of life instruments available and too many to all be included in this chapter.

Instrument should provide subjective data obtained via self-report of patients.

Several early studies of quality of life relied on caregivers, however, this proxy approach has not been found to be reliable [17]. Likewise, a poor correlation between doctors' and patients' HRQoL assessment was found in a study of 128 patients with chemo-resistant colorectal cancer [18], using the Spitzer Quality of Life Index (QLI) [19]. The physicians' scores of the visual analogue scale were 12% lower than the patients' ratings, a discrepancy also found in other studies [20, 21], including palliative medicine [22]. The Spitzer QLI is an example of an early generic HRQoL measure designed as an objective tool to measure quality of life in patients with advanced cancer. The Spitzer QLI questionnaire is comprised of five domains (activity, daily living, health, support, and outlook). Every item has three response categories indicating different levels of functional impairment. Although it was originally developed as an observer rated scale (QLI-*d*), it can also be used as a patient rated scale (QLI-*p*).

The Modular Approach to HRQoL Measures

Recently a trend has developed for more sensitive measures that will increase the capacity to capture small but, clinically important differences in quality of life. Cancer specific instruments address problems specific to a given cancer population.

For the greatest specificity and sensitivity, a modular approach to HRQoL measures is emerging. The modular approach is based on a core (patient self-report) questionnaire covering physical, emotional, and social health issues and symptoms/side effects which are relevant to a broad range of cancer patients. The most widely adopted instruments used in clinical trials involving cancer patients are the European Organization for Research and Treatment of Cancer (EORTC) core QL questionnaire (QLQ-C30) [23], and Functional Assessment of Cancer Therapy-General (FACT-G) [24]. The modular approach is an attempt to meet the competing requirements in oncology trials for outcome measures which are sufficiently generic to allow comparison of data across studies and sufficiently specific and sensitive to address the aspects of patients' experience relevant to specific clinical trial settings. Patients' self complete a core questionnaire, e.g. the QLQ-C30 or FACT-G, supplemented by additional disease or treatment specific modules for particular patient subgroups.

The European Organisation for Research and Treatment of Cancer (EORTC) Core QL Questionnaire (QLQ-C30)

The EORTC QLQ-C30 [23] is a 30 item multidimensional self-report measure of quality of life designed for clinical trials. It addresses the functional (physical, social, cognitive, and emotional) and financial aspects of quality of life as well as symptoms, global health, and global quality of life. Items are scaled from 0 (lowest functional and symptom items) to 100 (best functioning but most symptoms).

The Functional Assessment of Cancer Therapy-General (FACT-G)

The Functional Assessment of Cancer Therapy-General (FACT-G) Questionnaire [24] is a widely used QOL instrument. It comprises 27 questions that assess 4 primary dimensions of QOL: physical well being (PWB; 7 items), social and family well being (SFWB; 7 items), emotional well being (EWB; 6 items), and functional well-being (FWB; 7 items). It uses 5-point Likert-type response categories ranging from 0 = "not at all" to 4 = "very much". The total FACT-G score is the summation of the 4 subscale scores and ranges from 0 to 108.

Four similar phases are involved in the development process for both the EORTC and the FACT modules:

1. generation of relevant quality of life issues from the literature and interviews with appropriate health professionals and patients
2. operationalization of the issues into questionnaire items

3. international pre-testing of the provisional module in the target patient population to identify any revision needed in item content or layout
4. international field testing.

Development of a Questionnaire Module Specific to Patients with Colorectal Liver Metastases

For patients with colorectal liver metastases specific modules have been developed by both the EORTC QLQ-LMC21 and the FACT Hepatobiliary (Hep). Both modules include items concerning disease and treatment related symptoms and side effects, pain, fatigue, nutritional aspects, psychosocial issues, and items about the side effects of treatment. The development work for the EORTC QLQ-LMC21 has been published and the international reliability and validity testing is currently in progress [25]. The FACT Hep has recently been validated [26].

Which questionnaire will be most appropriate for patients with colorectal liver metastases, however, is still uncertain because few large studies have been published using either module. When considering which module is most appropriate for a new study, it has to be considered that the FACT Hep questionnaire has been developed in the United States of America for use in clinical trials with a range of hepatobiliary cancers and not just colorectal liver metastases. Alternatively, the EORTC QLQ-LMC21 has been developed specifically for patients with colorectal liver metastases. It may therefore have greater sensitivity in advanced colorectal cancer because it is focused upon a specific patient population and thus may have greater capacity to provide detailed information on how the different dimensions of an individuals' HRQoL is affected by their metastatic colorectal cancer and its treatment.

Methodological Issues in HRQoL: Implications for Advanced Colorectal Cancer Clinical Trials

Key aspects that need to be addressed when conducting and reporting HRQoL data in trials with colorectal cancer patients have been identified in a systematic review of the reported quality of HRQoL trial methodology [9]. Thirty-one randomised controlled trials involving 9,683 colorectal cancer patients were identified between 1980 and 2003. Nearly all studies involved patients with metastatic disease and principally compared chemotherapy regimes. Although studies were examined from 1980, none had been published before 1990 and most (71%)

had been published since 1998. Overall there was a lack of a uniform approach in terms of measurement and other related aspects of design, analysis, and interpretation.

Lack of A Priori Hypothesis About Possible QoL Changes Before Commencing The Trial

The two issues of stating an a priori *hypothesis* and the choice of a specific HRQoL measure are interwoven, as the choice of measure should be based upon the HRQoL hypothesis being tested. Domains to be explored by an instrument should reflect those which are expected to change in the trial [8, 9].

Rationale for Selecting a Specific Measure

When selecting a HRQoL measure, the most important considerations are the extent to which the selected instrument adequately covers the research question, has adequate psychometric properties (especially responsiveness), and whether it is feasible for use [8].

Baseline Data and Missing Data

Baseline assessment before randomisation is important because knowledge of their group assigned may influence their answers to the questionnaires. Missing data along with lack of baseline data reduce the ability to detect clinically meaningful differences and introduce bias which reduces any attempt at drawing conclusions. Furthermore, the reasons why patients do not complete HRQoL questionnaires could be a source of useful data in itself. Is the patient too ill to fill out the questionnaire or is it an administrative support problem? Whichever way, it creates a pattern of loss of information that is selective. Also, the concern that palliative care research is burdensome to patients has been refuted in a number of recent studies examining the ethical aspects of research [27] with most individuals willing to complete HRQoL measures.

Timing

Timing is a key issue as the methodological challenge of timing in HRQoL assessment in relation to the administration of chemotherapy can cause problems. For example exact timing is difficult to decide when two regimens differ in their time intervals. This is demonstrated in a trial comparing raltitrexed used at 3-week intervals with 5-FU/leucovorin every 4 weeks [28]. A statistically significant benefit in favour of raltitrexed at 2 weeks in several domains and overall HRQoL was described. In a similar trial [21], the EORTC QLQ-C30 was completed by patients at baseline and every 12 weeks thereafter. No differences in HRQoL were found, except a higher rate of perceived nausea/vomiting in the raltitrexed-treated group. These differences between these two similar trials are probably due to the timing of HRQoL distribution in relation to the administration of treatment and expression of toxicities [8].

Data Analysis and Interpretation

Whilst statistical methodology for analysing HRQoL data has developed rapidly over the last few years, there is no consensus on the most relevant way to analyse longitudinal studies. However, obtaining a statistical difference on HRQoL outcome does not necessarily imply a clinically meaningful difference from a patient's perspective [29]. Clinical significance from a patient's perspective is closely related to the difficulty in interpreting the HRQoL data from a given measure. Statistical significance is useful in understanding whether data can be accounted for by chance fluctuations (e.g. patient selection bias), but fails to help in understanding clinical relevance from a patient's perspective in terms of HRQoL changes. It has to be considered that when trials enroll large numbers of patients, small differences in HRQoL may be statistically significant despite apparently small numerical differences in scores of the questionnaire. The issue of whether small numerical differences have a clinical meaning from a patient's perspective has been highlighted as an important aspect for determining the impact of a given treatment [29, 30]. This concept appears to be relatively new in the clinical arena, but this issue should be addressed in future studies to help evaluate the value of HRQoL results.

Reporting Results

The methodological shortcomings identified demonstrate how essential it is to adopt a robust design when planning trials that incorporate HRQoL. However, an encouraging review of the quality of reports of QoL outcomes from Randomized Controlled Trials (RCTs) with an

Table 12.1 Minimum standard checklist for evaluating QoL outcomes in cancer clinical trials [31]

Conceptual:

- A priori hypothesis stated: have the authors identified a predefined QoL endpoint and/or stated expected changes due to the specific treatment
- Rationale for instrument reported: have the authors given a rationale for using a specific QoL measure

Measurement:

- Psychometric properties reported: has a previously validated measure been used or psychometric properties reported or referenced in the article
- Cultural validity verified: has the measure been validated for the specific study population
- Adequacy of domains covered: does the measure cover, at least, the main QoL dimensions relevant for a generic cancer population and/or according to the specific research question

Methodology:

- Instrument administration reported: have the authors specified who and/or in which clinical setting the QoL instrument was administered
- Baseline compliance reported: have the authors reported the number of patients providing a QoL assessment before the start of treatment
- Timing of assessment documented: have the authors specified the QoL timing of assessment during the trial
- Missing data documented: have the authors given some details on QoL missing data during the trial

Interpretation:

- Clinical significance addressed: has the patient's perspective on QoL data being clinically significant and not simply statistically significant been addressed
- Presentation of results in general: have the authors discussed the QoL outcomes, giving any comments regardless of results (either expected or not)

HRQoL end point published between 1990 and 2004, in four cancer types, (breast, colorectal, prostate, and non-small cell lung cancer), [10] does show some promising improvement in the reporting of HRQoL results.

One hundred and fifty-nine RCTs enrolling 58,635 patients were identified and were evaluated according to the "minimum standard checklist" for evaluating HRQoL outcomes in cancer clinical trials [31].

The quality of HRQoL reports, as measured by the overall checklist score was independently related to more recently published studies ($p < 0.0001$). This relationship was independent of industry funded, HRQoL endpoint (primary vs. secondary), cancer disease site, size of the study, and HRQoL differences between treatment arms.

While only 39.3% of studies published between 1990 and 2000 (89/159 RCTs) were identified as being probably robust, thus likely to support clinical decision making, this percentage was 64.3% for studies published after 2000 (70/159 RCTs). Unfortunately, only 4 of 29 randomised trials in colorectal cancer between 1990 and 2004 were robust for key HRQoL methodological factors.

A number of reasons have been suggested to account for the quality improvement of HRQoL reporting in the other cancers included in this study. Although some major guidelines on how to conduct and incorporate HRQoL as an endpoint into clinical trial protocols were published in the early 1990s, the majority of these were published in or after 1997 [32, 33, 34, 35]. Some of the frequently used HRQoL measures developed for a generic cancer population such as the EORTC QLQ-C30, or the FACT-G, whilst

psychometrically robust, were only published in 1993, and cancer site-specific modules such as the breast site specific module (e.g. EORTC QLQ-BR23 and the FACT-B) were published later in 1996 and 1997, respectively. This may have influenced the poor level of previously published reports due to the general unfamiliarity of clinical researchers in oncology with HRQoL issues as well as the lack of methodologically robust questionnaires.

Whilst there appears to have been a substantial quality improvement in the HRQoL reporting of RCTs over time, the impact of this may not be immediately apparent in clinical decision making and treatment policies. However, it is emerging [36] as illustrated in a review of surgical oncology trials where it was found that HRQoL outcomes influenced treatment decisions or provided valuable data for informed consent in 22 (67%) trials reviewed (Table 12.1).

Psychological Distress

Whilst the disease specific modules should improve the sensitivity of the core instrument to monitor the outcome effects of curative, palliative and adjuvant treatments, there has been concern expressed that measures of quality of life such as the EORTC QLQ-C30 and its modules have limited scope for specifically measuring psychological levels in patients with cancer [37]. However, from a methodological perspective the EORTC QLQ-C30 and its site specific modules have not been designed to specifically assess psychological distress, although responses in relation to social and psychological well-being may alert the clinician to undertake a more thorough psychological assessment.

Psychological distress is normal in advanced disease—tears are not a sign of pathology and should not be regarded as such. Hearing and coping with increasing bad news will cause distress which is better expressed, however, anxiety and depression are common concomitants of life-threatening illness and require as thorough an assessment and management as more overt physical symptoms.

It has been shown how psychological, social and spiritual concerns are less likely to be divulged by patients [38], but that these are important aspects of assessment as they are more associated with psychological distress. In a study examining the physical and psychological needs of patients dying from colorectal cancer [39] the prevalence of affective disorders in patients was 22%, which was lower than the 33% reported in studies of patients with advanced breast cancer [40]. Significantly, Maguire et al. [39] also found that caregivers had a greater prevalence of affective disorder than patients. Nevertheless, patients had unresolved problems with pain and several unresolved concerns including their illness, physical strength and inability to do things.

Anxiety

Anxiety following the diagnosis of a serious illness is normal. Most patients have a period of a few days to weeks where they are completely preoccupied by the diagnosis but with support from family and friends are able to adapt and to continue with their daily life. For others, anxiety is overwhelming and causes severe distress. Risk factors include previous anxious predisposition, poor social support and social isolation. Often the anxiety is related to fear of illness and death, but anxiety itself causes physical symptoms, which leads to a vicious circle of thought processes. Anxious patients, like depressed patients, tend to selectively remember the more "threatening" information given to them and often the process of explanation can be therapeutic in itself.

It is always worth considering medical causes in patients who present with anxiety—e.g. uncontrolled pain, medication, e.g. steroids; alcohol and benzodiazepine withdrawal and thyrotoxicosis.

Patients may be reluctant to give a true history of how they feel and history may need to obtained from friends or relatives. The examination often reveals that the patient has been tearful, unable to think of anything other than their illness. They will invariably have a disturbance of sleep and eating with autonomic disturbance, e.g. bowel

disturbance. Anxiety may be present all the time or come in episodes—so called panic attacks. Anxiety and depression have a high concordance and may be part of the same illness—symptoms of depression should also be uncovered and addressed.

Prevention is always better than cure—much anxiety could be prevented by better organisation of services for patients with cancer. Informing patients of the results of investigations as soon as possible, ensuring that all information is communicated between primary and secondary care and that those caring for patients with cancer possess good communication skills can all minimise morbidity. Explanation and information are essential components of treatment. All patients benefit from psychosocial support. An appropriately trained specialist nurse or psychologist can provide this. Often patients benefit from a short-acting benzodiazepine to relieve intense autonomic features of anxiety. Other medications, e.g. beta blockers may also help to remove some of the somatic symptoms while other measures are taking place. It is important that fears are addressed and that they are discussed with the patient. Anxiety management groups or individual anxiety management can also be therapeutic and are often offered under the supervision of a liaison psychiatry service. Complementary therapies, e.g. aromatherapy and massage and specific interventions, e.g. hypnosis, relaxation and imagery are all of benefit. Referral to a day centre can similarly reduce the sense of isolation of a patient and offer support for the family.

A persistently anxious patient is very demanding for the family and friends who may also need a lot of support in knowing how to encourage the patient. Other issues, e.g. spiritual fears may be a source of great anxiety and also need to be addressed.

Anxiety that does not resolve or that is persistent requires intervention from specialists who can offer advice to the patients and to others involved in their care. Most patients with a combination of approaches do respond and their anxiety improves. Anxiety and agitation during the last few weeks and days of life is distressing for the patient, relatives and staff. Even the very ill patient can derive great benefit from being encouraged to share their fears and anxieties with others. At this stage there may be concerns over previous experiences or rifts in the family and a visit from a family member who has not visited for months or even years is often found to ease the distress.

Depression

Depression is a common symptom in palliative care affecting one in four patients and can occur at any time during a cancer illness. The so-called crisis points are at diagnosis, recurrence and when patients are told that their illness is terminal—peaks in psychiatric morbidity occur at these points. Several factors are thought to be precipitant of depression, i.e. poor communication, social isolation, lack of social support, physical dependence and strained relationships within the family. Although it has always been thought that females are at a higher risk of depression, it appears that males and females are at equal risk. However, younger patients with cancer are at a greater risk of developing depression and other psychiatric morbidity.

Depression can present in a variety of ways, e.g. agitation, retardation and withdrawal. Patients are often reluctant to disclose their feelings of low mood for fear of being thought a "bad" or "difficult patient" or because they may fear troubling or upsetting their doctor. It is important therefore that depression is acknowledged and thought about in palliative care as much as the assessment of pain or nausea.

One of the main difficulties is distinguishing between depression and sadness—all patients can be expected to be sad at the end of life. What may be useful indicators that a patient is depressed? Feelings of overwhelming hopelessness and helplessness, guilt and thoughts of self-harm are all thought to be useful indicators of depression.

Assessing for depression is difficult when a patient has a terminal illness—asking patients how they have felt in their mood or their spirits over the last week or a general "How are you feeling in yourself?" may be the opening the patient needs. Asking about previous history of depression and also establishing the patient's fears should also be part of the examination.

The management of depression in palliative care patients is in many ways similar to other patients in primary care, but time is frequently shorter.

Explaining to the patients and their relatives that depression is common in cancer can itself be part of the healing process and many patients do feel they are somehow not coping as they should. Trying to uncover what is really bothering the patient, i.e. in terms of their families, their disease or mode of death can also help to lessen the feelings of isolation associated with depression. Whilst psychological support is of course vital, there is no evidence to suggest that counselling is effective for these patients, and antidepressant therapy is indicated.

The selective serotonin reuptake inhibitors (SSRIs) appear to cause fewer side effects in the terminally ill and are also safer in overdose. The main reason for antidepressant therapy to be ineffective is that it is commenced too late in the patient's illness or problems with compliance—considerable encouragement may be required to enable a patient to persevere with medication whilst waiting for a therapeutic benefit. It is suggested that, if possible, treatment should be maintained for at least 3 months. Patients may benefit from support from community nurses or palliative care specialist nurses and referral to a psychologist may be helpful. Complementary therapies, e.g. aromatherapy or relaxation can also enhance a feeling of well-being and be of benefit to the patient.

Screening for Depression

There are many tools available for screening depression in patients with advanced cancer. It must be remembered that tools can only serve to indicate which patients may be depressed and need to be further assessed. When considering which tool to use, there are four parameters which are useful to know. The *sensitivity* of a test is the probability that it will produce a true-positive result when a patient is depressed (as compared to a reference or "gold standard"). The *specificity* of a test is the probability that a test will produce a true-negative result when a patient is not depressed (as determined by a reference or "gold standard"). The *positive predictive value* (PPV) of a test is the probability that a person is depressed when a positive screening test result is observed. The *negative predictive value* (NPV) of a test is the probability that a person is not depressed when a negative test result is observed. Most often these results are given as percentages and clearly for a test to be applicable it needs to have values for these parameters which are as high as possible.

Hospital Anxiety and Depression Scale (HADS)

This scale was devised to be used with patients who had a medical illness. It has 14 items, 7 relating to anxiety and 7 to depression; each response is given a score of 0–3, with the most negative response gaining the highest score [41]. The HADS is widely used in clinical trials and in patients with early cancer but it is not so discriminating in patients with more advanced disease. Studies have shown that in patients with advanced cancer the scale should be used as a combined scale with a cut-off of 19 which has a sensitivity of 68% and specificity of 67% [42].

Edinburgh Depression Scale (EDS)

The Edinburgh depression scale (EDS) [43] contains questions on worthlessness, subjective sadness and suicidal ideation. A study in a population of palliative care patients using the EDS found that a cut-off threshold of 13 had a sensitivity of 79% and specificity of 81% [44, 45].

More recently work has been carried out to abbreviate the Edinburgh scale into a six-item Brief Edinburgh Depression Scale (BEDS). The most valid cut-off for defining a case, using a psychiatric interview as the "gold-standard", was a score of 6 out of 18 on the BEDS which gave a sensitivity of 72% and a specificity of 83% with a PPV of 65.1% and NPV of 87.1% [46].

Social Functioning and Quality of Life

Several social factors give life meaning and purpose—relationships, home, occupation, family, income, role within community. Life threatening illness is a series of losses and each of these can impact on QoL. The impact of serious illness on relationships often pulls couples and families together but equally can pull them apart, especially if illness is accompanied by loss of income. How can social issues that impinge on quality of life be addressed—being open to them—enquiring gently and sensitively to issues such as how a family is managing financially; offering referral to social worker or someone who can help ensure that family are coping financially. Working albeit in a part-time capacity can also help maintain social integrity and self-esteem. Many people feel compelled to give up work upon the diagnosis of serious illness when perhaps with some encouragement and negotiation with their employer they could have retained some sort of link with their place of employment. Social isolation—for some people this can cause the greatest pain. Everyone is out at work during the day and they are stuck at home or in yet another outpatient appointment. Referral to hospice day care or to hospice drop-ins can do much to lessen this isolation and give much peer support to the patient and their families.

Spiritual Aspects of Quality of Life

There is increasing acknowledgement of the importance of recognising spiritual needs in all people regardless of whether they profess a faith. Spiritual care is engaging with a patient to find what in their life gives them meaning. This may be identified as the closeness of family relationships, the friendships with another, walking in the countryside on a beautiful spring day or regular attendance at their place of worship. Spiritual care is not solely the role of the chaplain—patients frequently disclose their most intimate spiritual concerns to those who they feel closest to and this can include the chemotherapy nurse, the health care support worker who is helping them wash or the person who is delivering their meals on wheels.

Being open, showing acceptance and a willingness to be alongside whilst acknowledging that there are no answers to the big questions—Why me? Why now? in itself can be so comforting and affirming at times of great distress.

Predictive Value of Qol Parameters: The Emergence of Social Functioning

Evidence is beginning to show that baseline HRQoL scores may be a prognostic factor for survival. One of the largest multivariate analyses, conducted on 3,825 patients with metastatic colorectal cancer [47], recently identified four key biomedical variables (performance status, white blood cell count, alkaline phosphatase and the number of involved metastatic sites) as clinical determinants of survival. This study, however, did not take into account patient-reported HRQoL data as possible prognostic factors. Using this latter evidence as a benchmark against which to test the possible independent prognostic value of baseline HRQoL data, Efficace et al. investigated this issue in 299 advanced colorectal patients undergoing 5-FU-based chemotherapy [48].

In addition to HRQoL data, a number of traditional clinical indicators were also analysed. It was found that the final multivariate Cox regression model retained four variables as independent prognostic factors for survival. These were as follows:

- white blood cell count (WBC) with a hazard ratio (HR) of 1.961 (95% CI, 1.439–2.672; $p < 0.001$),
- alkaline phosphatase with $HR = 1.509$ (95% CI, 1.126–2.022; $p = 0.005$),
- number of sites involved with $HR = 1.108$ (95% CI, 1.024–1.198; $p = 0.01$),
- the patient's score on the social functioning scale of the EORTC QLQ-C30 with $HR = 0.991$ (95% CI, 0.987–0.996; $p < 0.001$) which translates into a 9% decrease in the patient's hazard of death for any 10 point increase.

The independent prognostic importance of social functioning and the stability of the final Cox regression model were also internally validated, thus lending further credit to this evidence. In an attempt to validate this model on an independent sample of advanced colorectal cancer patients with similar clinical characteristics, Efficace et al. confirmed previous results [49]. Overall, this evidence suggests that social functioning is a very sensitive HRQoL parameter in this population. This finding is important when taking into account that colorectal cancer patients may specifically experience long-lasting pain and a reduction in functional and social well-beings [50]. However, further research is needed to confirm this finding in other groups.

In a recent large population-based study using the EORTC QLQ-C30 to compare long-term HRQoL issues between colorectal cancer patients and the general population, social functioning was the most impaired functioning scale [51]. It could be argued that these data could lend support to the sensitivity of the social functioning scale as measured by the EORTC QLQ-C30 in picking up key HRQoL aspects in colorectal cancer patients.

However, the issue of the prognostic value of patients' reported HRQoL parameter is still challenging as the mechanism underlying the association between HRQoL parameters and length of survival in advanced cancer patients is not yet entirely clear. At present, the most plausible explanation is that underlying severity of the disease is better reflected by patients' own health status judgment than by a number of previously known traditional prognostic biomedical indicators [52]. Within this framework, patients' scores on HRQoL questionnaires might reflect an early perception of the severity of the disease, thus, patients who report worse HRQoL scores are simply those with worse underlying disease [53]. This hypothesis is supported by prognostic studies in patients with upper gastrointestinal cancer, where baseline fatigue scores and physical function predict both short- and long-term survivals after adjusting for known clinical and HRQoL baseline variables [54, 55].

Whilst the evidence of the independent prognostic value of HRQoL parameters is emerging in the advanced disease setting, further research will definitely have to focus on how this information can be integrated into routine clinical practice and clinical research. As an example, this information can potentially be used to facilitate clinical decision making in palliative treatment settings (e.g. to provide more tailored and timely interventions) and could also have important implications for the stratification of patients into risk groups for future trials with patients with advanced colorectal cancer [48].

Inclusion of other relevant modules in future research such as those currently under development which assess for example levels of fatigue (e.g. EORTC QLQ-FA-R15) may contribute to a greater understanding of the wider dimensions of social functioning.

Liver Metastases and Palliative Care: Advanced Stages

When cancer is first detected, about half of all patients will have evidence of metastatic disease, with a probable high incidence of undiagnosed, occult metastases.

Treatment available depends on the primary cancer, and this is an important information issue for patients and their caregivers; it needs to be actively addressed by healthcare professionals, to ensure that patients understand why oncological palliative treatment options might, or might not, be available to them. For example, surgery is not a treatment option for liver metastases in the presence of pancreas cancer or breast cancer, but may be considered in colorectal cancer or for lung metastases in soft tissue sarcoma.

In advanced stages treatment may not be appropriate and efforts are directed at symptom control. Some patients with extensive liver metastases and profound jaundice are remarkably symptom free. In some cases, there are no symptoms, but when symptoms occur, they may include:

- Weight loss
- Pain, usually in the right upper quadrant of the abdomen
- Jaundice
- Nausea
- Poor appetite
- Pruritus

Pain

Pain is caused by stretching of the liver capsule and can usually be palliated effectively by the use of either nonsteroidals (e.g. Ibuprofen) or with steroids (e.g. Dexamethasone). Dexamethasone is prescribed at a dose of 6 mg with efforts made to reduce the dose where possible. The advantages of Dexamethasone is that it also relieves nausea and poor appetite and may actually improve jaundice by reducing some of the oedema associated with liver metastases which encroach on the common bile duct. Opiates can also be effective for liver capsule pain.

Jaundice

Symptomatic jaundice can sometimes be relieved by biliary stenting which is a relatively noninvasive procedure and can give effective palliation for some months.

Jaundice can be very distressing for the patient and their family—it is a constant and very frightening reminder that their disease is progressing.

Nausea

Nausea with liver metastases is mainly due to biochemical disturbance. The most effective antiemetic in this case is

Haloperidol—there is no benefit in splitting the dosage so a single night time dose of 1.5—5 mg depending on the age and weight of the patient can be prescribed. Dexamethasone also is very effective in the palliation of nausea as stated above. For resistant nausea and vomiting, Methotrimeprazine 6.25– 12.5 mg nocte can also be very effective and as with Haloperidol can also be given in a syringe driver. Antiemetics should be prescribed regularly as well as "as needed" and the route of administration should be considered. If oral absorption is likely to be affected by persistent vomiting, a continuous subcutaneous infusion (CSCI) is most appropriate.

Pruritus

The accumulation of bile salts often causes persistent pruritus. Again, the treatment of this is symptomatic but always consider whether the patient is well enough to be assessed for biliary stenting. Antihistamines can be prescribed for pruritus and are sometimes very effective. Cholestyramine is also used but in patients who are already very unwell and have a poor appetite may find cholestyramine impossible to tolerate. Dexamethasone can relieve some of the obstruction and help the pruritus. A topical preparation of 2% menthol crystals in aqueous cream is an excellent relief for many patients—it can be used whenever required and the cooling action of the menthol provides instant relief from the pruritus. General advice to patients to try to keep cool and to wear loose cotton clothing can also be of help.

Poor Appetite

Most patients with liver metastases complain of poor appetite. The accumulation of toxins and general deterioration and debility contribute to this symptom. Poor appetite is often a cause of friction between patient and their family who believe that if the patient is not eating this will precipitate their deterioration. It is important to explain to both patients and their relatives that it is the deterioration that is causing the poor appetite and not the other way around. General advice on diet can also help. Advising patients to consider taking four–six small meal type snacks a day rather than conventional three meals can help. Taste may well change so patients may prefer eating more spicy or sharper foods and again reassuring that it does not matter what is eaten or when as long as the patient is enjoying some food intake. Relatives may try to overload patients with food therefore suggesting that a

tea plate or dessert plate is used instead of the conventional dinner plate for a meal thereby giving smaller portions and also giving patient the satisfaction of being able to possibly enjoy a small meal in this way. Steroids (e.g. Dexamethasone) can improve appetite as can, for example, Megace. It is common practice to prescribe nutritional drinks but in our experience patients rarely tolerate such drinks and they are seldom used by patients. To try to improve calorific intake, suggest to relatives that they use full cream milk, butter and add cream, for example, to soups/puddings, etc. High-calorie powders which are very soluble and can be added to normal food, e.g. Maixjul super soluble can also be helpful in these situations.

Confusion and the Terminal Phase

Invariably, as the liver metastases progress, patients become confused: this is often more disturbing for their relatives than for the patient themselves who may be unaware. Confusion is often accompanied by difficulty in taking oral medication and it is important to consider using a syringe driver sooner rather than later to ensure that patients are kept comfortable and that symptoms are well managed. Diamorphine together with Methotrimeprazine which is an effective antiemetic as well as anxiolytic can be used. At this stage there is no value in continuing with Dexamethasone subcutaneously. Information needs to be given honestly, but always with the assurance that symptoms can be palliated. "There is nothing more that can be done to help you" is both cruel and untrue and should never be said. In addition to communicating with patients and relatives, it is also important to communicate what has been told to patients and management decisions, both within the hospital team and to primary care colleagues to ensure that patients receive a consistent message.

Caregivers and Palliative Care in Liver Metastases

There is a need to involve family members and caregivers at all stages of the patient's cancer journey with consequences for their psychological health if excluded. Evidence is emerging that caregivers' information needs may be different to patients, and that understanding details related to the patient's illness can help caregivers cope. Fear of not knowing what to do or expect seems to increase caregiver stress, as does poor coordination of care [56]. Acknowledging and anticipating caregivers' needs through information and education seem to be key issues.

In the final stages, caregivers will often be very fearful of what may happen and it is important to inform them that the body is shutting down and that over a period of time the patient will not want to take any food, and will be spending increasing amounts of time in bed. Most patients with liver metastases become comatose and die very peacefully. It is also important to ask the relatives how they are coping and what can be done to help them. If the patient is at home, they should be offered daily visits by the district nurses who can also advise on equipment that may be required.

Summary

The assessment, measurement and reporting of HRQoL in clinical trials in advanced colorectal cancer do appear to be improving, with new insights into the positive and negative aspects of various palliative treatments not previously provided by traditional outcomes. However, assessment of HRQoL as a valid outcome in advanced colorectal cancer is in need of further methodological refinement before this parameter can be regarded as being fully established with respect to its ability to provide useful data unequivocally.

It is anticipated that developments such as the liver metastases module EORTC (QLQ-LMC21) questionnaire will increase the sensitivity to change and will provide essential HRQoL information regarding the use of treatments in both the curative and palliative settings. It is also encouraging to see that evidence is emerging that social functioning is a very sensitive HRQoL parameter in this palliative population. This finding is important when taking into account that colorectal cancer patients may specifically experience long-lasting pain and a reduction in functional and social well-beings. However, further research is needed and the inclusion of other measures such as fatigue (e.g. EORTC QLQ-FA-R15), and measures of psychological distress (e.g. Brief Edinburgh Depression Scale [BEDS] 2007) may confirm the sensitivity of this finding and contribute further to our knowledge about HRQoL.

As illustrated, the inclusion of HRQoL assessment in a clinical trial setting requires important methodological planning. Thus, easy-to-use, simple tools such as shown in Table 12.1 might be of great help in guiding investigators on the basis of minimum criteria and may promote this improved standard of reporting which may in turn further bridge the gap between HRQoL research and clinical practice.

In advanced colorectal cancer, time may be limited and the palliative care needs of caregivers should be included in any assessment of quality of life. Increasing evidence demonstrates the need to involve family members and caregivers at all stages of the patient's cancer journey with consequences for their psychological health if excluded.

References

1. Stewart BW, Kleihues P. World Health Organisation. World Cancer Report. Lyon: IARC Press; 2003.
2. Hugh TJ, Kinsella AR, Poston GJ. Management strategies for colorectal liver metastases Part I. Surg Oncol. 1997; 6(1): 19–30.
3. Poston GJ. Surgical strategies for colorectal liver metastases. Surg Oncol. 2004; 13: 125–136.
4. Meyerhardt JA, Mayer RJ. Systemic therapy for colorectal cancer. New Eng J Med. 2005; 352: 476–87.
5. Poston GJ. Radiofrequency ablation of colorectal liver metastases: where are we really going? J Clin Oncol. 2005; 23: 1342–1344.
6. Simmonds PC. Palliative chemotherapy for advanced colorectal cancer: systematic review and meta-analysis. Colorectal Cancer Collaborative Group. Br Med J. 2000; 341: 531–535.
7. Levine MN, Ganz PA. Beyond the development of quality of life instruments: where do we go from here? (Editorial) J Clin Oncol. 2001; 19: 4224–4237.
8. Conroy T, Bleiberg H, Glimelius B. Quality of life in patients with advanced colorectal cancer: what has been learnt? Eur J Cancer. 2003; 39: 287–294.
9. Efficace F, Bottomley A, Vanvoorden V, Blazeby JM. Methodological issues in assessing health related quality of life in colorectal cancer patients in randomised controlled trials. Eur J Cancer. 2004; 40: 187–197.
10. Efficace F, Osoba D, Gotay C, et al. Has the quality of health-related quality of life reporting in clinical trials improved over time? Towards bridging the gap with clinical decision making. Ann Oncol. 2007; 18: 775–781.
11. Martin RCG, Studts JL, McGuffin SA, et al. Method of presenting oncology treatment outcomes influences patient treatment decision-making in metastatic colorectal cancer. Ann Surg Oncol. 2006; 13: 86–95.
12. Sanders T, Skevington S. Participation as an expression of patient uncertainty: an exploration of bowel cancer consultations. Psycho-oncology. 2004; 13: 675–88.
13. Beaver K, Bogg J, Luker KA. Decision making role preferences and information needs: a comparison of colorectal and breast cancer. Health Expectations. 1999; 2: 266–276.
14. Beaver K, Jones D, Susnerwala S, et al. Exploring decision making preferences of people with colorectal cancer Health Expectations. 2005; 8: 103–13.
15. World Heath Organisation. Definition of Palliative Care WHO: Geneva; 2002.
16. Frank-Stromberg M. Single instruments for measuring quality of life. In: Frank-Stromberg M, ed. Instruments for Clinical Nursing Research. Norwalk, Conn: Appleton and Lange; 1988.
17. Macmillan S, Mahon M. Measuring quality of life in hospice patients using a newly developed Hospice Quality of life Index. Qual Life Res. 1994; 3: 437–447.
18. Sloan JA, Loprinzi CL, Kuross SA, et al. Randomised comparison of four tools measuring overall quality of life in patients with advanced cancer. J Clin Oncol. 1998; 16: 3662–3673.
19. Spitzer WO, Dobson, AJ, Hall J. Measuring the quality of life in cancer patients. A concise QL-index for use by physicians. J Chron Dis. 1981; 34: 585–597.

20. Glimelius B, Hoffman K, Graf W, et al. Quality of life during chemotherapy in patients with symptomatic advanced colorectal cancer. The Nordic Gastrointestinal Tumour Adjuvant Therapy Group. Cancer. 1994; 73: 556–562.

21. Cunningham D, Zalcberg JR, Rath U, et al. Final results of a randomised trial comparing "Tomudex" (raltitrexed) with 5-fluorouracil plus leucovorin in advanced colorectal cancer. Ann Oncol. 1996; 7: 961–965.

22. Petersen MA, Larsen H, Pedersen L, et al. Assessing health-related quality of life in palliative care: comparing patient and physician assessments. Eur J Cancer. 2006 May; 42(8): 1159–66.

23. Aaronson NK, Ahmedzai S, Bergman B, et al. The European Organisation for Research and Treatment of Cancer QLQ-C30: a quality-of-life instrument for use in international clinical trials in oncology. J Natl Cancer Inst. 1993; 85: 365–376.

24. Cella DF, Tulsky DS, Gray G, et al. The Functional Assessment of Cancer Therapy scale: development and validation of the general measure. J. Clin Oncol. 1993; 11: 570–579.

25. Kavadas V, Blazeby J, Conroy T, et al. Development of an EORTC disease-specific quality of life questionnaire for use in patients with liver metastases from colorectal cancer. Eur J Cancer. 2003; 39: 1259–1263.

26. Heffernan N, Cella D, Webster K, et al. Measuring health related quality of life in patients with hepatobiliary cancers: the functional assessment of cancer therapy-hepatobiliary questionnaire. J Clin Oncol. 2002; 20(9): 2229–39.

27. Woods S, Beaver K, Luker K. User's views of palliative care services: ethical implications. Nursing Ethics. 2002; 7: 314–326.

28. Cocconi G, Cunningham D, Van Cutsem E, et al. Open, randomised, multicentre trial of raltitrexed versus fluorouracil plus high dose leucovorin in patients with advanced colorectal cancer. J Clin Oncol. 1998; 16: 2943–2952.

29. Osoba D, Rodrigues G, Myles J, et al. Interpreting the significance of changes in health-related quality-of-life scores. J Clin Oncol. 1998; 16: 139–144.

30. Osoba D. A taxonomy of the uses of health-related quality-of-life instruments in cancer care and the clinical meaningfulness of the results. Med Care. 2002; 40(suppl.): III31–III38.

31. Efficace F, Bottomley A, Osoba D, et al. Beyond the development of health-related quality of life (HRQoL) measures. A checklist for evaluating HRQoL outcomes in cancer clinical trials- does HRQoL in prostate cancer research inform clinical decision making? J Clin Oncol. 2003; 21: 3502–3511.

32. Fayers P, Hopwood PM, Harvey A, et al. Quality of life assessment in clinical trials—guidelines and a checklist for protocol writers: the UK Medical Research Council experience. MRC Cancer Trials Office. Eur J Cancer. 1997; 33: 20–28.

33. Osoba D. Guidelines for measuring health related quality of life in clinical trials. Methods and practice. In: Staquet MJ, Hays RD, Fayers PM, eds. Quality of Life Assessment in Clinical Trials. Oxford: Oxford University Press; 1998: 19–35.

34. Sprangers MA, Moinpour CM, Moynihan TJ, et al. Assessing meaningful change in quality of life over time: a users guide for clinicians. Mayo Clin Proc. 2002; 77: 561–571.

35. de-Haes J, Curran D, Young T. et al. Quality of life evaluation in oncological clinical trials—the EORTC model. The EORTC Quality of Life Study Group. Eur J Cancer. 2000; 36: 821–825.

36. Blazeby JM, Avery K, Sprangers M, et al. Health related quality of life measurement in randomised clinical trials in surgical oncology. J Clin Oncol. 2006; 24: 3178–3186.

37. Skarstein J, Aass N, Fossa SD, et al. Anxiety and depression in cancer patients: relation between the Hospital Anxiety and Depression Scale and the European Organization for Research and Treatment of Cancer Core Quality of Life Questionnaire. J Psychosom Res. 2000; 49(1): 27–34.

38. Heaven CM, Maguire P. Disclosure of concerns by hospice patients and their identification by nurses. Palliat Med. 1997; 11: 283–90.

39. Maguire P, Walsh S, Keeling F, et al. Physical and psychological needs of patients dying from colo-rectal cancer. Palliat Med. 1999; 13: 45–50.

40. Hopwood P, Howell A, Maguire P. Psychiatric morbidity in patients with advanced cancer of the breast: prevalence measured by two self-rating questionnaires. Br J Cancer. 1991; 64: 349–352.

41. Zigmund AS, Snaith RP. The Hospital Anxiety and Depression Scale. Acta Psychiatr Scand. 1983; 67: 361–370.

42. Lloyd-Williams M, Friedman T, Rudd N. An analysis of the validity of the Hospital Anxiety and Depression scale as a screening tool in patients with advanced metastatic cancer. J Pain Symptom Management. 2001; 22(6): 990–6.

43. Cox J, Holden J, Sagovsky R. Detection of postnatal depression: development of 10 item Edinburgh Postnatal Depression Scale. Brit J Psychiatr. 1987; 150: 782–786.

44. Lloyd-Williams M, Friedman T, Rudd N. The criterion validation of the EPDS for the assessment of depression in patients with advanced metastatic disease. J Pain Symptom Management. 2000; 20: 259—265.

45. Lloyd-Williams M, Dennis M, Taylor F, Baker I. A prospective study to determine whether it is appropriate to ask palliative care patients "Are you depressed?" BMJ. 2003; 327: 372–373.

46. Lloyd-Williams M, Shiels C, Dowrick C. The development of the Brief Edinburgh Depression Scale (BEDS) to screen for depression in patients with advanced cancer. J Affect Disord. 2007; 99(1–3): 259–64.

47. Kohne CH, Cunningham D, Di Costanzo F, et al. Clinical determinants of survival in patients with 5-fluorouracil-based treatment for metastatic colorectal cancer: results of a multivariate analysis of 3825 patients. Ann Oncol. 2002; 13: 308–17.

48. Efficace F, Bottomley A, Coens C, et al. Does a patient's self-reported health related quality of life predict survival beyond key biomedical data in advanced colorectal cancer? Eur J Cancer. 2006; 42: 42–49.

49. Efficace F, Innominato PF, Bjarnason G, et al. Proceedings of the 14th Annual Conference of the International Society for Quality of Life Research, Toronto, Canada. Qual Life Res. (in press).

50. Ramsey SD, Andersen MR, Etzioni R, et al. Quality of life in survivors of colorectal carcinoma. Cance.r 2000; 88: 1294–303.

51. Arndt V, Merx H, Stegmaier C, et al. Quality of life in patients with colorectal cancer 1 year after diagnosis compared with the general population: a population based study. J Clin Oncol. 2004; 22: 4777–84.

52. Efficace F, Bottomley A. Towards a clearer understanding (HRQoL) parameters in breast cancer. J Clin Oncol. 2005; 23: 1335–6.

53. Coates AS, Hurny C, Peterson HF, et al. Quality of life scores predict outcome in metastatic but not early breast cancer. J Clin Oncol. 2000; 18: 3768–74.

54. Blazeby JM, Williams MH, Brookes ST, et al. Quality of life measurement in patients with oesophageal cancer. Gut. 1995; 37(4): 505–8.

55. Blazeby JM, Metcalf C, Nicklin J, et al. Association between quality of life scores and short-term outcome after surgery for cancer of the oesophagus or gastric cardia. Br J Surg. 2005; 92(12): 1502–7.

56. Beaver K, Luker KA, Woods S. Primary care services received during terminal illness. Int J Palliative Nursing. 2000; 6(5): 220–7.

John Bendelow, Louise Jones, and Graeme J. Poston

Introduction

The clinical course of patients with metastatic carcinoid is highly variable and largely unpredictable [1, 2, 3]. Patients with high tumour burden can remain relatively asymptomatic for years, while others with minimal residual (but non-resectable) disease in the small bowel mesentery can suffer all the symptoms of the carcinoid syndrome without having liver metastases. However, the majority of patients with carcinoid metastatic to the liver will exhibit at least some symptoms of the carcinoid syndrome [1, 2, 3]. These symptoms include facial and sometimes torso flushing which may progress to rosacea and scleroderma [4], and may include the cutaneous manifestations of pellagra [4]. Other symptoms include diarrhoea, breathlessness, and wheezing.

Advanced carcinoid syndrome is characterised by the manifestation of fibrosis [5], which is most significant when affecting the right-sided heart valves [5]. As carcinoid patients are surviving longer, cardiac manifestations now affect two thirds of patients and are proving increasingly to cause the terminal events [1, 5, 6, 7]. Valve replacement surgery can offer significant improvement in both symptoms and quality of life [8, 9].

Detecting Metastatic Carcinoid Disease

Metastatic carcinoid disease frequently presents symptomatically or is found during investigations or laparotomy for the primary tumour. Following apparently curative surgery for primary carcinoid tumour(s), it is good practice to establish radiologic and biochemical baseline parameters to which comparisons can be made as future symptoms evolve.

Ultrasound scanning is relatively cheap, non-invasive, and widely available but operator dependent. Endoscopic ultrasound is useful in planning treatment for primary luminal gut carcinoids [10] and locating pancreatic neuroendocrine tumours [11]. Recent technological advances in computed tomography (CT) and magnetic resonance imaging (MRI), coupled with developments in scinti-graphy using somatostatin analogues (Fig. 13.1), *meta*-iodobenzylguanidine (MIBG) (Fig. 13.2) and positron emission tomography (PET), now allow very precise radiologic evaluation of disease staging [12].

Radiolabelled somatostatin analogue scintigraphy remains presently the gold standard in confirming the location of functioning neuroendocrine tumour tissue [13, 14]. All neuroendocrine tumours possess the ability to express functioning somatostatin receptors of the various receptor sub-groups [15, 16], and radiolabelled identification of such functioning tissue will predict response to treatment using somatostatin analogues [13] (vide infra). Mid-gut carcinoids (by far the commonest) predominantly express somatostatin receptors from sub-group 2 (sst2) [17]. Data now exist to show at least equivalence of technetium-99 [18, 19] and yttrium-86 [20] labelled somatostatin analogues in localisation and treatment planning in advanced carcinoid disease. Nearly 70% of carcinoid tumours will also take up [131]I-*meta*-iodobenzylguanidine (MIBG) [21]. MIBG is a biogenic amine precursor, which is actively taken up by tumours derived from the neural crest and stored in neurosecretory granules [22]. In direct scintigraphy comparisons, MIBG is inferior (50–70% sensitivity) to radiolabelled octreotide (90% sensitivity) in localisation of carcinoid tumours [23].

The role of PET–CT in both localising disseminated cancer, and also in monitoring the disease response to systemic therapies is increasing [24, 25]. Carcinoid-specific

G.J. Poston (✉)
Division of Surgery, Digestive Diseases, Critical Care and Anaesthesia, Centre for Digestive Diseases, University Hospital Aintree, Liverpool, UK

J.-N. Vauthey et al. (eds.), *Liver Metastases*, DOI 10.1007/978-1-84628-947-7_13,
© Springer-Verlag London Limited 2009

130   J. Bendelow et al.

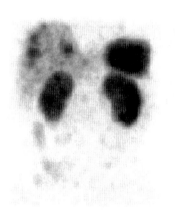

Fig. 13.1 Indium-labelled octreoscan showing active uptake in three carcinoid liver metastases

agents such as 5-hydroxy-ʟ-tryptophan (5-HTP) [24, 25, 26]; 64Cu-1, 4, 8, 11-tetra-azacyclo-tetradecane-*N*, *N'*, *N''*, *N'''*-tetra-acetic acid (TETA-OC) [26] and ^{18}F-dopa [27] have replaced the use of ^{18}F-labelled deoxyglucose (FDG); however when compared, none appears superior to somatostatin analogue scintigraphy in tumour localisation [28, 29].

Treatment of Carcinoid Liver Metastases

Resection

Like many malignant neuroendocrine tumours, carcinoid metastases are mostly indolent, although hepatic metastases commonly present can potentially lead to incapacitating endocrinopathies, pain, and even death [30]. The appropriate timing and efficacy of interventions remain controversial and should always remain within the domain of the multi-disciplinary team [30, 31, 32]. Associated endocrinopathies (and in particular cardiac co-morbidity) result in a higher operative mortality than that seen after resection of typical colorectal metastases [30, 31, 32, 33]. Peri-operative complications can be reduced by the routine administration of continuous octreotide infusion [34].

Five-year survival after liver resection for carcinoid ranges between 47% and 82% [30, 34, 35, 36, 37]. Factors influencing long-term survival after hepatectomy in these patients include size of metastases, radicality of resection, localisation of primary tumour, and extent of liver replacement (Figs. 13.3, 13.4, and 13.5) [30, 34, 35, 36]. Cytoreductive (R2 resection) surgery (using either resectional [38, 39] or ablative [40, 41, 42] techniques) has been advocated for both symptomatic liver [38, 39, 40, 41, 42] and peritoneal disease [43] where resection with curative intent (R0) is not possible. Median symptom-free survival of up to 5 years has been reported following cytoreductive

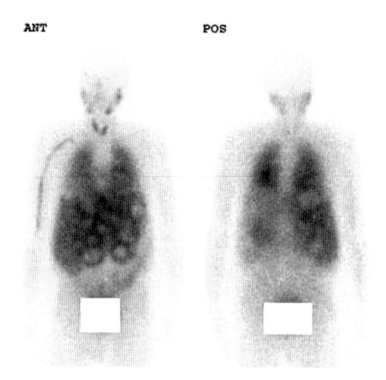

Fig. 13.2 ^{131}I-MIBG scan showing active uptake in multiple neuroendocrine liver metastases with gross hepatomegaly

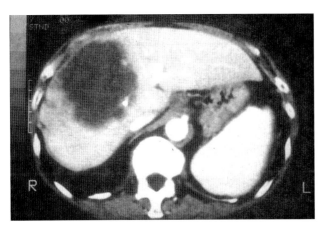

Fig. 13.3 Solitary, giant carcinoid liver metastasis; resectable with curative intent

surgery [38, 39, 44, 45, 46, 47, 48, 49, 50], but it is still too early to interpret survival data objectively from these reports of ablative treatment [40, 41, 42, 43, 44, 45, 46, 47, 48, 49, 50].

Liver transplantation continues to be advocated as a treatment for liver only carcinoid metastases [51, 52]. There have been some recent improvements in operative mortality for this procedure in these patients [51, 52, 53, 54].

Lastly, remains the question of the management of the very rare primary carcinoids of the liver and biliary tract. If technically feasible then resection with curative intent remains the object of treatment [55, 56]. When not feasible, there are anecdotal case reports of long-term survival following orthotopic liver transplantation [56].

Chemoembolisation

Carcinoid liver metastases derive their blood supply exclusively from the hepatic artery. Hepatic artery embolisation (HAI), especially when complemented by the addition of regional chemotherapy (trans-arterial chemoembolisation or TACE), therefore offers a theoretically attractive therapeutic treatment strategy (Fig. 13.6). With comparison to surgical resection in the same centre, outcomes after HAI, a symptomatic improvement [57–59], are not concordant with improved survival [60].

Chemotherapy agents employed during TACE include streptozotocin [61], doxorubicin [62], or various combinations of cytotoxic regimens including ^{90}Y-microspheres [63, 64]. When TACE is compared directly to HAI, the addition of chemotherapy to the procedure does not confer any survival benefit over HAI alone in carcinoid patients [65].

Somatostatin Analogues

The gold standard of care for inoperable symptomatic carcinoid patients remains the long-term therapy using somatostatin analogues [66]. Two analogues, octreotide and lanreotide are now widely available commercially, and both can be administered as depot long-acting preparations [67].

Symptomatic response to long-term octreotide correlates closely with radiolabelled octreotide scintigraphy positivity [68]. There are now a number of reports of good long-term (up to 5 year) compliance (with good symptomatic improvement) of patients on long-acting (LAR) octreotide [69], although patients need to be monitored regularly to

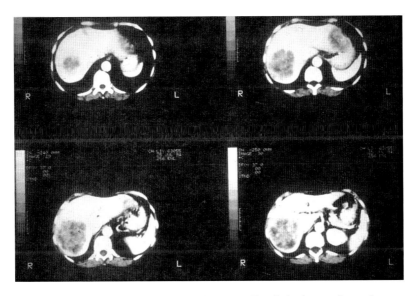

Fig. 13.4 Multiple, but resectable (R2) carcinoid liver metastases. Surgery offers little chance of cure, but a good prospect for long-term symptom-free survival

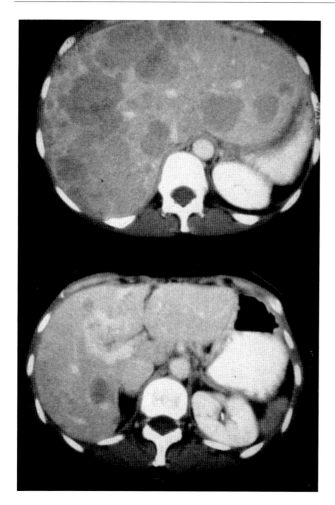

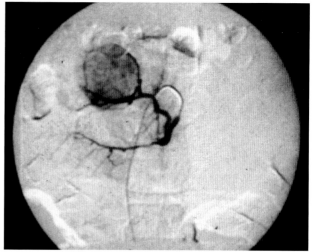

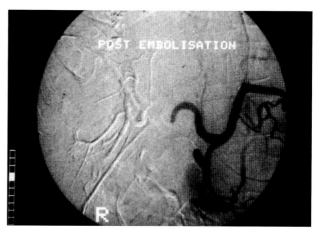

Fig. 13.5 Unresectable, multiple carcinoid liver metastases where there is no role for surgical resection

Fig. 13.6 Unresectable carcinoid liver metastases at angiography, before (**A**) and after (**B**) chemoembolisation

confirm their ongoing dosage requirements [70]. Interestingly, patients with gastric type 1 carcinoids associated with CAG-A do show a decrease in gastric enterochromaffin-like cell (ECL) hyperplasia (which predisposes to type 1 gastric carcinoid) with commensurate falls in serum chromogranin A, despite no fall in the putative driving force of the ECL hyperplasia, the patients' elevated endogenous serum gastrin levels [71].

Similar results with good symptom control are seen with lanreotide therapy [72, 73]. In prospective crossover evaluations to compare efficacy, patient acceptability, and tolerance no differences were found between octreotide and lanreotide [74].

Targeted Nuclear Treatments

Between 50% and 70% of carcinoid patients have tumours that will actively take up (therefore positive to) MIBG (see Fig. 13.2) [20, 21, 75, 76]. The exact mechanism of MIBG

therapy in the treatment of carcinoid remains unclear. Guanidine is a precursor of dopa in the adrenergic catecholamine synthetic pathway [20]. The uptake of MIBG by neuroendocrine tumours is probably mediated by vesicular monoamine transporters into the tumour cells [77], and interestingly the response to ^{131}I-labelled MIBG is enhanced by pre-treatment with non-labelled MIBG [75]. Good long-term symptomatic control, with decreased demand for somatostatin analogue treatment has now been reported in a number of series [75, 76, 78, 79]. Toxicities include pancytopaenia, thrombocytopaenia, nausea, emesis, and hypothyroidism (as a consequence of ^{131}I treatment) [75, 76, 78, 79].

Targeted labelled-somatostatin analogue therapy (Fig. 13.1) has been limited by difficulties producing a stable association between the analogues and isotopes, which would be effective therapeutically. Currently DOTA-D-Phe1-Tyr3-octreotide (DOTATOC) labelled with either [90]Y [80, 81, 82] or ^{177}Lu appears to be much more stable in clinical use, and early reports indicate a higher response rate than that seen after MIBG therapy [80, 81, 82]. Toxicities include lymphocytopaenia, anaemia, renal impairment, and carcinoid crisis [80, 81, 83].

Systemic Therapies

Somatostatin analogues have proven to be the only systemic therapy effective in the treatment of carcinoid syndrome. Interferon treatment alone [84, 85, 86], or in combination with MIBG [87, 88], has failed to show clinical benefit despite some anecdotal evidence [89]. Outcomes following conventional cytotoxic chemotherapy regimens are limited to phase II studies showing little survival benefit from conventional chemotherapy [90] or taxol derivatives [91, 92, 93].

Recently, interest has turned to the use of the newer targeted biological therapies. Gefitinib (an inhibitor of epidermal growth factor receptor (EGFR)-sensitive tyrosine kinase) inhibits the growth of human carcinoid cells in vitro [94] and along with SU11248 [95], another tyrosine kinase inhibitor, has been demonstrated to stabilise advanced carcinoid tumours in small phase II clinical trials [96]. Preliminary phase II studies of bevacizumab (a human monoclonal antibody to vascular endothelial growth factor) look promising [97, 98], but side effects include increased rates of hypertension and thrombotic events [99]. Lastly, there are preliminary data on the use of imatinib (Gleevec), an inhibitor of platelet derived growth factor [100], bortezomib, a proteosome inhibitor [101], and temsirolimus, a small-molecule inhibitor of the mammalian target of rapamycin (mTOR) [102].

Quality of Life

Quality of life is a multidimensional concept that is increasingly being used as an outcome variable in the evaluation of cancer treatments, with assessments based on subjective evaluations by the patient [103, 104]. While some of the treatments for carcinoid syndrome have been shown to prolong life, the subsequent effect on quality of life is not clear. Quality of survival for these patients who may have to endure years of debilitating symptoms should be considered as important as quantity of survival, and both of these factors should be considered when decisions are made on treatment strategies.

The improving overall prognosis associated with carcinoid tumours, together with complex symptoms and use of multiple treatment modalities, reinforces the need to address quality of life issues in this patient group. The aim of many treatments is to palliate symptoms, or prolong time without symptoms, and so comprehensive assessment of quality of life is often as important as evaluation of symptoms. The absence of a large evidence base of treatment outcomes and resulting side effects specific for this disease indicates the importance of the contribution of quality of life data in aiding decision-making.

The involvement of patients in the decision-making process has emphasised the need to address quality of life in order for the patients to make informed decisions. Survival figures combined with an understanding of how patients perceive symptoms, and how treatment choices and disease progression will affect their quality of life, will greatly assist in the holistic management of this disease.

There is currently no disease specific quality of life score questionnaire for patients with carcinoid disease. Comparatively few reports have been published examining this specific patient group and quality of life [105, 106], with no general conclusion drawn. The only cancer specific questionnaire used in some studies is the EORTC QLQ-C30, but this questionnaire is limited as it does not cover specific carcinoid disease issues such as flushing, abdominal pain, worry that the family cannot cope with the illness, worry that the illness will get worse, and worry about recurrence [107]. In order to address this deficit a disease specific quality of life score questionnaire for patients with neuroendocrine tumours is currently under development by the EORTC quality of life group. This study aims to develop a module for patients with neuroendocrine tumours of the gastro-intestinal tract, in adherence with the modular approach to quality of life (QoL) assessment and guidelines proposed by the EORTC QoL group [103, 108, 109]. Once validated, the module will be an extremely useful tool in measuring the quality of life for this patient group, and will play a valuable part in the future management of carcinoid disease.

References

1. Kulke MH, Mayer RJ. Carcinoid tumors. N Engl J Med. 1999; 340: 858–67.
2. Modlin IM, Sandor A. An analysis of 8305 cases of carcinoid tumors. Cancer. 1997; 79: 813–29.
3. Williams ED, Sandler M. The classification of carcinoid tumours. Lancet. 1963; 1: 238–9.
4. Bell HK, Poston GJ, Vora J, Wilson NJE. Cutaneous manifestations of the malignant carcinoid syndrome. Br J Dermatol. 2005; 152: 71–5.
5. Modlin IM, Shapiro MD, Kidd M. Carcinoid tumors and fibrosis: an association with no explanation. Am J Gastroenterol. 2004; 99: 2466–78.

6. Moller JE, Pellikka PA, Bernheim AM, et al. Prognosis of carcinoid heart disease: analysis of 200 cases over two decades. Circulation. 2005; 112: 3320–7.

7. Connolly HM, Pellikka PA. Carcinoid heart disease. Curr Cardiol Rep. 2006; 8: 96–101.

8. Robiolio PA, Rigolin VH, Harrison JK, et al. Predictors of outcome of tricuspid valve replacement in carcinoid heart disease. Am J Cardiol. 1995; 75: 485–8.

9. Connolly HM, Nishimura RA, Smith HC, et al. Outcomes of cardiac surgery for carcinoid disease. J Am Coll Cardiol. 1995; 25: 410–6.

10. Kobayashi K, Katsumata T, Yoshizawa S, et al. Indications for endoscopic polypectomy for rectal carcinoids and clinical usefulness of endoscopic ultrasonography. Dis Colon Rectum. 2005; 48: 285–91.

11. Anderson MA, Carpenter S, Thompson NW, et al. Endoscopic ultrasound is highly accurate and directs management in patients with neuroendocrine tumors of the pancreas. Am J Gastroenterol. 2000; 96: 2271–7.

12. Kaltsas G, Rockall A, Papdogias D, et al. Recent advances in radiological and radionuclide imaging and therapy of neuroendocrine tumours. Eur J Endocrinol. 2004; 151: 15–27.

13. Janson ET, Westlin JE, Eriksson B, et al. [^{111}In-DTPA-D-Phe1] octreotide scintigraphy in patients with carcinoid tumours: the predictive value for somatostatin analogue treatment. Eur J Endocrinol. 1994; 131: 577–81.

14. Savelli G, Lucignani G, Seregni E, et al. Feasibility of somatostatin receptor scintigraphy in the detection of occult primary gastro-entero-pancreatic (GEP) neuroendocrine tumours. Nucl Med Commun. 2004; 25: 445–9.

15. Bousquet C, Guillermet J, Vernejoul F, et al. Somatostatin receptors and regulation of cell proliferation. Dig Liver Dis. 2004; 36(S1): S2–7.

16. Kulaksiz H, Eissele R, Rossler D, et al. Identification of somatostatin receptor subtypes 1, 2A, 3 and 5 in neuroendocrine tumours with specific antibodies. Gut. 2002; 50: 52–60.

17. Hashemi SH, Benjegard SA, Ahlman H, et al. ^{111}In-labelled octreotide binding by the somatostatin receptor subtype 2 in neuroendocrine tumours. Br J Surg. 2003; 90: 549–54.

18. Decristoforo C, Mather SJ, Cholewinski W, et al. 99mTc-EDDA/HYNAC-TOC: a new 99mTc-labelled radiopharmaceutical for imaging somatostatin receptor-positive tumours; first clinical results and intra-patient comparison with 111In-labelled octreotide derivatives. Eur J Nucl Med. 2000; 27: 1318–25,

19. Gabriel M, Decristoforo C, Maina T, et al. 99mTc-N4-[Tyr3]-octreotate versus 99mTc-EDDA/HYNIC-[Tyr3]octreotide: an interpatient comparison of two novel technetium-99m labelled tracers for somatostatin receptor scintigraphy. Cancer Biother Radiopharm. 2004; 19: 73–9.

20. Forster GJ, Engelbach MJ, Brockmann JJ, et al. Preliminary data on biodistribution and dosimetry for therapy planning of somatostatin receptor positive tumours: comparison of (86)Y-DOTATOC and (111)In-DTPA-octreotide. Eur J Nucl Med. 2001; 28: 1743–50.

21. Otte A, Mueller-Brand J, Dellas S, et al. Yttrium-90-labelled somatostatin analogue for cancer treatment. Lancet. 1998; 351: 417–8.

22. Hoefnagel CA, Lewington VJ. MIBG therapy. In: Murray IPC, Ell PJ, eds. Nuclear Medicine, V01.2. Edinburgh: Churchill Livingstone; 1994: 851–64.

23. Kaltsas G, Korbonits M, Heintz E, et al. Comparison of somatostatin analog and meta-iodobenzylguanidine radionuclides in the diagnosis and localization of advanced neuroendocrine tumors. J Clin Endocrinol Metab. 2001; 86: 895–902.

24. Sundin A, Eriksson B, bergstrom M, et al. PET in the diagnosis of neuroendocrine tumors. Ann NY Acad Sci. 2004; 1014: 246–57.

25. Orlefors H, Sundin A, Garske U, et al. Whole-body (11)C-5-hydroxytryptophan positron emission tomography as a universal imaging technique for neuroendocrine tumors: comparison with somatostatin receptor scintigraphy and computed tomography. J Clin Endocrinol Metab. 2005; 90: 3392–400.

26. Anderson CJ, Dehdashti F, Cutler PD, et al. ^{64}Cu-TETA-octreotide as a PET imaging agent for patients with neuroendocrine tumors. J Nucl Med. 2001; 42: 213–21.

27. Koopmans KP, de Vries EG, Kema IP, et al. Staging of carcinoid tumours with 18F-DOPA PET: a prospective, diagnostic accuracy study. Lancet Oncol 2006; 7: 728–34.

28. Virgolini I, Patri P, Novotny C, et al. Comparative somatostatin receptor scintigraphy using in-111-DOTA-lanreotide and in-111-DOTA-Tyr3-octreotide versus F-18-FDG-PET for evaluation of somatostatin receptor-mediated radionuclide therapy. Ann Oncol. 2001; 12(2): S41–5.

29. Kowalski J, Henze M, Schuhmacher J, et al. Evaluation of positron emission tomography imaging using [^{68}Ga]-DOTA-D Phe(1)-Tyr(3)-octreotide in comparison to [^{111}In]-DTPAOC SPECT. First results in patients with neuroendocrine tumors. Mol Imaging Biol. 2003; 5: 42–8.

30. Chamberlain RS, Canes D, Brown KT, et al. Hepatic neuroendocrine metastases: does intervention alter outcomes? J Am Coll Surg. 2000; 190: 432–45.

31. Sutcliffe R, Maguire D, Ramage J, et al. Management of neuroendocrine liver metastases. Am J Surg. 2004; 187: 39–46.

32. Sarmiento JM, Que FG. Hepatic surgery for metastases from neuroendocrine tumors. Surg Oncol Clin N Am. 2003; 12: 321–42.

33. Kinney MA, Warner ME, Nagorney DM, et al. Perianaesthetic risks and outcomes of abdominal surgery for metastatic carcinoid tumours. Br J Anaesth. 2001; 87: 447–52.

34. Touzios JG, Kiely JM, Pitt SC, et al. Neuroendocrine hepatic metastases: does aggressive management improve survival? Ann Surg. 2005; 241: 776–83.

35. Norton JA, Warren RS, Kelly MG, et al. Aggressive surgery for metastatic liver neuroendocrine tumors. Surgery. 2003; 134: 1057–63.

36. Sarmiento JM, Heywood G, Rubin J, et al. Surgical treatment of neuroendocrine metastases to the liver: a plea for resection to increase survival. J Am Coll Surg. 2003; 197: 29–37.

37. Knox CD, Feurer ID, Wise PE, et al. Survival and functional quality of life after resection for hepatic carcinoid metastases. J Gastrointest Surg. 2004; 8: 653–9.

38. Chung MH, Pisegna J, Spirt M, et al. Hepatic cytoreduction followed by a novel long-acting somatostatin analog: a paradigm for intractable neuroendocrine tumors metastatic to the liver. Surgery. 2001; 130: 954–62.

39. Gulec SA, Mountcastle TS, Frey D, et al. Cytoreductive surgery in patients with advanced-stage carcinoid tumors. Am Surg. 2002; 68: 667–71.

40. Dick EA, Joarder R, de Jode M, et al. MR-guided laser thermal ablation of primary and secondary liver tumours. Clin Radiol. 2003; 58: 112–20.

41. Gillams A, Cassoni A, Conway G, Lees W. Radiofrequency ablation of neuroendocrine liver metastases—the Middlesex experience. Abdom Imaging. 2005; 30: 435–41.

42. Atwell TD, Charboneau JW, Que FG, et al. Treatment of neuroendocrine cancer metastatic to the liver: the role of ablative techniques. Cardiovasc Intervent Radiol. 2005; 28: 409–21.

43. Elias D, Sideris L, Liberale G, et al. Surgical treatment of peritoneal carcinomatosis from well-differentiated digestive endocrine carcinomas. Surgery. 2005; 137: 411–6.

44. Jensen EH, Kvols L, McLaughlin JM, et al. Biomarkers predict outcomes following cytoreductive surgery for hepatic metastases

from functional carcinoid tumors. Ann Surg Oncol. 2007; 14: 780–5.

45. Hirai I, Kimura W, Fuse A, et al. Surgical management for metastatic liver tumors. Hepatogastroenterology. 2006; 53: 757–63.

46. Musunuru S, Chen H, Rajpal S, et al. Metastatic neuroendocrine hepatic tumors: resection improves survival. Arch Surg. 2006; 141: 1000–4.

47. Veenendaal LM, Rinkes IH, Lips CJ, van Hillegersberg R. Liver metastases of neuroendocrine tumours; early reduction of tumour load to improve life expectancy. World J Surg Oncol. 2006; 4: 35.

48. Osborne DA, Zervos EE, Strosberg J, et al. Improved outcome with cytoreduction versus embolization for symptomatic hepatic metastases of carcinoid and neuroendocrine tumors. Ann Surg Oncol. 2006; 13: 572–81.

49. Hodul P, Malafa M, Choi J, Kvols L. The role of cytoreductive surgery as an adjunct to the management of metastatic neuroendocrine carcinomas. Cancer Control. 2006; 13: 61–71.

50. Givi B, Pommier SJ, Thompson AK, et al. Operative resection of primary carcinoid neoplasms in patients with liver metastases yields significantly better survival. Surgery. 2006; 140: 891–8.

51. Ahlman H, Friman S, Cahlin C, et al. Liver transplantation for treatment of metastatic neuroendocrine tumors. Ann NY Acad Sci. 2004; 1014: 265–9.

52. Florman S, Toure B, Kim L, et al. Liver transplantation for neuroendocrine tumors. J Gastrointest Surg. 2004; 8: 208–12.

53. Frilling A, Malago M, Weber F, et al. Liver transplantation for patients with metastatic endocrine tumors: single-center experience with 15 patients. Liver Transpl. 2006; 12: 1089–96.

54. van Vilsteren FG, Baskin-Bey ES, Nagorney DM, et al. Liver transplantation for gastroenteropancreatic neuroendocrine cancers: Defining selection criteria to improve survival. Liver Transpl. 2006; 12: 448–56.

55. Knox CD, Anderson CD, Lamps LW, et al. Long-term survival after resection for primary hepatic carcinoid tumor. Ann Surg Oncol. 2003; 10: 1171–5.

56. Fenwick SW, Wyatt JI, Toogood GJ, Lodge JP. Hepatic resection and transplantation for primary carcinoid tumors of the liver. Ann Surg. 2004; 239: 210–9.

57. Gupta S, Johnson MM, Murthy R, et al. Hepatic arterial embolization and chemoembolization for the treatment of patients with metastatic neuroendocrine tumors: variables affecting response rates and survival. Cancer. 2005; 104: 1590–602.

58. Meij V, Zuetenhorst JM, van Hillegersberg R, et al. Local treatment in unresectable hepatic metastases of carcinoid tumors: Experiences with hepatic artery embolization and radiofrequency ablation. World J Surg Oncol. 2005; 3: 75.

59. Strosberg JR, Choi J, Cantor AB, Kvols LK. Selective hepatic artery embolization for treatment of patients with metastatic carcinoid and pancreatic endocrine tumors. Cancer Control. 2006; 13: 72–8.

60. Yao KA, Talamonti MS, Nemcek A, et al. Indications and results of liver resection and hepatic chemoembolization for metastatic gastrointestinal neuroendocrine tumors. Surgery. 2001; 130: 677–82.

61. Dominguez S, Denys A, Madeira I, et al. Hepatic arterial chemoembolization with streptozotocin in patients with metastatic digestive endocrine tumours. Eur J Gastroenterol Hepatol. 2000; 12: 151–7.

62. Roche A, Girish BV, de Baere T, et al. Trans-catheter arterial chemoembolization as first-line treatment for hepatic metastases from endocrine tumors. Eur Radiol. 2003; 13: 136–40.

63. Fiorentini G, Rossi S, Bonechi F, et al. Intra-arterial chemoembolization in liver metastases from neuroendocrine tumors: a phase II study. J Chemother. 2004; 16: 293–7.

64. Dong XD, Yin X, Zeh HJ, et al. Long-term outcome in patients with liver metastases from neuroendocrine tumors treated with chemoembolization. Proc ASCO. 2005; 23: 349S (abstract 4167).

65. Gupta S, Johnson MM, Murthy R, et al. Hepatic arterial embolization and chemoembolization for the treatment of patients with metastatic neuroendocrine tumors. Cancer. 2005; 104(8): 1590–602.

66. Oberg K, Kvols L, Caplin M, et al. Consensus report on the use of somatostatin analogs for the management of neuroendocrine tumors of the gastrointestinal system. Ann Oncol. 2004; 15: 966–73.

67. Rubin J, Ajani J, Schirmer W, et al. Octretide acetate long-acting formulation versus open-labelled subcutaneous octreotide acetate in malignant carcinoid syndrome. J Clin Oncol. 1999; 17: 600–6.

68. Filosso PL, Ruffini E, Oliaro A, et al. Long-term survival of atypical bronchial carcinoids with liver metastases, treated with octreotide. Eur J Cardiothorac Surg. 2002; 21: 913–7.

69. Welin SV, Janson ET, Sundin A, et al. High-dose treatment with a long-acting somatostatin analogue in patients with advanced midgut carcinoid tumours. Eur J Endocrinol. 2004; 151: 107–12.

70. Woltering E, Mamikunian PM, Zeitz S, et al. Octreotide acetate (LAR) dose effect on plasma octreotide levels: impact on neuroendocrine tumor management. Proc ASCO. 2005; 23: 235S (abstract 3177).

71. Fykse V, Sandvik AK, Qvigstad G, et al. Treatment of ECL cell carcinoids with octreotide LAR. Scand J Gastroenterol. 2004; 39: 621–8.

72. Ducreux M, Ruszniewski P, Chayvialle JA, et al. The antitumoral effect of the long-acting somatostatin analog lanreotide in neuroendocrine tumors. Am J Gastroenterol. 2000; 95: 3276–81.

73. Ricci S, Antonuzzo A, Galli L, et al. Long-acting depot lanreotide in the treatment of patients with advanced neuroendocrine tumors. Am J Clin Oncol. 2000; 23: 412–5.

74. O'Toole D, Ducreux M, Bommelaer G, et al. Treatment of carcinoid syndrome: a prospective crossover evaluation of lanreotide versus octreotide in terms of efficacy, patient acceptability, and tolerance. Cancer. 2000; 88: 770–6.

75. Hoefnagel CA, Taal BG, Sivro F, et al. Enhancement of ^{131}I-MIBG uptake in carcinoid tumours by administration of unlabelled MIBG. Nucl Med Commun. 2000; 21: 755–61.

76. Mukherjee JJ, Kaltsas GA, Islam N, et al. Treatment of metastatic carcinoid tumours, phaeochromocytomas, paraganglionoma and medullary carcinoma of the thyroid with (131)I-meta-iodobenzylguanidine [(131)I-mIBG]. Clin Endocrinol. 2001; 55: 47–60.

77. Kolby L, Bernhardt P, Levin-Jakobsen AM, et al. Uptake of meta-iodobenzylguanidine in neuroendocrine tumours is mediated by vesicular monoamine transporters. Br J Cancer. 2003; 89: 1383–8.

78. Sywak MS, Pasieka JL, McEwan A, et al. ^{131}I-meta-iodobenzylguanidine in the management of midgut carcinoid tumors. World J Surg. 2004; 28: 1157–62.

79. Safford SD, Coleman RE, Gockerman JP, et al. Iodine-131 metaiodobenzylguanidine treatment for metastatic carcinoid. Results in 98 patients. Cancer. 2004; 101: 1987–93.

80. Valkema R, Kvols LK, Pawels S, et al. Peptide receptor radiotherapy (PRRT) with [Y-90-DOTA, Tyr3]octreotide: toxicity and efficacy of 4-cycle and single-cycle regimens. Proc ASCO. 2004; 23: 206 (abstract 3046).

81. Kwekkeboom DJ, Teunissen JJ, Bakker WH, et al. Radiolabelled somatostatin analog [177Lu-DOTA0, Tyr3] octreotate in patients with endocrine gastroenteropancreatic tumors. J Clin Oncol. 2005; 23: 2754–62.

82. Kwekkeboom DJ, Mueller-Brand J, Paganelli G, et al. Overview of results of peptide receptor radionuclide therapy with 3 radiolabelled somatostatin analogs. J Nucl Med. 2005; 46: 62S–66S.

83. Davi MV, Bodei L, Francia G, et al. Carcinoid crisis induced by receptor radionuclide therapy with 90Y-DOTATOC in a case of liver metastases from bronchial neuroendocrine tumor (atypical carcinoid). J Endocrinol Invest. 2006; 29: 563–7.

84. Kolby L, Persson G, Franzen S, Ahren B. Randomized clinical trial of the effect of interfer90n alpha on survival in patients with disseminated carcinoid tumours. Br J Surg. 2003; 90: 687–93.

85. Stuart K, Levy DE, Anderson T, et al. Phase II study of interferon gamma in malignant carcinoid tumors (E9292): a trial of the Eastern Cooperative Oncology Group. Invest New Drugs. 2004; 22: 75–81.

86. Wirth LJ, Carter MR, Janne PA, Johnson BE. Outcome of patients with pulmonary carcinoid tumors receiving chemotherapy or chemoradiotherapy. Lung Cancer. 2004; 44: 213–20.

87. Hopfner M, Sutter AP, Huether A, et al. A novel approach in the treatment of neuroendocrine gastrointestinal tumors: additive antiproliferative effects of interferon-gamma and meta-iodobenzylguanidine. BMC Cancer. 2004; 4: 23.

88. Zuetenhorst JM, Valdes Olmos RA, Muller M, et al. Interferon and meta-iodobenzylguanidin combinations in the treatment of metastatic carcinoid tumours. Endocr Relat Cancer. 2004; 11: 553–61.

89. Pape UF, Wiedenmann B. Adding interferon-alpha to octreotide slows tumour progression compared with octreotide alone but evidence is lacking for improved survival in people with disseminated midgut carcinoid tumours. Cancer Treat Rev. 2003; 29: 565–9.

90. Sun W, Lipsitz S, Catalano P, et al. Phase II/III study of doxorubicin with fluorouracil compared with streptozotocin with fluorouracil or dacarbazine in the treatment of advanced carcinoid tumors: Eastern Cooperative Oncology Group study E1281. J Clin Oncol. 2005; 23: 4897–904.

91. Kulke MH, Kim H, Stuart K, et al. A phase II study of decetaxel in patients with metastatic carcinoid tumors. Cancer Invest. 2004; 22: 353–9.

92. Kegel T, Grothe A, Jordan M, et al. Paclitaxel, carboplatin and etoposid (TCE) in the treatment of advanced neuroendocrine tumours. Proc ASCO. 2005; 23: 373S (abstract 4263).

93. Miranda FT, Spigel DR, Hainsworth JD, et al. Paclitaxel/carboplatin/etoposide (PCE) therapy for advanced poorly differentiated neuroendocrine (PDNE) carcinoma: a Minnie Pearl Cancer Network phase II trial. Proc ASCO. 2005; 23: 322S (abstract 4058).

94. Hopfner M, Sutter AP, Berst B, et al. A novel approach in the treatment of neuroendocrine gastrointestinal tumours. Targeting the epidermal growth factor receptor by gefitinib (ZD1839). Br J Cancer. 2003; 89: 1766–75.

95. Kulke M, Lenz HJ, Meropol NJ, et al. A phase 2 study to evaluate the efficacy and safety of SU11248 in patients with unresectable neuroendocrine tumors. Proc ASCO. 2005; 23: 310S (abstract 4008).

96. Hobday TJ, Mahoney M, Erlichman C, et al. Preliminary results of a phase II trial of gefitinib in progressive metastatic neuroendocrine tumors (NET): a phase II Consortium (P2C) study. Proc ASCO. 2005; 23: 328S (abstract 4084).

97. Yao JC, Charnsangavej S, Faria SC, et al. Rapid decrease in blood flow, blood volume and vascular permeability in carcinoid patients treated with bevacizumab. Proc ASCO. 2004; 23: 198 (abstract 3013).

98. Yao JC, Ng C, Hoff PM, et al. Improved progression free survival, and rapid, sustained decrease in tumor perfusion among patients with advanced carcinoid treated with bevacizumab. Proc ASCO. 2005; 23: 309S (abstract 4007).

99. Mares JE, Worah S, Mathew SV, et al. Increased rate of hypertension among patients with advanced carcinoid treated with bevacizumab. Proc ASCO. 2005; 23: 329S (abstract 4087).

100. Carr K, Yao JC, Rashid A, et al. A phase II trial of imatinib in patients with advanced carcinoid tumor. Proc ASCO. 2005; 23: 343 (abstract 4124).

101. Shah MH, Young D, Kindler HL, et al. Phase II study of the proteasome inhibitor bortezomib (PS-341) in patients with metastatic neuroendocrine tumors. Clin Cancer Res. 2004; 10: 6111–8.

102. Duran I, Le L, Saltman D, et al. A phase II trial of temsirolimus in metastatic neuroendocrine carcinomas. Pro ASCO. 2005; 23: 215S (abstract 3096).

103. Aaronson NK, Cull A, Kaasa S, Sprangers M. The EORTC modular approach to quality of life assessment in oncology. Int J Mental Health. 1994; 23: 75–96.

104. Shumaker SA, Naughton MJ. The international assessment of health-related quality of life: a theoretical perspective. In: Schumaker SA, Bernzon R, eds. The International Assessment of Health-Related Quality of Life: Theory, Translation, Measurement and Analysis. Oxford: Rapid Communications of Oxford; 1995: 3–10.

105. Larsson G, Haglund K, Von Essen L. Distress, quality of life and strategies to 'keep a good mood' in patients with carcinoid tumours: patient and staff perceptions. Eur J Cancer Care (Engl). 2003; 12: 46–57.

106. O'Toole D, Ducreux M, Bommelaer G, et al. Treatment of carcinoid syndrome: a prospective crossover evaluation of lanreotide versus octreotide in terms of efficacy, patient acceptability, and tolerance. Cancer. 2000; 88: 770–6.

107. Davies AH, Larsson G, Ardill J, et al. Development of a disease-specific Quality of Life questionnaire module for patients with gastrointestinal neuroendocrine tumours. Eur J Cancer. 2006; 42: 477–84.

108. Aaronson NK, Bullinger M, Ahmedzai S. A modular approach to quality of life assessment in cancer clinical trials. Recent Results Cancer Res. 1988; 111: 231–49.

109. Sprangers MA, Cull A, Groenvold M, et al. The European Organisation for Research and Treatment of Cancer approach to developing questionnaire modules: an update and overview. EORTC Quality of Life Study Group. Qual Life Res. 1998; 7(4): 291–300.

Gastrointestinal Stromal Tumors

14

Dan Byrd and Charles Blanke

Introduction

Gastrointestinal stromal tumors (GISTs) are mesenchymal tumors that can arise anywhere in the GI tract. Stromal tumors of the gastrointestinal tract were formerly thought to be of smooth muscle or neural origin at least partly due to their light microscopic appearance, but more sophisticated microscopy and improved immunohistochemical and molecular techniques have demonstrated that these tumors are a unique pathologic entity arising from the interstitial cells of Cajal (ICC), the pacemaker cells of the gut. Historically, surgery was the only effective therapy for patients diagnosed with GISTs, as these tumors are highly refractory to chemotherapy and probably irradiation. However, GISTs often have oncogenic activating mutations of select receptor tyrosine kinases and drugs that target these receptors have demonstrated marked activity in both the adjuvant and metastatic settings. Despite therapeutic advances to date, however, GIST management needs further enhancement. Areas in question include timing and agent selection for neoadjuvant and adjuvant treatment planning and the role of combined modality therapies such as surgery plus systemic biologic agents in the setting of imatinib resistance. Finally, remaining unanswered is the question of whether other locally directed therapies, particularly those addressed at liver metastases, should be offered to patients up front or in the salvage setting.

Pathology

GISTs may display a wide variety of histologic and cytologic features, though making a specific diagnosis by light microscopy remains relatively straightforward in the

hands of an experienced pathologist. Early pathologic studies described gastrointestinal mesenchymal tumors as originating from smooth muscle [1]. However, electron microscopy showed that most of these tumors lacked smooth muscle differentiation while simultaneously demonstrating that some had neuronal features [2]. Immunohistochemical techniques later defined common, specific staining patterns, including both neuronal and smooth muscle arrangements [3]. With rare exceptions, usually occurring in the esophagus or rectum, mesenchymal tumors of the GI tract often turn out to be GISTs, once appropriate immunohistochemical stains are performed (see below). This has presented a dilemma when examining older data regarding stromal tumors of the gastrointestinal tract, as many tumors previously classified as leiomyosarcomas would likely be described as GISTs using modern techniques.

GISTs appear to arise from the ICC, which form a complex network in the wall of the GI tract associated with Auerbach's plexus, and which give rise to peristalsis through autonomous pacemaker activity [4, 5]. Because of the anatomic location of the ICCs, GISTs tend to arise extraluminally in the GI tract.

Light Microscopy and Immunohistochemistry

By light microscopy GISTs can be classified as epithelioid, spindle cell, or mixed. The differential for tumors with similar appearance includes leiomyomas/leiomyosarcomas, schwannomas, fibroid polyps, and desmoid fibromatosis. In 1998 Sarlomo-Rikala and colleagues noted that almost all GISTs stain positively for KIT (CD117), a receptor tyrosine kinase [6]. Ninety-five percent of GISTs stain positively for KIT, 60–70% for CD34, 30–40% for smooth muscle actin, and virtually 100% have strong expression of PKC-theta. However, immunostaining should be interpreted with caution, as

D. Byrd (✉)
Department of Medicine, OHSU Cancer Institute, Vancouver, BC, Canada

J.-N. Vauthey et al. (eds.), *Liver Metastases*, DOI 10.1007/978-1-84628-947-7_14,
© Springer-Verlag London Limited 2009

melanomas, angiosarcomas, germ cell tumors, and some other carcinomas can be KIT positive, though they typically have morphology and cell surface markers distinct from GIST [7]. Recently, a unique upregulated gene, FLJ10261, was described [8]. FLJ10261 encodes a protein named discovered-on-GIST-1 (DOG-1) [8]. West and colleagues recently assessed samples from 460 soft tissue tumors and 149 GISTs for the presence of DOG-1. Staining for DOG-1 was found in 136 of 139 scorable GIST samples. Only 4 of 438 scorable soft tissue tumor samples were positive for DOG-1. The function of DOG-1 remains unknown.

Molecular Pathology

GISTs tend to have relatively simple cytogenetics. Deletion of chromosome 14 is the most frequent karyotypic abnormality, followed by deletions of chromosomes 22q, 1p, 9p, and 11p [9]. Studies using loss of heterozygosity and comparative genomic hybridization have demonstrated loss of regions 14q11.2-q12 and 14q22-q24, as well as 22q11.21–22, 22q12.3, and 22q13.3 [9]. Additionally, loss of chromosome 9p is associated with both loss of function of p16Ink4a, a cyclin dependent kinase inhibitor, and aggressive behavior [10].

The c-kit gene has 21 exons, coding an extracellular ligand-binding domain, a transmembrane domain, and an intracellular split-kinase domain [11]. The ligand for the encoded protein, KIT, is stem cell factor (SCF) [11]. Binding of SCF to KIT induces receptor dimerization and autophosphorylation, resulting in activation of multiple intracellular signaling cascades including PI-3-K, Jak-STAT, mTOR, Ras-Erk, and phospholipase C [12]. These pathways promote cell growth and survival. Hirota and associates reported that the majority of GISTs harbor activating mutations of c-kit [13]. They collected 58 mesenchymal GI tumors (4 esophageal, 36 gastric, 14 small intestinal, 4 colonic) and demonstrated that 8 definitively identified leiomyomas and 1 schwannoma did not express KIT. Of the remaining tumors, 94% expressed KIT, 82% CD34, and 78% both. c-kit mutations were then found in the juxtamembrane domain of five of six GISTs. Later work has shown that roughly 75% of GISTs have constitutively activating mutations of c-kit, while the 5–7% have activating mutations in a related receptor tyrosine kinase PDGFR-A (see below), and 10% have no detectable mutations.

There are at least five defined sets of c-kit mutations [11]. Most commonly seen are exon 11 mutations, which affect the juxtamembrane domain of the protein and occur in 60–70% of GISTs. Exon 9 mutations affect the extracellular domain, occurring in roughly 10% of cases. Exons 13 and 17 mutations, which affect the kinase domains, are rare. Exon 8 mutations occur in familial GIST, and are exceedingly rare. Roughly one-third of GISTs with non-mutated c-kit have mutations of a homologous receptor tyrosine kinase, the alpha polypeptide of the platelet derived growth factor receptor (PDGFR-A) [14]. PDGFR-A mutations are more common in epithelioid or mixed histologies. Two PDGFR-A mutations have been defined in GIST, which almost never occur in untreated tumors possessing c-kit mutations. Activating mutations in exon 12 affect the juxtamembrane portion of the receptor. Exon 18, which codes the receptor activation loop, is a second, commonly mutated site.

Mutated c-kit is common even in small, incidentally discovered GISTs, which may indicate that mutation is an early event in tumor pathogenesis [15]. Corless and associates sampled 120 GISTs, identifying 13 incidentally discovered tumors less than 1 cm in diameter, all of which lacked mitoses and were morphologically likely to be benign. Tumor lysate DNA was screened for KIT exons 11 and 9 mutations. Ten tumors with exon 11 mutations, and one with an exon 9 mutation were identified. All mutations were similar to documented deletions and point mutations from studies of larger, clinically relevant GISTs. Additionally, transgenic mice expressing mutated constitutively activated KIT develop ICC hyperplasia and cecal tumors morphologically identical to GIST [16]. Thus, c-kit—or by extension PDGFR-A—mutation clearly underlies most GIST oncogenesis.

Epidemiology

GISTs occur at a peak age of 60, and males comprise slightly more than one-half of cases. Most GISTs arise in the stomach (60%), or small intestine (25%); the others originate mostly in the large intestine or rectum, with a small minority scattered throughout the remainder of GI tract, including the retroperitoneum. Most GISTs are sporadic; however, they may be associated with neurofibromatosis type I, Carney triad, and familial gastrointestinal stromal tumor syndrome. However, there are no demonstrated consistent associations between GISTs and other malignancies.

Familial cases result from autosomal-dominant heritable mutations in exons 8, 11, 13, or 17 of c-kit, or exon 12 of PDGFR-A; exon 11 mutations are most common [17]. Familial patients tend to present during their teens, with multifocal GISTs of the stomach and small bowel, as well as hyperpigmented skin lesions. The majority of non-familial pediatric GIST cases lack c-kit or PDGFR-A mutation [18]. Females are predominately affected, and they tend to develop tumors before the age of 20. Carney triad is a clinical association of extra-adrenal paragangliomas, pulmonary chondromas, and multifocal gastric GISTs [19]. Typically this syndrome occurs in young females. Presence of all three tumor types in one patient is rare; most common is the combination of pulmonary chondromas and GIST. Finally, patients with neurofibromatosis type I have a disproportionately high rate of GISTs which tend to strongly express KIT, but lack c-kit mutations [20].

Little historical epidemiological data regarding the incidence and prevalence of GISTs exist. This is partly due to a poor understanding of these tumors' unique identifying features, making a precise classification of GIST difficult until very recently. A retrospective study by Nilsson and colleagues did report data on GIST epidemiology in western Sweden prior to the widespread use of imatinib, the first effective systemic treatment for these tumors [21]. Comprehensive pathology data were gathered from three hospitals covering the period from 1983 to 2000, and from one hospital covering 1993 to 2000. Search indices included all patients with potential GISTs, including GI tract tumors coded as benign or malignant mesenchymal lesions, autonomic or peripheral nervous system lesions, or benign or malignant lesions not otherwise classified. One thousand four hundred and sixty potential cases were initially identified, and 288 were study-defined GIST. The annual incidence of GIST in this study was 14.5 per million inhabitants, which did not vary with time. The prevalence was estimated at 129 cases per million.

Tryggvason and associates reported another major epidemiologic study of GIST performed in Iceland [22]. The records of the two hospital-based pathology programs in the country were searched for all mesenchymal tumors in the digestive tract, mesentery, and omentum. After excluding cases obviously not GIST, each remaining case had one representative block selected for immunohistochemical analysis for CD 117 (c-kit), CD34, desmin, S-100, and SMA. All KIT positive tumors were included in the subsequent analysis. Fifty-seven cases were identified. Based on well-defined population figures, an annual incidence of 1.1 case per 100,000 population was found, which did not vary with time.

Organ Specific Studies

Miettinen and colleagues have cataloged clinicopathologic experience with GISTs arising from throughout the GI tract [23, 24, 25]. They also recently summarized results on pathology and prognosis [26]. Esophageal GISTs are actually quite rare, and leiomyomas represent a far greater fraction of connective tissue tumors. True esophageal GISTs are actually quite aggressive, but this may be because most are quite large and/or have a high-mitotic rate. Gastric tumors are the most common (representing ~50% of GISTs), and they tend to have the best prognosis overall following resection. Indeed, tumors less than 5 cm in size tend not to recur at all. Small bowel GISTs represent about 35% of the total tumors. Small bowel primaries are histologically more homogenous, and they tend to have a higher risk of recurrence, even following complete resection. While exon 11 mutations are still the most common type seen in small bowel GISTs, tumors with exon 9 mutations, which differ prognostically and in response to therapy (see below), arise predominantly in the small intestine (and right colon). Approximately 10% of GISTs arise in the large bowel, and more than half recur if large or if their mitotic rate is high. GISTs have also been described as arising from gall bladder, appendix, esophagus, pancreas, and mesentery/omentum. GISTs arising outside the upper GI tract tend to have spindle cell morphology, but site-specific behavior for these primaries is poorly defined. Omental GISTs can be aggressive, particularly when mitotically active.

Clinical Disease

GIST patients may present with a variety of gastrointestinal symptoms, including abdominal pain, bloating, early satiety, or rarely outright bowel obstruction. Bleeding is most common, and patients commonly present with iron deficiency anemia and fatigue. A significant minority of GISTs are incidentally detected. Additionally, very large tumors can rupture. GISTs tend to metastasize within the abdominal compartment to peritoneum and to the liver. Lymph node spread is rare except in cases of childhood GIST, which comprises a clinical disease distinct from adult cases; adult lymph node involvement occurs in less than 5% of cases. Very advanced disease may eventually spread to the lungs or bones, but this typically occurs in fewer than 1% of cases.

Diagnosis

Imaging

Radiologic examination may aid in GIST diagnosis, as well as assessment following therapy. On CT, GISTs may appear as large heterogeneous masses with non-enhanced areas typically representing necrosis [27]. Additionally, mesenteric and omental implants tend not to enhance with contrast. However, hepatic GIST metastases are hypervascular, and do tend to enhance with contrast; three-phase CT scanning is felt to be the best imaging modality for their assessment.

PET can be used to stage patients, as well as to monitor response to systemic therapy. Its use in surveillance following complete resection of GIST is less clear. Untreated GISTs are exquisitely FDG-PET avid, and PET is felt to be more sensitive than CT in GIST [28, 29]. Indeed, effectively treated tumors may lose FDG uptake within 24 h of effective therapy (likely too soon to represent true cell death). New activity in a treated patient with a formerly non-avid PET may signal drug resistance, and these PET changes usually occur significantly earlier than would changes be visible on CT.

Biopsy

Surgical resection with pathologic assessment has been the standard of care for abdominal malignancies felt likely to be soft-tissue sarcomas. However, less invasive modalities have been investigated for obtaining tissue from suspected stromal tumors of the GI tract (see below). Diagnosis of GIST by fine needle aspirate remains difficult, as large tumors tend to have necrotic cores, and samples can thus be devoid of cellular material. Additionally, percutaneous biopsies can rupture the tumor and scatter malignant cells throughout the peritoneum. Thus, complete surgical resection with careful pathologic analysis is often recommended when GIST is suspected, though pretherapeutic tissue remains necessary when considering neoadjuvant systemic treatments.

Endoscopic Ultrasound

Endoscopic ultrasound (EUS) has potential utility in GISTs arising in the luminal GI tract. By EUS, GIST appears as a round or oval lesion with a ground-glass echotexture which is hypoechoic relative to surrounding structures. Although other tumors, including neuromas, carcinoid, and metastases may have similar EUS appearance, Nickl and colleagues showed that roughly half of resected hypoechoic intramural tumors turned out to be GIST [30]. Ando and colleagues found the diagnostic accuracy of EUS for GIST with a mitotic rate of 3 mitoses per 10 hpf compared to surgical specimen analysis of 78%, while standard histopathologic analysis of

FNA-obtained specimens improved sensitivity to 91% [31]. Addition of Ki-67 staining improved diagnostic sensitivity for GIST with the same mitotic rate to 100%.

Treatment

Complete surgical resection remains the only therapy felt to be potentially curative for GISTs. Nonetheless, surgical results are less than optimal, and the use of effective systemic agents, preceding or following resection, is increasingly becoming common. Targeted agents remain the sine qua non for disseminated or locally advanced, unresectable disease.

Surgery

Despite widespread use, both primary and salvage surgeries for GIST frequently fail, particularly as patients are followed for longer periods of time. A modern series have assessed risk, the true benefit of resection. DeMatteo and associates examined surgical outcomes for 200 GIST patients referred to the Memorial Sloan-Kettering Cancer Center from 1982 to 1998 [32]. Only cases regarded as malignant were included. Primary tumor sites included stomach in 78 patients (39%), small intestine in 63 (32%), rectum in 21 (10%), large intestine in 11 (5%), unspecified in 9 (5%), and other sites including mesentery, omentum, esophagus or diaphragm in 18 (9%). Ninety-four patients presented with metastases, of which 61 had liver metastases, and 50 liver-only metastases. All patients were considered for surgical resection, and complete resection was achieved in 80 patients with de novo local disease (86%), 28 patients with metastatic disease (30%), and 6 patients with local recurrence (46%). The remaining 86 patients (43%) had residual disease after surgical resection, or disease which was primarily surgically unresectable.

For the population as a whole the disease-free survival was 69% at 1 year, 44% at 3 years, and 35% at 5 years. Median survival was 60 months for those with primary tumors only, 22 months for patients with primary disease plus metastases, 12 months for locally recurrent disease, and 9 months for locally recurrent disease with metastases. In a multivariate analysis, male gender, tumor size greater than 5 cm, and incomplete resection or unresectable tumor status were statistically significant poor prognostic indicators for survival.

Additional analysis for this study was performed on the 80 patients whose primary treatment was at MSKCC and who had complete resection with prospective follow-up.

This group comprises 54% gastric tumors, 16% rectal cancers, and 15% small intestinal primaries. With median follow-up of 24 months, disease-free survival was 80% at 1 year, 67% at 2 years, and 45% at 5 years. Thirty-two patients (40%) recurred. Seventeen of these patients (63%) had recurrence in the liver, with 12 cases (44%) of liver-only recurrence. The median survival of these 80 patients was 66 months, with the statistically significant prognostic variable being tumor size greater than 10 cm.

This series suggests that GIST patients in the modern era do have some potential for long-term survival with resection alone, but cure rates remain low.

Risk of Recurrence

Specifically predicting risk of recurrence following complete resection depends on a number of factors. In 2002, an NIH consensus panel suggested elimination of the terms "benign" and "malignant," since all GISTs have the possibility of metastasizing [33]. A risk stratification table was devised, based solely on tumor size and mitotic rate. Miettinien and colleagues expanded on this, adding site of primary as a variable (Table 14.1) [26]. As broad concepts, tumors less than 2 cm in size rarely recur unless they arise from the duodenum and have a high-mitotic rate. Tumors greater than 10 cm in size represent much higher risk, particularly if they arise outside the stomach or have a high-mitotic rate.

Laparoscopy

Laparoscopy remains controversial in GIST. Theoretically, manipulated tumors might be prone to rupture, particularly if they are large. Recent NCCN guidelines call for the same principles observed during laparotomy: complete gross resection with an intact pseudocapsule and avoidance of tumor rupture [34]; additionally tumor should be removed in a protective bag to minimize port site recurrence. In expert hands, laparoscopic resections are not associated with higher rates of local recurrence.

Cytotoxic Chemotherapy

Several different chemotherapy agents have been tried in GIST, as single-agents or in combination regimens. Many trials focused on sarcoma-specific regimens based on successful use of ifosfamide and adriamycin for soft-tissue sarcomas [35, 36]. Results of cytotoxic chemotherapy for GIST have been disappointing, demonstrating response rates less than 10% and no survival benefit. Standard cytotoxic agents have no role in the treatment of GIST.

Imatinib Mesylate

The discovery that the majority of GISTs harbor activating mutations in c-kit eventually led to the development of an effective systemic therapy. Imatinib is a small molecule tyrosine kinase inhibitor which targets the ATP binding domains of KIT, PDGFR-A, and ABL, among others [37, 38, 39]. The inhibition of ATP binding abrogates the constitutive activation of potentially mutated receptor tyrosine kinases. Imatinib was initially developed to treat chronic myelogenous leukemia, due to its targeting of the BCR–ABL fusion tyrosine kinase and proved highly effective in that disease. Preclinical data demonstrated that imatinib could block the in vitro kinase activity of both wild-type and the mutant forms of KIT, and that the drug could inhibit the growth of a GIST cell line containing a c-kit gene mutation [39, 40].

Table 14.1 Rates of metastases related to size, mitotic rate, and location of primary

Mitotic index	Size	Gastric (n = 1055)	Duodenum (n = 144)	Jejunum/ileum(n = 629)	Rectum (n = 111)
≤ 5 per 50 hpf	≤ 2 cm	0%	0%	0%	0%
	> 2 ≤ 5 cm	1.9%	8.3%	4.3%	8.5%
	> 5 ≤ 10 cm	3.6%	Insuff. data	24%	Insuff. data
	>10 cm	10%	34%	52%	57%
>5 per 50 hpf	≤ 2 cm	None	Insuff. data	High	54%
	> 2 ≤ 5 cm	16%	50%	73%	52%
	> 5 ≤ 10 cm	55%	Insuff. data	85%	Insuff. data
	>10 cm	86%	86%	90%	71%

Adapted from Miettinen M, Lasota J. Gastrointestinal stromal tumors: pathology and prognosis at different sites. Semin Diag Pathol. 2006; 23: 70–83. Copyright Elsevier, 2006. Courtesy Dr. Christopher Corless.

Imatinib for the Treatment of Locally Advanced and Metastatic GIST

Imatinib was initially proven to have clinical activity in a single GIST patient with widely metastatic disease [41]. Subsequently, a series of more formal phase I/II trials were conducted. van Oosterom and colleagues tested four dosing schedules of imatinib, starting with 400 mg daily, and progressing to 300, 400, and 500 mg twice daily [42]. Forty patients were enrolled, 36 of whom had GIST and 4 of whom had non-GIST soft tissue sarcomas. Main toxicities included edema (30 patients), skin rashes (22), nausea (17), diarrhea (14), periorbital edema, (12), conjunctivitis (5), and neutropenic fever (1). The maximum tolerated dose was felt to be 400 mg twice daily. Twenty-five of 36 GIST patients had responses, and only 4 GIST patients had progressive disease. Twenty-four of 27 GIST patients with tumor symptoms at entry into the study experienced symptomatic relief. Eight of 14 patients with positive baseline PET scans had complete PET responses by day 8, and 2 had partial responses at day 8 but complete PET responses by day 28. No non-GIST patient responded.

The B2222 study was an international multicenter randomized phase II trial of imatinib 400 mg versus 600 mg daily, in patients with surgically incurable GIST [43]. It included 147 patients and was recently updated with 64-month median follow-up [44]. Ninety-eight patients overall (67%) demonstrated partial responses and 2 (1.4%) demonstrated complete responses for an overall objective response rate of 68% (95% CI: 59.8–75.5%). Twenty-three other patients (16%) had prolonged stable disease, the majority of them for greater than 1 year. Seventeen (12%) exhibited progression. Response rates were similar between arms, though the complete responses came from the high-dose arm. Median time to response for all patients was 13 weeks, and median time to progression was 24 months. Estimated median overall survival was 57 months, and 31% of patients were alive at most recent follow-up.

The European Organization for Research and Treatment of Cancer (EORTC) also conducted a phase II study of imatinib for GIST using 400 mg BID [45]. Entry criteria and response assessments were similar to their phase I trial. Side effects (all severities/grades III and IV) included anemia (92%/12%), edema including periorbital edema (84%/12%), fatigue (76%/12%), skin rash (69%/14%), nausea (57%/4%), granulocytopenia (47%/6%), diarrhea (47%/4%) and vomiting (43%/6%). No patients discontinued therapy due to side effects. The complete and partial response rates in GIST patients were 4% and 67%, respectively. Nineteen percent experienced stable disease. Seventy-three percent were free from progression at 1 year.

Two phase III trials, one conducted by the EORTC and the other by SWOG, compared two dosing schedules, 400 mg daily versus twice daily [46, 47, 48]. The trials had similar eligibility and statistical endpoints and were designed to have results combined into a preplanned meta-analysis [49]. The SWOG trial (B0033) enrolled 746 patients and achieved a 43% overall response rate with estimated 2 year progression-free survival of 50% (CI: 76–85%), and overall survival of 78% (CI: 88–94%), with no significant efficacy differences between arms [48]. The EORTC trial enrolled 946 patients and achieved a 52% response rate overall, with an estimated 2 year overall survival of 69% [46, 47]. Again, no differences between doses were seen in terms of progression-free survival, or overall survival.

The meta-analysis of these trials, which collectively contain 1,640 patients, has been preliminarily reported [49]. The overall response rates were similar for both dosing schedules, with disease control rates of 70–85%. In comparing the daily to twice-daily dosing, progression-free survival was 1.58 versus 1.95 years, HR 0.89, $p = 0.041$. The overall survival was 4.05 versus 4.08 years, $p = 0.97$. The entire benefit in PFS appeared to derive from patients with exon 9 mutations. PFS for the exon 9 mutant cases was markedly longer in the high-dose group (1.59 years vs. 0.5 years in those treated once daily, HR 0.58, $p = 0.017$). Overall survival appeared better for high-dose therapy in this subgroup, but the difference did not reach statistical significance, likely due to small numbers. On multivariate analysis, male sex, poor performance status, GIST of bowel origin, low hemoglobin and high-baseline neutrophil counts were associated with worse PFS. Four hundred milligrams daily remains the standard starting dose for imatinib mesylate in incurable GIST patients.

Mutational Assessment and Use of Imatinib

As discussed above, the vast majority of GISTs harbor oncogenic mutations in KIT, allowing ligand-independent receptor dimerization and activation of downstream signaling cascades. Common KIT mutations are exquisitely sensitive to imatinib preclinically, though this is not true across the board for PDGFR mutants. These mutations have prognostic value, as untreated patients with exon 11 mutations have a worse outcome than those with other KIT or PDGFR mutations or wild-type KIT. However, the true value in identifying mutations is in predicting outcome from therapy with tyrosine kinase inhibitors. Multiple phase II and III studies have demonstrated that patients with exon 11 mutations have the highest chance of responding to imatinib, as well as the best progression-free survival and overall survival [44, 48, 49]. Studies to date have been mixed on the relative drug benefit in exon 9 and patients with wild-type tumors, and there are no statistically clear differences between these groups. While patients with exon 9 tumors may benefit more from higher doses of imatinib than with standard dosing, mutation analysis is not of sufficient specificity to exclude upfront advanced disease patients from imatinib therapy.

Results from Escalating Doses of Imatinib

On the phase II and III studies, patients progressing on 400 mg of daily imatinib responded or at least stabilized in 25–33% of cases, when switched to an 800-mg daily dose [43, 48, 50]. The benefit on cross-over was also seen preferentially in exon 9 patients, at least on the EORTC phase III study. Regardless, all patients failing standard dosing, regardless of mutational status, may reasonably be tried on 800 mg daily as the initial new intervention, provided they were tolerating the lower dose without significant toxicities.

Duration of Therapy

As GIST patients live longer and occasionally achieve complete responses, the question has arisen as to whether individuals may stop safely imatinib (i.e., are they cured?). An extremely novel trial tested the question of duration of imatinib dosing in incurable patients. The French BFR-14 phase III study examined continuation versus discontinuation of imatinib at 1 and 3 years [51, 52]. Patients who were not progressing after 1 (first phase of study) or 3 (second phase) years of treatment with imatinib 400 mg daily, were randomized to continuation or discontinuation of imatinib. Patients allocated to the interruption arm could restart drug in the setting of progression. After both 1 and 3 years, patients stopping drug had markedly higher rates of progression than those continuing, though re-starting drug again achieved tumor control in the vast majority with no differences seen in overall survival. Despite this latter finding, the authors suggested that dosing should not be interrupted, even in those achieving complete remissions.

Surgery Plus Imatinib

Given the propensity for GIST to recur following even a complete resection, coupled with the efficacy of imatinib in advanced disease, the use of imatinib either before or following complete resection is theoretically attractive. The American College of Surgeons Oncology Group (ACOSOG) Z9001 adjuvant imatinib study randomized 708 people with completely resected GIST measuring at least 3 cm and expressing KIT to placebo or 1 year of imatinib 400 mg daily [53]. A planned interim analysis showed 1-year recurrence-free survival of 97% for the imatinib arm, versus 83% for the placebo arm, a statistically and clinically significant difference. No overall survival differences were seen between the arms. Subset analysis demonstrated a progression-free survival advantage (imatinib treatment vs. none) only for patients with tumors at least 6 cm in size.

Despite the strength of the initial findings, numerous questions related to Z9001 remain, including what the optimal duration of therapy is, which patients truly benefit, and whether the lack of an overall survival change should temper enthusiasm for use of the drug before recurrence. Data collection continues, with a planned correlation with patient mutational status. Additionally, European studies are trying to pin down optimal duration of adjuvant therapy (including trial designs with 0 vs. two, or 1 vs. 3 years of postoperative imatinib).

Neoadjuvant Imatinib or Surgery

Data are limited regarding the preoperative use of imatinib mesylate for tumors that are potentially resectable. Certainly the use of systemic therapy before resection is not mandated. New information is emerging, however. The Radiation Therapy Oncology Group (RTOG) has completed a trial of 2 months of neoadjuvant imatinib (600 mg daily), followed by surgery, followed by 2 years of postoperative drug [54]. Preliminary data reveal the use of imatinib in this setting to be safe, with no increase in operative complications. Intact tumors have the potential for bleeding that can be exacerbated by imatinib use; additionally, tumors that are borderline resectable can progress on imatinib (though this is admittedly rare) and become truly incurable. In general preoperative imatinib is reserved for situations where tumor down-sizing might lead to organ-sparing surgery (e.g., wedge resection of the stomach vs. total gastrectomy), or for locally advanced, unresectable GISTs.

Data involving the use of surgery as an adjuvant to imatinib or other tyrosine kinase inhibitors are also just now emerging from major GIST centers. Surgery preliminarily appears most effective in those with stable or responding disease. Those operated on with generalized progression, or even progressive disease limited to a few easily respectable areas does not appear to improve progression-free survival or overall survival and cannot be recommended outside of a clinical trial.

On multivariate analysis, presence of extrahepatic disease, greater extent of hepatic involvement, no use of imatinib, and lack of response to HACE were significantly associated with worsened survival.

The authors concluded that HACE is potentially superior to systemic chemotherapy and that HACE is an effective palliative therapy for imatinib-resistant GIST. Whether resistant patients with liver-predominant GIST should receive sunitinib versus undergoing HACE remains unknown. Given GISTs' propensity for liver metastases, new trials investigating focused therapy for liver disease should be undertaken.

Conclusions

The successful treatment of GIST with tyrosine kinase inhibitors is a model for the development of rational, molecularly targeted therapy in solid tumors. The characterization of its molecular biology has allowed ideal dose selection of one particular drug (imatinib) and holds the promise of eventually picking the best agent for the individual patient. However, many questions remain regarding GIST biology and best clinical therapy, particularly in regard to optimally utilizing multimodality setting and treating locally problematic resistant tumors, such as liver metastases which have progressed on imatinib and sunitinib. Future clinical trials should focus on the development of new targeted therapies, as well as the best scheduling of surgery or other locally directed therapies, as well as systemic adjuvant treatment. This path should lead to additional prolongation in median and long-term survival for patients suffering from GISTs.

References

1. Appelman HD. Smooth muscle tumors of the gastrointestinal tract. What we know now that Stout didn't know. Am J Surg Pathol. 1986; 10(Suppl. 10): 83–99.
2. Mazur MT, Clark HB. Gastric stromal tumors. Reappraisal of histogenesis. Am J Surg Pathol. 1983; 7: 507–519.
3. Newman PL, Wadden C, Fletcher CG. Gastrointestinal stromal tumours: correlation of immunophenotype with clinicopathological features. J Pathol. 1991; 164: 107–117.
4. Kindblom L, Remotti H, Aldenborg F, et al. Gastrointestinal pacemaker cell tumor (GIPACT): gastrointestinal stromal tumors show phenotypic characteristics of the interstitial cells of Cajal. Am J Pathol. 1998; 152: 1259–69.
5. Sanders KM. A case for interstitial cells of Cajal as pacemakers and mediators of neurotransmission in the gastrointestinal tract. Gastroenterology. 1996; 111: 492–515.
6. Sarlomo-Rikala M, Kovatich A, Barusevicius A, et al. CD117: a sensitive marker for gastrointestinal stromal tumors that is more specific than CD34. Mod Pathol. 1998; 11: 728–34.

7. Rubin B.P. Gastrointestinal stromal tumors: an update. Histopathology. 2006; 48: 83–96.
8. West RB, Corless CL, Chen X, et al. The novel marker, DOG1, is expressed ubiquitously in gastrointestinal stromal tumors irrespective of KIT of PDGFRA mutation status. Am J Pathol. 2004; 165: 107–113.
9. Heinrich M, Rubin B, Longley B, et al. Biology and genetic aspects of gastrointestinal stromal tumors: KIT activation and cytogenetic alterations. Hum Pathol. 2002; 33: 484–95.
10. Sabah M, Cummins R, Leader M, et al. Loss of heterozygosity of chromosome 9p and loss of p16INK4A expression are associated with malignant gastrointestinal stromal tumors. Mod Pathol. 2004; 7: 1364–1371.
11. Heinrich MC, Corless CL, Demetri GD, et al. Kinase mutations and imatinib response in patients with metastatic gastrointestinal stromal tumor. J Clin Oncol. 2003; 21: 4342–49.
12. Duensing A, Medeiros F, McConarty B, et al. Mechanisms of oncogenic KIT signal transduction in primary gastrointestinal tumors (GISTs). Oncogene. 2004; 23: 3999–4006.
13. Hirota S, Koji I, Yasuhiro M, et al. Gain of function mutations of c-kit in human gastrointestinal stromal tumors. Science. 1998; 279: 577–580.
14. Corless CL, Schroeder A, Griffith D, et al. PDGFRA mutations in gastrointestinal stromal tumors: frequency, spectrum and in vitro sensitivity to imatinib. J Clin Oncol. 2005; 23: 5357–5364.
15. Corless CL, McGreevey L, Haley A, et al. KIT mutations are common in incidental gastrointestinal stromal tumors one centimeter or less in size. Am J Pathol. 2002; 160: 1567–1572.
16. Rubin BP, Antonescu CR, Scott-Browne JP, et al. A knock-in mouse model of gastrointestinal stromal tumor harboring kit K641E. Cancer Res. 2005; 65: 6631–6639.
17. Li FP, Fletcher JA, Heinrich MC, et al. Familial gastrointestinal stromal tumor syndrome: phenotypic and molecular features in a kindred. J Clin Oncol. 2005; 23: 2735–2743.
18. Price VE, Zielenska M, Chilton-MacNeill S, et al. Clinical and molecular characteristics of pediatric gastrointestinal stromal tumors (GISTs). Ped Blood Cancer. 2005; 45: 20–24.
19. Carney JA. Gastric stromal sarcoma, pulmonary chondroma, and extra-adrenal paraganglioma (Carney Triad): natural history, adrenocortical component, and possible familial occurrence. Mayo Clin Proc. 1999; 74: 543–552.
20. Yantiss RK, Rosenberg AE, Sarran L, et al. Multiple gastrointestinal stromal tumors in type I neurofibromatosis: a pathologic and molecular study. Mod Pathol. 2005; 18: 475–84.
21. Nilsson B, Bumming P, Meis-Kindblom JM, et al. Gastrointestinal stromal tumors: the incidence, prevalence, clinical course, and prognostication in the preimatinib mesylate era—a population-based study in western Sweden. Cancer. 2005; 103: 821–29.
22. Tryggvason G, Gislason H, Magnusson M, et al. Gastrointestinal stromal tumors in Iceland, 1990–2003: the Icelandic GIST study, a population-based incidence and pathologic risk stratification study. Int J Cancer. 2005; 117: 289–293.
23. Miettinen M, Sarlomo-Rikala M, Sobin L, et al. Gastrointestinal stromal tumors and leiomyosarcomas in the colon: a clinicopathologic, immunohistochemical, and molecular genetic study of 44 cases. Am J Surg Pathol. 2000; 24(10): 1339–1352.
24. Miettinen M, Makhlouf H, Sobin L, et al. Gastrointestinal stromal tumors of the jejunum and ileum: a clinicopathologic, immunohistochemical, and molecular genetic study of 906 cases before imatinib, with long-term follow-up. Am J Surg Pathol. 2006; 30: 477–489.
25. Miettinen M, Sobin L, Lasota J. Gastrointestinal stromal tumors of the stomach: a clinicopathologic, immunohistochemical, and molecular genetic study of 1765 cases with long-term follow-up. Am J Surg Pathol. 2005; 29(1): 52–68.

26. Miettinen M, Lasota J. Gastrointestinal stromal tumors: pathology and prognosis at different sites. Semin Diag Pathol. 2006; 23: 70–83.

27. Chen MY, Bechtold RE, Savage PD. Cystic changes in hepatic metastases from gastrointestinal stromal tumors (GISTs) treated with Gleevec (imatinib mesylate). Am J Roent. 2002; 179: 1059–1062.

28. Gayed I, Vu T, Iyer R, et al. The role of FDG-PET in staging and early prediction of response to therapy of recurrent gastrointestinal stromal tumors. J Nucl Med. 2004; 45: 17–21.

29. Blodgett TM, Meltzer CC, Townsend DW. PET/CT: Form and function. Radiol. 2007; 242: 360–385.

30. Nickl N, Gress F, McClave S, et al. Hypoechoic intramural tumor study: final report. Gastrointest Endosc. 2002; 55: AB98.

31. Ando N, Goto H, Niwa Y, et al. The diagnosis of GI stromal tumors with EUS-guided fine needle aspiration with immunohistochemical analysis. Gastrointest Endosc 2002; 56:3: 7–43.

32. DeMatteo R, Lewis J, Leung D, et al. Two hundred gastrointestinal stromal tumors: recurrence patterns and prognostic factors for survival. Ann Surg. 2002; 231(1): 51–58.

33. Fletcher C, Berman J, Corless CC, et al. Diagnosis of gastrointestinal stromal tumors: a consensus approach. Hum Pathol. 2002; 33: 459–465.

34. Demetri GD, Benjamin RS, Blanke CD, et al. NCCN task force report: management of patients with gastrointestinal stromal tumor (GIST)—update of the NCCN clinical practice guidelines. J Natl Comp Cancer Net. 2007; 5(suppl 2): S1-S29.

35. Le Cesne A, Judson I, Crowther D, et al. Randomized phase III study comparing conventional-dose doxorubicin plus ifosfamide versus high-dose doxorubicin plus ifosfamide plus recombinant human granulocyte-macrophage colony-stimulating factor in advanced soft tissue sarcomas: a trial of the European Organization for Research and Treatment of Cancer/Soft Tissue and Bone Sarcoma Group. J Clin Oncol. 2000; 18(14): 2676–84.

36. Nielsen OS, Judson I, van Hoesel Q, et al. Effect of high-dose ifosfamide in advanced soft tissue sarcomas. A multicentre phase II study of the EORTC Soft Tissue and Bone Sarcoma Group. Eur J Cancer. 2000; 36(1): 61–7.

37. Dewar AL, Cambareri AC, Zannettino AC, et al. Macrophage colony-stimulating factor receptor c-fms is a novel target of imatinib. Blood. 2005; 105: 3127–32.

38. Okuda K, Weisberg E, Gilliland DG, et al. ARG tyrosine kinase activity is inhibited by STI571. Blood. 2001; 97: 2440–8.

39. Heinrich MC, Griffith DJ, Druker BJ, et al. Inhibition of c-kit receptor tyrosine kinase activity by STI 571, a selective tyrosine kinase inhibitor. Blood. 2000; 96: 925–32.

40. Tuveson DA, Willis NA, Jacks T, et al. STI571 inactivation of the gastrointestinal stromal tumor c-KIT oncoprotein: biological and clinical implications. Oncogene. 2001; 20: 5054–5058.

41. Joensuu H, Roberts PJ, Sarlomo-Rikala M, et al. Effect of the tyrosine kinase inhibitor STI571 in a patient with a metastatic gastrointestinal stromal tumor. N Engl J Med. 2001; 344: 1052–6.

42. Van Oosterom AT, Judson I, Verweij J, et al. Safety and efficacy of imatinib (STI571) in metastatic gastrointestinal stromal tumors: a phase I study. Lancet. 2001; 358(9291): 1421–3.

43. Demetri G, von Mehren M, Blanke C, et al. Efficacy and safety of imatinib mesylate in advanced gastrointestinal stromal tumors. N Engl J Med. 2002; 347(7): 472–478.

44. Byrd DM, Demetri GD, Joensuu H, et al. Evaluation of imatinib mesylate in patients with large volume gastrointestinal stromal tumors (GISTs). Proc Am Soc Clin Oncol. 2007; 25: 558s(abstr 10054).

46. Verweij J, Casali PG, Zalcberg J, et al. Progression-free survival in gastrointestinal stromal tumors with high-dose imatinib: randomized trial. Lancet. 2004; 364: 1127–1134.

47. Casali PG, Verweij J, Kotasek D, et al. Imatinib mesylate in advanced gastrointestinal stromal tumors (GIST): survival analysis of the Intergroup EORTC/ISG/AGITG randomized trial in 946 patients. Eur J Cancer. 2005; 3 (suppl): 201(abstr 711).

48. Blanke C, Rankin C, von Mehren M, et al. Phase III randomized, intergroup trial assessing imatinib mesylate at two dose levels in patients with unresectable or metastatic gastrointestinal stromal tumors expressing the KIT receptor tyrosine kinase: S0033. J Clin Oncol. 2008; 26: 626–632.

49. Van Glabbeke MM, Owzar K, Rankin C, et al. Comparison of two doses of imatinib for the treatment of unresectable or metastatic gastrointestinal stromal tumors (GIST): a meta-analysis based on 1,640 patients. Proc Am Soc Clin Oncol. 2007; 25: 546s(abstr 10004).

50. Zalcberg JR, Verweij J, Casali PG, et al. Outcome of patients with advanced gastro-intestinal stromal tumours crossing over to a daily imatinib dose of 800 mg after progression on 400 mg. Eur J Cancer. 2005; 41: 1751–1757.

51. Blay JY, Le Cesne A, Ray-Coquard I, et al. Prospective multicentric randomized phase III study of imatinib in patients with advanced gastrointestinal stromal tumors comparing interruption versus continuation of treatment beyond 1 year: the French Sarcoma Group. J Clin Oncol. 2007; 25: 1107–13.

52. Le Cesne I, Ray-Coquard B, Bui M, et al. Continuous versus interruption of imatinib (IM) in responding patients with advanced GIST after three years of treatment: a prospective randomized phase III trial of the French Sarcoma Group. Proc Am Soc Clin Oncol. 2007; 25: 546s(abstr 10005).

53. DeMatteo R, Owzar K, Maki R, et al. Adjuvant imatinib mesylate increases recurrence free survival (RFS) in patients with completely resected localized primary gastrointestinal stromal tumor (GIST): North American Intergroup phase III trial ACOSOG Z9001. Proc Am Soc Clin Oncol. 2007; 25(abstr 10079).

54. Eisenberg B. (personal communication).

55. Choi H, Charnsangavej C, Faria S, et al. Correlation of computed tomography and positron emission tomography in patients with metastatic gastrointestinal stromal tumors treated at a single institution with imatinib mesylate: Proposal of new computed tomography response criteria. J Clin Oncol. 2007; 25(13): 1753–59.

56. Benjamin RS, Choi H, Macapinlac HA, et al. We should desist using RECIST, at least in GIST. J Clin Oncol. 2007; 25: 1760–1764.

57. Prenen H, Cools J, Mentens N, et al. Efficacy of the kinase inhibitor SU11248 against gastrointestinal stromal tumor mutants refractory to imatinib mesylate. Clin Cancer Res. 2006; 12: 2622–2627.

58. Heinrich MC, Maki RG, Corless CL, et al. Sunitinib response in imatinib-resistant GIST correlates with KIT and PDGFRA mutation status. Proc Am Soc Clin Oncol. 2006; 24: 520s(abstr 9502).

59. Demetri GD, van Oosterom AT, Garrett CR, et al. Efficacy and safety of sunitinib in patients with advanced gastrointestinal stromal tumour after failure of imatinib: a randomised controlled trial. Lancet. 2006; 368: 1329–1338.

60. Casali G, Garrett CR, Blackstein ME, et al. Updated results from a phase III trial of sunitinib in GIST patients (pts) for whom imatinib (IM) therapy has failed due to resistance or intolerance. Proc Am Soc Clin Oncol. 2006; 24: 523s(abstr 9513).

61. George S, Blay JY, Casali PG, et al. Continuous daily dosing of sunitinib malate compares favorably with intermittent dosing in patients with advanced GIST. Proc Am Soc Clin Oncol. 2007; 25: 548s(abstr 10015).

62. Heinrich MC, Corless CL, Blanke CD, et al. Molecular correlates of imatinib resistance in gastrointestinal stromal tumors. J Clin Oncol. 2006; 24: 4764–4774.

63. von Mehren M, Reichardt P, Casali PG, et al. A phase I study of nilotinib alone and in combination with imatinib in patients with imatinib-resistant gastrointestinal stromal tumors-Study update. Proc Am Soc Clin Oncol. 2007; 25: 550s (abstr 10023).

64. Reichardt P, Pink D, Lindner T, et al. A phase I/II trial of the oral PKC-inhibitor PKC412 in combination with imatinib mesylate in patients with gastrointestinal stromal tumors refractory to imatinib mesylate. Proc Am Soc Clin Oncol. 2006; 24: 124s (abstr 3016).

65. Kobayashi K, Gupta S, Trent JC, et al. Hepatic artery chemoembolization for 110 gastrointestinal stromal tumors: Response, survival, and prognostic factors. Cancer. 2006; 107(12): 2833–2841.

Surgery for Breast Cancer Liver Metastases

15

Georges Vlastos and Daria Zorzi

Introduction

Breast cancer is the most common cancer among women. It has been estimated that one in eight women will develop breast cancer during her lifetime [1]. Approximately 50% of all breast cancer patients will present with distant metastases during the course of their disease [2, 3], accounting for breast cancer's ranking as a leading cause of cancer-related mortality in women [1].

Despite significant progress made in the multidisciplinary management of breast cancer patients, including prevention and early diagnosis, the use of more effective systemic chemotherapy regimens (anthracyclines and taxanes), hormonal therapies (tamoxifen and aromatase inhibitors), and novel approaches such as targeted therapies (trastuzumab) [4], the development of distant metastases continues to be associated with a very poor prognosis [5].

Metastatic breast cancer patients have a median survival period of 2–3 years [1], with few (2%) surviving 20 years after the diagnosis of metastasis [6]. As liver metastases occur in the setting of widely disseminated disease, systemic treatments are usually indicated for this condition but are palliative, with a median survival of only 2–14 months [3, 7, 8]. However, in light of advances made in the treatment of colorectal as well as neuroendocrine tumors, consideration has now been given to identify a subset of patients with limited liver metastases from breast cancer who might be considered viable candidates for surgical approaches.

In this chapter, we will present the published series on this topic and clarify selection criteria for patients who may be candidates for surgical resection or ablation.

Metastatic Disease

Metastatic breast cancer is considered an incurable disease. Despite the use of modern systemic treatments, median survival time ranges from 3 to 15 months [4, 9, 10]. Survival depends upon sites of metastases. For instance, breast cancer patients with bone metastases have a better survival (2–4 years) compared to patients with other metastatic disease sites such as the liver (less than 4–6 months) [11]. The liver is the third most common site of distant metastases in breast cancer patients, after bones and lungs. In general, liver metastases occur in the setting of widely disseminated disease associated with other metastatic disease sites. At the time of diagnosis, 5–10% of patients have hepatic metastases, and at a more advanced stage of the disease, more than 50% of breast cancer patients will develop systemic disease including liver metastases. Liver metastases are found in 12–15% of patients newly diagnosed with metastatic breast cancer and are the only site of distant disease in one third of these patients [7, 12]. Liver failure secondary to metastases is an important cause of death in more than 20% of these patients [3].

The presence of metastatic disease isolated to the liver is a rare finding, occurring in only 4–5% of the cases [13]. This situation with disease limited to the liver is different from a situation with disseminated disease. In case of disseminated disease, "cure" is not the goal of treatment; instead, most conservative treatments are preferred to obtain maximum control of symptoms, prevent serious complications, and prolong life with minimal toxicities and disruption of quality of life. Treatments are systemic and include combinations of chemo-endocrine treatments. Typically, metastatic breast cancer is treated by a combination of chemotherapy regimens including cyclophosphamide, methotrexate, 5-fluorouracil or doxorubicin. In first-line regimens, response is reported in 30–80% of cases, with higher responses when anthracyclines are used. Alternative regimens are used during the progression of disease. Cytotoxic agents such as alkaloids,

G. Vlastos (✉)
Department of Gynecology and Obstetrics, Division of Gynecology, Senology and Surgical Gynecologic Oncology Unit, Geneva University Hospitals, Geneva, Switzerland

Table 15.1 Recent series on liver resection for breast cancer metastases

Studies	Date	Patients, n	Follow-up (months)	Overall survival% at 3 years	Overall survival% at 5 years
Maksan [19]	1984–1998	9	29	51	51
Adam [23]	1984–2004	85	38	47	37
Seifert [25]	1985–1997	15	12	54	NA
Yoshimoto [26]	1985–1998	25	NA	71*	27
Sakamoto [24]	1985–2003	34	72	52	21
Raab [27]	1986–1997	34	27	50	18
Elias [18]	1986–2000	54	32	50	34
Selzner [21]	1987–1999	17	24	35	22
Pocard [20]	1988–1999	65	41	71	38
Santoro [28]	1990–1998	15	NA	NA	38
Kondo [29]	1990–1999	6	36	60	40
Vlastos [30]	1991–2002	31	63	75	61
Okaro [31]	1996–2002	6	2–62	NA	NA
Carlini [32]	2002	17	NA	NA	46
Arena [33]	2003	17	NA	52	41
Thelen [22]	1988–2006	39	24	50	42
Adam [34] (multicenter)	1983–2004	454 (41 centers)	31	NA	41

*Two-year survival, not 3-year.
NA: Not available.

mitomycin or taxanes are used with only 25% response rates. Newer combinations using drugs such as docetaxel, doxorubicin or gemcitabine as part of the treatment have demonstrated responses rates of up to 83% [14]. These high response rates are reported in limited series and need to be confirmed with larger numbers of patients, emphasizing the limitation of available treatments and the importance of alternative therapeutic approaches for metastatic breast cancer patients. Hormonal treatments can be proposed to these patients. However, these treatments are less effective against liver metastases, which tend to be hormone-receptor negative [15]. Thus, chemotherapy is usually proposed as first-line treatment of visceral metastases. And liver metastases are considered to be less responsive to chemotherapy than metastases of other sites. This may partly explain why breast cancer patients with liver metastases have a shorter survival compared to patients with metastases at other sites [16, 17].

The strategy is different for metastatic disease isolated to the liver. Isolated liver metastases in breast cancer patients are rare (1–3% of patients with hepatic metastases), but occasionally such limited hepatic disease becomes stable on systemic therapy. Liver resection should be considered if chemotherapy yields response or control of tumor progression. These differing strategies highlight the importance of multidisciplinary evaluation for patients with breast cancer as well as for those with limited liver-only metastatic disease with response to systemic therapy.

Retrospective, single-institution studies demonstrated 3-year overall survival rates of 50–75% [18, 19, 20] and showed a 5-year survival of 18–61% after liver resection (Table 15.1). In one of these studies, a disease-free interval (DFI) between resection of the primary tumor and development of liver metastases of greater than 48 months was associated with a 82% 3-year survival compared to only 45% for a shorter DFI [20]. For highly selected patients with breast cancer who have prolonged DFI, stability on systemic therapy, and isolated liver metastases, hepatic resection can be considered as a component of multimodality therapy.

Patient Selection

All patients who are candidates for surgical therapeutic approaches need to have complete diagnostic work-up including thoraco-abdominal CT scan, bone scan and in selected cases, a PET scan. Less than 20% of patients with liver metastases from breast cancer who are treated in a multidisciplinary approach are candidates for hepatectomy; the majority of patients are not suitable for resection because of multiple extrahepatic metastatic sites at the time of diagnosis [22]. Patient selection is based on several factors including biological characteristics of the primary tumor such as TNM stage, grade, estrogen and progesterone receptor status, and response to systemic treatments. Characteristics of liver metastases such as number and size, location within the liver, extrahepatic metastases, or lymph nodes involvement in hepatic pedicles need to be carefully studied before surgery. Also, response to chemotherapy correlates significantly with survival after liver resection [23], demonstrating the important role of systemic therapy in the multimodal treatment of patients with metastatic breast cancer.

In an attempt to identify selection criteria for patients who benefit from liver resection for metastatic breast cancer, many studies have addressed prognostic factors after hepatectomy. Pocard et al. [20] found that a short DFI between treatment of the primary tumor and onset of liver metastasis significantly correlated with poor survival. This may be explained by more aggressive biology of tumors in patients with a short DFI. Sakamoto et al. [24] described extrahepatic disease prior to liver resection to predict poor survival. The poorer outcome in these patients might be explained by the more advanced stage of the cancer. Another explanation may be limited chemotherapeutic options. Chemotherapy represents a major tool in the treatment and control of primary and recurrent breast cancer. Patients suffering from metastatic manifestation prior to liver resection mostly have had multiple chemotherapeutic protocols, reducing the treatment options after hepatectomy. Thelen et al. [22] also reported vascular invasion of the liver metastases to correlate significantly with poor patient survival. This was not described previously for liver metastases from breast cancer, but it is known to be an independent prognostic factor in primary liver cancers [35]. Vascular invasion is mostly diagnosed histologically so its use as a selection criterion may be restricted. Nonetheless, it might be a useful selection parameter in patients with macroscopically detectable vascular invasion and for the decision about further adjuvant chemotherapy.

Studies in the literature do not uniformly consider completeness of surgical resection as an independent prognostic factor, [18, 22, 23, 27] perhaps because of the slow growth pattern of breast cancer, which causes prolonged survival even after palliative resection in some patients. However, most of the larger series describe a curative resection to significantly correlate with superior survival [22, 23, 27]. (Fig. 15.1) Therefore, the achievement of a macroscopic complete resection represents an important selection criterion for patients suitable for liver resection. If there is doubt on the ability to achieve a complete resection, in particular regarding extrahepatic metastases, diagnostic laparoscopy should be performed.

Hormone-receptor status is another key variable when determining the treatment for breast cancer [7]. However, the studies on the prognostic impact of hormone-receptor status demonstrate equivocal results [18, 24, 36]. Also, the expression of erb B2 showed influence on survival in one series [22] but was not described as prognostic factor in another study [36]. The differences between the studies are most likely due to small patient numbers. Further investigation may clarify the importance of receptor status

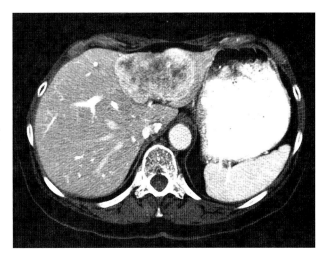

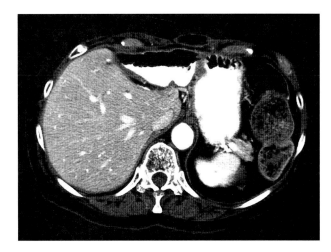

Fig. 15.1 A 66-year-old female patient with a solitary metachronous breast cancer liver metastasis. The primary breast cancer was resected 7 years prior to presentation. A: The preoperative computed tomography of the liver shows an 8 cm mass in segments II, III and IV. B: A follow-up computed tomography of the liver shows no evidence of recurrent disease 5 years later. The patient is currently disease-free

for prognosis after liver resection for metastatic breast cancer.

Liver Resection Of Breast Cancer Metastases

Liver resection offers the only chance of cure in patients with a variety of primary and secondary liver tumors. For breast cancer, the natural history of this condition is poorly defined and the management remains controversial. Most physicians view liver metastases from breast cancer with resignation or attempt palliation with hormones and chemotherapy. But a decade ago, some advocated more aggressive management, proposing liver resections when feasible with the hope of increasing survival. Recent data suggest a role for surgical resection of isolated breast cancer metastases not only in the liver but also in the lung, bone, or brain [37].

Proper patient selection is crucial to ensure favorable long-term results. In addition, liver surgery has to be performed by experienced and specialized liver surgeons practicing in highly specialized centers with high caseloads. Although results of hepatic resection for metastatic colorectal cancer have been reported extensively, the experience with liver resection of metastases from breast cancer is limited. In 1991, the first series reporting hepatectomy for breast cancer patients was published [38]. Since then, reports on the role of hepatic resection in patients with breast cancer liver metastases contain very few cases (Table 15.1). In these retrospective, heterogeneous and single-institution series, the patient numbers range from 9 to 85. The literature contains only three reports that examine the outcomes following hepatic resection in more than 50 patients [18, 20, 23]. Overall survival at 5 years is 18–61% depending on the series (Table 15.1). Recurrence-free survival, when reported, varies between 16% and 31%. Median survival after resection varies from 25 to 63 months. The results are particularly difficult to interpret and do not allow clear conclusions to be drawn regarding the true indications for hepatectomy in patients with metastatic breast cancer.

With aggressive staging using systematic intraoperative ultrasound scan and preoperative and intraoperative biopsy of all suspicious extrahepatic sites, investigators at the University of Texas M.D. Anderson Cancer Center (UT-MDACC) found a 61% 5-year overall survival with a median overall survival of 25 months in patients who underwent resection of breast cancer liver metastases [30]. Importantly, 80% of patients in this series received systemic chemotherapy, and 45% received hormonal therapy in conjunction with hepatic resection. A subsequent series of resected breast cancer liver metastases from Adam et al. [23] complemented these findings. In 85 patients, some of whom had known extrahepatic disease and clinical response to prehepatectomy chemotherapy, the 5-year overall survival rate was 37%, and median overall survival was 34 months; 83% of patients received chemotherapy, and 34% received hormonal therapy. Analysis of outcome predictors from these two studies showed that a disease-free interval of less than 1 year from breast primary to liver metastases diagnosis and a positive hepatic resection margin diminished the probability of long-term survival. Patients with relatively limited hepatic burden and long disease-free intervals are likely to benefit from hepatic resection.

An objection against the inclusion of liver resection in the multidisciplinary treatment approach of metastatic breast cancer patients may be the perioperative risk. However, favorable perioperative results have been reported with morbidity of 13% and zero mortality [18, 22, 23]. Minimization of toxicity represents a goal in the treatment of metastatic breast cancer. The low morbidity and mortality indicate the safety of this procedure when appropriate patient selection is applied. Therefore, liver resection represents a therapeutic tool with low risk in these patients. The results of the recently published studies indicate that liver resection should be considered in the multimodal treatment approach of patients with breast cancer liver metastases.

A large series by Adam et al. [34] reported the experience of 41 French centers regarding liver resection for noncolorectal, nonendocrine liver metastases. Among the 1452 patients who were studied, 454 (32%) were breast cancer patients. Mean age was 52 years (range 27–80 years). Most patients received adjuvant chemotherapy (58%), as few were downstaged by neoadjuvant chemotherapy. Delay between the treatment of the primary breast tumor and metastases was 54 months, with metachronous metastases in more than 90% of cases. There was a single metastasis in 56% of cases and less than three metastases in 84%. Only 8% were nonresectable. Most patients (77% of cases) underwent anatomical major resections (>3 segments). Negative margins were obtained in 82% of cases. Operative mortality was 0.2% during the 2 months following surgery. Fewer than 10% of the patients developed a local or systemic complication. With a median follow-up of 31 months, the overall survival was 41% at 5 years and 22% at 10 years, with a median of 45 months. Five- and 10-year recurrence-free survival rates were 14% and 10%, respectively. Poor survival was associated with four factors determined by multivariate analysis: time to metastases, extrahepatic location, progression under chemotherapy treatment, and incomplete resection.

At the UTMDACC, breast cancer patients who present with isolated synchronous liver metastases are treated initially with systemic chemotherapy. In responders, hepatic resection is only contemplated if no other disease becomes evident during initial systemic treatment (Fig. 15.1). Most candidates for hepatic resection undergo treatment for metachronous disease and only undergo resection for metastatic disease confined to the liver.

Liver Ablation Of Breast Cancer Metastases

Published studies on ablative therapies, such as radiofrequency ablation (RFA) show disappointing results with high recurrence at short-term follow-up. Prior clinical series of radiofrequency ablation in the management of breast hepatic metastasis had small number of patients

(14–24 patients), most of whom had metastatic disease confined to the liver [39, 40].

A recent report from Memorial Sloan-Kettering Cancer Center [41] describes the results in a group of 12 breast cancer patients with hepatic metastases, most of whom presented with extrahepatic disease at the time of RFA; only in 50% of the patients the treated lesions remained necrotic, this resulted in a median primary local progression-free interval of 12 months.

The largest RFA series, from Livraghi et al. [39], reported on 24 patients with breast cancer who underwent percutaneous RFA for liver metastases. Despite complete ablation in 59 of 64 lesions by post-procedure imaging, 58% of the patients developed recurrence at short-term follow-up, with 71% of all recurrences confined to the liver.

Data from the UTMDACC experience with solitary metastases from colorectal cancer [42] show that 37% of the patients had a local recurrence after RFA, while only 5% recurred locally in the resected group after a median follow-up of 31 months.

Outcomes for RFA are not comparable to liver resection; therefore, RFA must be considered as a palliative procedure in breast cancer liver metastases.

Conclusion

Metastatic breast cancer is considered an incurable disease. Recent studies suggest that with careful patient selection, resection of breast cancer liver metastases is associated with long-term survival.

Liver resection of metastatic breast cancer is considered in the context of a multimodality approach including chemotherapy and/or hormonal therapy. While cure is rare in metastatic breast cancer, complete resection provides the meaningful option of a chemotherapy-free, progression-free interval.

Liver surgery is indicated if metastatic disease is well controlled after chemotherapy, and resection is macroscopically complete, with a DFI from treatment of the primary tumor to diagnosis of liver metastases of more than 1 year and without extrahepatic disease. RFA is an inferior alternative treatment option for high-risk patients and those with stable extrahepatic disease who are not candidates for resection.

References

1. Jemal A, Siegel R, Ward E, et al. Cancer statistics, 2007. CA Cancer J Clin 2007; 57: 43–66.
2. Hoe AL, Royle GT, Taylor I. Breast liver metastases—incidence, diagnosis and outcome. J R Soc Med 1991; 84: 714–6.
3. Zinser JW, Hortobagyi GN, Buzdar AU, et al. Clinical course of breast cancer patients with liver metastases. J Clin Oncol 1987; 5: 773–82.
4. Goldhirsch A, Wood WC, Gelber RD, et al. Progress and promise: highlights of the international expert consensus on the primary therapy of early breast cancer 2007. Ann Oncol 2007; 18: 1133–44.
5. Sledge GW, Neuberg D, Bernardo P, et al. Phase III trial of doxorubicin, paclitaxel, and the combination of doxorubicin and paclitaxel as front-line chemotherapy for metastatic breast cancer: an intergroup trial (E1193). J Clin Oncol 2003; 21: 588–92.
6. Greenberg PA, Hortobagyi GN, Smith TL, et al. Long-term follow-up of patients with complete remission following combination chemotherapy for metastatic breast cancer. J Clin Oncol 1996; 14: 2197–205.
7. Insa A, Lluch A, Prosper F, et al. Prognostic factors predicting survival from first recurrence in patients with metastatic breast cancer: analysis of 439 patients. Breast Cancer Res Treat 1999; 56: 67–78.
8. Fossati R, Confalonieri C, Torri V, et al. Cytotoxic and hormonal treatment for metastatic breast cancer: a systematic review of published randomized trials involving 31,510 women. J Clin Oncol 1998; 16: 3439–60.
9. O'Reilly SM, Richards MA, Rubens RD. Liver metastases from breast cancer: the relationship between clinical, biochemical and pathological features and survival. Eur J Cancer 1990; 26: 574–7.
10. Wyld L, Gutteridge E, Pinder SE, et al. Prognostic factors for patients with hepatic metastases from breast cancer. Br J Cancer 2003; 89: 284–90.
11. Goldhirsch A, Gelber RD, Castiglione M. Relapse of breast cancer after adjuvant treatment in premenopausal and perimenopausal women: patterns and prognoses. J Clin Oncol 1988; 6: 89–97.
12. Clark GM, Sledge GW Jr, Osborne CK, McGuire WL. Survival from first recurrence: relative importance of prognostic factors in 1,015 breast cancer patients. J Clin Oncol 1987; 5: 55–61.
13. Diaz R, Santaballa A, Munarriz B, Calderero V. Hepatic resection in breast cancer metastases: should it be considered standard treatment? Breast 2004; 13: 254–8.
14. Hortobagyi GN. Treatment of breast cancer. N Engl J Med 1998; 339: 974–84.
15. Samaan NA, Buzdar AU, Aldinger KA, et al. Estrogen receptor: a prognostic factor in breast cancer. Cancer 1981; 47: 554–60.
16. Sherry MM, Greco FA, Johnson DH, Hainsworth JD. Metastatic breast cancer confined to the skeletal system. An indolent disease. Am J Med 1986; 81: 381–6.
17. Koizumi M, Yoshimoto M, Kasumi F, Ogata E. Comparison between solitary and multiple skeletal metastatic lesions of breast cancer patients. Ann Oncol 2003; 14: 1234–40.
18. Elias D, Maisonnette F, Druet-Cabanac M, et al. An attempt to clarify indications for hepatectomy for liver metastases from breast cancer. Am J Surg 2003; 185: 158–64.
19. Maksan SM, Lehnert T, Bastert G, Herfarth C. Curative liver resection for metastatic breast cancer. Eur J Surg Oncol 2000; 26: 209–12.
20. Pocard M, Pouillart P, Asselain B, Salmon R. Hepatic resection in metastatic breast cancer: results and prognostic factors. Eur J Surg Oncol 2000; 26: 155–9.
21. Selzner M, Morse MA, Vredenburgh JJ, et al. Liver metastases from breast cancer: long-term survival after curative resection. Surgery 2000; 127: 383–9.

22. Thelen A, Benckert C, Jonas S, et al. Liver resection for metastases from breast cancer. J Surg Oncol 2008; 97: 25–9.

23. Adam R, Aloia T, Krissat J, et al. Is liver resection justified for patients with hepatic metastases from breast cancer? Ann Surg 2006; 244: 897–907.

24. Sakamoto Y, Yamamoto J, Yoshimoto M, et al. Hepatic resection for metastatic breast cancer: prognostic analysis of 34 patients. World J Surg 2005; 29: 524–7.

25. Seifert JK, Weigel TF, Gonner U, et al. Liver resection for breast cancer metastases. Hepatogastroenterology 1999; 46: 2935–40.

26. Yoshimoto M, Sugitani I, Iwase T, et al. [Therapeutic efficacy of hepatectomy in the treatment of hepatic metastases from breast cancer]. Nippon Geka Gakkai Zasshi 1995; 96: 174–9.

27. Raab R, Nussbaum KT, Behrend M, Weimann A. Liver metastases of breast cancer: results of liver resection. Anticancer Res 1998; 18: 2231–3.

28. Santoro E, Vitucci C, Carlini M, et al. [Live metastasis of breast carcinoma. Results of surgical resection. Analysis of 15 operated cases]. Chir Ital 2000; 52: 131–7

29. Kondo S, Katoh H, Omi M, et al. Hepatectomy for metastases from breast cancer offers the survival benefit similar to that in hepatic metastases from colorectal cancer. Hepatogastroenterology 2000; 47: 1501–3.

30. Vlastos G, Smith DL, Singletary SE, et al. Long-term survival after an aggressive surgical approach in patients with breast cancer hepatic metastases. Ann Surg Oncol 2004; 11: 869–74.

31. Okaro AC, Durkin DJ, Layer GT, et al. Hepatic resection for breast cancer metastases. Ann R Coll Surg Engl 2005; 87: 167–70.

32. Carlini M, Lonardo MT, Carboni F, et al. Liver metastases from breast cancer. Results of surgical resection. Hepatogastroenterology 2002; 49: 1597–601.

33. Arena E, Ferrero S. Surgical treatment of liver metastases from breast cancer. Minerva Chir 2004; 59: 7–15.

34. Adam R, Chiche L, Aloia T, et al. Hepatic resection for non-colorectal nonendocrine liver metastases: analysis of 1,452 patients and development of a prognostic model. Ann Surg 2006; 244: 524–35.

35. Vauthey JN, Lauwers GY, Esnaola NF, et al. Simplified staging for hepatocellular carcinoma. J Clin Oncol 2002; 20: 1527–36.

36. Martinez SR, Young SE, Giuliano AE, Bilchik AJ. The utility of estrogen receptor, progesterone receptor, and Her-2/neu status to predict survival in patients undergoing hepatic resection for breast cancer metastases. Am J Surg 2006; 191: 281–3.

37. Singletary SE, Walsh G, Vauthey JN, et al. A role for curative surgery in the treatment of selected patients with metastatic breast cancer. Oncologist 2003; 8: 241–51.

38. Elias D, Lasser P, Spielmann M, et al. Surgical and chemotherapeutic treatment of hepatic metastases from carcinoma of the breast. Surg Gynecol Obstet 1991; 172: 461–4.

39. Livraghi T, Goldberg SN, Solbiati L, et al. Percutaneous radio-frequency ablation of liver metastases from breast cancer: initial experience in 24 patients. Radiology 2001; 220: 145–9.

40. Gunabushanam G, Sharma S, Thulkar S, et al. Radiofrequency ablation of liver metastases from breast cancer: results in 14 patients. J Vasc Interv Radiol 2007; 18: 67–72.

41. Sofocleous CT, Nascimento RG, Gonen M, et al. Radiofrequency ablation in the management of liver metastases from breast cancer. AJR Am J Roentgenol 2007; 189: 883–9.

42. Aloia TA, Vauthey JN, Loyer EM, et al. Solitary colorectal liver metastasis: resection determines outcome. Arch Surg 2006; 460–67.

Debashish Bose and Timothy M. Pawlik

Introduction

Melanoma is the fifth most common malignancy among males and the seventh most common malignancy among females in the United States. The incidence of cutaneous melanoma is approximately 55,100 cases per year [1], while ocular melanoma occurs at a frequency of 4,000 cases per year [2]. Depending on the clinicopathologic characteristics of the primary tumor, up to one-third of patients with melanoma may develop distant metastasis [3, 4]. A common site for distant metastasis, particularly for ocular melanoma, is the liver. In fact, up to 40% of patients with ocular melanoma have hepatic metastasis present at initial diagnosis, and the liver becomes involved in up to 95% of individuals who develop metastatic disease [5]. Although cutaneous melanoma metastasizes to the liver less frequently, it still occurs in 15–20% of patients with metastatic disease [6, 7]. In one prospective analysis of over 26,000 patients with melanoma from the United States and Australia, approximately 1,700 (6.7%) developed metastatic disease to the liver, which represented 10–20% of metastatic disease in terms of all sites of recurrence/metastasis [8].

Patients with stage IV melanoma have traditionally been deemed to have an abysmal prognosis. The 5-year survival rate of most patients has been reported to be in the range of 6% with a mean survival time between 4 and 6 months [8]. Because of the poor prognosis for such patients, the benefit of treatment for melanoma metastases to the liver has been somewhat controversial. There is some evidence, however, that surgical treatment

of select patients with melanoma metastasis to other anatomic sites—specifically the lung, spleen, and adrenal—may result in increased survival in the range of 24–49 months [9, 10, 11, 12, 13]. Based on this, some investigators have advocated for more aggressive therapeutic approaches for patients with melanoma liver metastasis. Treatment of metastatic melanoma to the liver, however, remains poorly defined. Therapeutic options for liver-based metastatic melanoma include systemic chemotherapy, locoregional chemotherapy/chemoembolization, isolated hepatic perfusion, and liver resection. The role, as well as efficacy, of each of these treatments continues to evolve. In this chapter we review the relative indications, feasibility, and efficacy of those treatment options most likely to benefit patients with metastatic melanoma to the liver.

Melanoma: Primary Tumor Site

Ocular

Ocular melanoma includes melanoma of the uveal tract and the conjunctiva. Eighty-five percent of ocular melanoma is, however, uveal in origin. Uveal melanoma is a disease of uveal tract melanocytes in the eye which may primarily involve the iris (anterior uveal tract), the choroid plexus or the ciliary body (both posterior uveal tract) [14]. Most uveal tract melanomas originate in the choroids. The ciliary body is less commonly a site of origin, and the iris is the least common. Compared to cutaneous melanoma, uveal melanoma demonstrates a much greater propensity to metastasize primarily to the liver. In fact, for most patients with hepatic metastasis from a uveal primary melanoma, the liver is the only organ involved at the time of detection of systemic metastases [15]. Specifically, once metastases occur, the liver is the sole site of organ involvement in 70–80% of cases [16, 17]. The specific anatomic origin of the uveal melanoma also dictates, to some degree, a patient's propensity to metastasize. Uveal

D. Bose (✉)
Fellow, Department of Surgical Oncology, The University of Texas M.D. Anderson Cancer Center, Houston, TX, USA

T.M. Pawlik (✉)
Assistant Professor of Surgery Department of Surgery, Division of Surgical Oncology, Johns Hopkins Hospital, Johns Hopkins University School of Medicine, Baltimore, MD, USA

J.-N. Vauthey et al. (eds.), *Liver Metastases*, DOI 10.1007/978-1-84628-947-7_16,
© Springer-Verlag London Limited 2009

melanoma confined to the iris generally has a better overall prognosis with most patients having localized disease on diagnosis. Only a small fraction of patients (3–5%) with melanoma completely confined to the iris will develop metastatic disease within a 10-year period [18]. In contrast, involvement of the choroid and/or ciliary body is associated with a significantly worse overall prognosis. Up to 40% of patients with posterior uveal melanoma will develop metastatic disease to the liver within the 10-year period following diagnosis and treatment of their primary tumor [19].

The propensity of uveal melanoma to metastasize to the liver may be related both to embryologic and anatomic considerations. The uveal tract often develops embryologically within the liver. Perhaps more importantly, since the uveal tract is devoid of lymphatics, metastasis from uveal melanoma is purely hematogenous. Unlike cutaneous melanoma, patients with ocular melanoma seldom—if ever—develop locoregional metastatic recurrence.

While the site of metastatic spread is somewhat predictable (e.g., liver), the time from diagnosis of the primary tumor to the development of metastatic disease is highly variable. Metastasis from uveal melanoma has been reported to develop many years after treatment of the primary ocular tumor. While most patients develop metastatic disease from uveal melanoma between 2 and 5 years following eye treatment [20, 21, 22, 23], up to one-third of patients develop metastasis after 5 years [16]. Some investigators have even reported hepatic metastasis from a uveal melanoma 4 decades following treatment of the primary tumor [24]. Of note, Sato et al. [25] have reported that age older than 60 years, male gender, and larger dimension of the primary melanoma were associated with a shorter time to systemic metastasis.

The Collaborative Ocular Melanoma Study Group reported on 2,320 patients who had no evidence of metastatic disease at the time of diagnosis of choroidal melanoma [26]. Seven hundred and thirty-nine patients developed metastasis, primarily to the liver (89%). Of those patients with metastasis, the 1- and 2-year mortality rates were 80% and 92%, respectively. In this series, the risk of metastasis was directly related to the size of the initial primary tumor. Interestingly, 46% of patients had liver-only metastatic disease, while 43% of patients had liver plus other sites of disease. Only 11% of patients had metastatic disease without liver involvement. Of note, only about half of patients who were diagnosed with metastatic disease received treatment. The relatively low rate of treatment may reflect the nihilism that often accompanies this disease. Traditionally, most studies have reported a median survival for patients with ocular liver metastasis of 2 months without treatment and 5–9 months with treatment [22]. Overall, 1-year survival historically ranges from 13% to 20% [20, 22].

Cutaneous

Based on the Surveillance, Epidemiology and End Results (SEER) database, 62,190 Americans were diagnosed with cutaneous melanoma in 2006, and 7,910 patients succumbed to cutaneous melanoma that year [27]. Eighty percent of individuals diagnosed with melanoma present with disease that is localized to the primary tumor site, while about 12–20% will have locoregional metastatic disease to the lymph nodes. In contrast, only about 5% of patients with melanoma present with metastatic or stage IV disease.

Regarding the metastatic pattern of cutaneous melanoma, the liver is the third most common site of metastatic disease after the lymph nodes and the lungs. Cutaneous melanoma is generally believed to spread via both the lymphatics to lymph nodes as well as hematogeneously to any organ, including the liver [28]. Unlike ocular melanoma, patients with hepatic metastasis from a cutaneous primary are more likely to harbor other sites of systemic disease. The Eastern Cooperative Oncology Group (ECOG) compared the characteristics of a large cohort of patients ($n = 713$) with either metastatic ocular or cutaneous melanoma [29]. Patients with ocular melanoma tended to be older and had a distinct pattern of metastasis as compared with patients who had cutaneous melanoma [29]. Specifically, the ECOG study noted that patients with ocular melanoma were significantly more likely to have isolated liver metastasis. Pawlik et al. [30] recently confirmed these findings. Specifically, Pawlik et al. [30] reported that whereas patients with ocular melanoma presented with isolated liver metastasis, patients with cutaneous melanoma were more likely to present with liver metastasis in conjunction with extrahepatic disease.

Primary tumor location on the trunk, lymph node metastasis, increasing tumor thickness, and male gender are associated with an increased risk of distant metastasis. No prognostic factor, however, is known to be associated with a particular pattern of distant metastasis (e.g., liver predominant). Similar to ocular melanoma, patients with cutaneous melanoma can present with metastasis to the liver after prolonged disease-free intervals. In one series of patients undergoing hepatic resection [30], the median disease-free interval from the time of wide local excision of the primary cutaneous melanoma to the time of hepatic metastasis was 63.1 months (range, 13.6 months–31 years).

As expected, prognosis for patients with cutaneous melanoma is dictated by disease extent. Specifically, 5-year survival is roughly 99% for local-only disease, 40–65% for regional disease, and 5–15% for distant disease. Patients with melanoma liver metastases have a reported mean survival of 4–5 months [8]. As such, patients with hepatic metastases from cutaneous melanoma have traditionally been considered poor candidates for liver-directed therapy.

Therapeutic Options for Melanoma Hepatic Metastases

Despite the general poor prognosis of patients with either ocular or cutaneous melanoma to the liver, several therapeutic options have emerged. Traditionally, patients with advanced stage melanoma have been treated with systemic chemotherapy. More recently, therapeutic regimens directed specifically at the liver have been investigated as a possible option for metastatic melanoma of the liver. Such therapies as the infusion of chemotherapy or immunotherapy directly into the hepatic artery either with or without concomitant embolization have been described. In addition, hepatic resection of metastatic melanoma to the liver has been advocated for a very select group of patients.

Systemic Chemotherapy

Metastatic melanoma is largely unresponsive to systemic chemotherapeutic agents, with systemic chemotherapy offering little or no chance of cure. Despite this, in an attempt to extend survival, chemotherapy is frequently employed for patients with metastatic disease—including those with hepatic metastasis. Single-agent chemotherapy remains the standard of care for systemic chemotherapy in patients with metastatic melanoma. Dacarbazine is the drug of choice, with a response rate of 16%. Other drugs, including cisplatin, paclitaxel, docetaxel, and the dacarbazine analogue temozolomide, have also shown activity. Based on observed single-agent activity, several combination regimens have been investigated. The Dartmouth regimen (dacarbazine, cisplatin, carmustine, and tamoxifen) was initially reported to have an overall response rate of 55% and complete response rate of 20% [31]. However, subsequent multicentre trials have failed to corroborate these favorable results. In fact, in randomized phase III trials, the two most active combination chemotherapy regimens, the Dartmouth regimen and cisplatin, vinblastine, and dacarbazine, have not proven to be superior to single-agent dacarbazine in terms of overall survival [32]. Other combinations, such as temozolomide and cisplatin, have not been shown to have clear benefits in terms of response rates but may be associated with a

higher incidence of grade 3 or 4 emesis. Biologic therapy with interferon-alpha and interleukin-2 is also associated with low complete response rates and survival rates of less than 5%. While biochemotherapy has been shown to produce higher response rates (~50%), only a small portion of patients will derive a long-term benefit [33]. In general, even when metastatic melanoma responds to systemic chemotherapy, the duration of the response is usually short, in the range of 3–6 months.

Interestingly, there appears to be a differential response to chemotherapy in patients with ocular versus cutaneous melanoma. For example, ECOG [29] noted that response to chemotherapy was significantly different between patients with ocular versus cutaneous melanoma. In the ECOG study, none of the 51 patients with metastatic ocular melanoma responded to therapy, compared with 74 responders in the cutaneous melanoma group ($p = 0.03$) [29]. Among the subgroup of 218 patients with liver metastases, no patient with an ocular primary tumor responded to therapy while the response rate was 9% for cutaneous primary tumors. Nathan et al. [34] reported on the results of patients with ocular or cutaneous melanoma who were treated with cisplatin, dacarbazine, carmustine, and tamoxifen. Of the 16 patients with ocular melanoma who had hepatic metastasis, only one (6%) achieved a partial response. In contrast, of the 57 patients with cutaneous melanoma who had liver metastases, 19 (33.3%) achieved an objective response ($p = 0.05$).

Pawlik et al. [30] similarly noted that chemotherapy may have a more substantial role in the treatment of patients with metastatic cutaneous melanoma as compared with ocular melanoma. In that series of 40 patients who underwent resection of liver metastases from melanoma, chemotherapy was a significant predictor of prolonged survival in patients with cutaneous melanoma but not in patients with ocular melanoma. Specifically, patients with cutaneous melanoma who were treated with chemotherapy had over a fivefold increase in their median survival as compared to patients who did not receive chemotherapy. Data from this study are, however, difficult to interpret. Given the retrospective nature of the study, it is not possible to comment definitively on the ultimate role of chemotherapy. Clearly a selection bias exists when evaluating the outcome of patients treated with systemic therapy versus those who underwent resection alone, and this selection bias alone could potentially explain the differences encountered in the outcome.

Data from several other groups have, however, corroborated the finding that uveal melanoma is particularly resistant to most systemic chemotherapy, as well as immunotherapy regimens [5, 35, 36]. Becker et al. [5] reported on 48 patients with metastatic uveal melanoma with interferon alpha, interleukin-2, and fotemustine (administered either intravenously or intra-arterially if the metastatic disease was restricted to the liver). Unfortunately, the response rate was 14.5% and only one patient achieved a complete response.

Because of the limited efficacy of systemic chemotherapeutic agents to treat patients with metastatic disease—including those with liver metastasis—there has been increased interest in regional treatment strategies for those patients with melanoma metastasis confined to the liver.

Locoregional Therapies

Locoregional therapies for metastatic melanoma to the liver continue to evolve. For patients with liver-only or liver-predominant disease, a liver-directed locoregional therapeutic approach has intuitive appeal. Patients with hepatic metastases can theoretically be treated with concentrated doses of chemotherapeutic or immunologic agents directed to the site of disease while sparing them of systemic toxicity. Such locoregional approaches have come to include hepatic artery chemotherapy/immunotherapy, hepatic artery chemoembolization, as well as isolated hepatic perfusion (Table 16.1) [37, 38, 39, 40, 41, 42, 43, 44, 45, 46, 47, 48, 49, 50, 51, 52, 53, 54, 55].

Hepatic Artery Infusion Therapy

Whereas systemic chemotherapy is limited by the ability to deliver high doses of drug, direct hepatic artery infusion offers the possibility of delivering cytotoxic drugs to the tumor without systemic morbidity. By directly infusing the drug to the hepatic metastasis, both the normal hepatic parenchyma and the systemic circulation can be spared. Such a therapy can be delivered via a totally implantable catheter surgically placed into the hepatic artery through the gastroduodenal artery that is connected to a subcutaneous access chamber. Ideally, to maximize local drug effect relative to systemic exposure, one would want to administer a chemotherapeutic agent that has a high hepatic extraction rate. Fotemustine, a third-generation nitrosourea, has a high plasma clearance that approximates hepatic blow flow and has a 0.4–0.9 first-pass liver extraction ratio [38, 56]. Because of fotemustine's known activity in treating melanoma, as well as its favorable pharmacokinetic profile, fotemustine has been investigated in several studies evaluating the efficacy of hepatic arterial chemotherapy to treat melanoma metastatic to the liver.

In 1997, Leyvraz et al. [38, 39] reported the feasibility and good tolerance of the hepatic arterial chemotherapy approach for patients with ocular melanoma metastatic to the liver. In that study, the investigators subjected 31 patients to laparotomy and placed a totally implantable catheter into the hepatic artery. Fotemustine (100 mg/m^2) was administered via the catheter as a 4-h infusion, first once a week for four times and then, after a 5-week rest period, every 3 weeks until progression or toxicity. The authors reported an objective response rate of 40% with a median response duration of 11 months. The median overall survival time was 14 months. Importantly, toxicity was minimal and treatment could be administered on an outpatient basis. More recently, the same investigative group [39, 40] reported on an extended and multicentre experience of 101 patients treated with intra-arterial hepatic fotemustine. A median of eight fotemustine infusions per patient were delivered (range, 1–26). Catheter-related complications occurred in 23% of patients; however, this required treatment discontinuation in only 10% of patients. The overall response rate was 36%; median and 2-year survival were 15 months and 29%, respectively [40]. Gender, lactase dehydrogenase level, and time between diagnosis and treatment start were all associated with survival. The investigators concluded that locoregional treatment with fotemustine was well-tolerated and may improve outcome in patients with uveal melanoma metastatic to the liver. The EORTC Melanoma Group has recently undertaken a phase III randomized study of fotemustine administered as an intravenous infusion versus an intra-arterial hepatic perfusion in patients with surgically incurable or unresectable liver metastases secondary to uveal melanoma.

Little data exist on the effect of intra-arterial fotemustine therapy for liver metastases from cutaneous melanoma. Siegel et al. [40, 41] reported a retrospectively analyzed observational study of 36 consecutive patients with hepatic metastases from ocular or cutaneous melanoma who had surgical hepatic port-catheter implantation. Fotemustine was delivered weekly for a 4-week period, followed by a 5-week rest and a maintenance period every 3 weeks until progression. A total of 30 patients (18 with ocular and 12 with cutaneous melanoma) were ultimately treated. Patients received a median of eight infusions per patient (range, 3–24). Nine out of 30 patients had a partial remission, 10 had stable disease, and 11 patients had progressive disease. Overall, the median survival was 14 months; partial remission and stable disease were associated with a survival advantage compared to progressive disease (19 months vs. 5 months). Of note, no significant difference in survival was observed for ocular versus cutaneous melanoma.

Table 16.1 Results of select studies investigating hepatic artery infusion, chemoembolization, or isolated hepatic perfusion of metastatic melanoma to the liver

Author	Number of patients	Therapeutic modality	Primary tumor site	Median survival (months)	Response rate (%)	Five-year survival(%)
Leyvraz et al. [38]	31	HAI, fotemustine	Ocular	14	40	–
Peters et al. [39]	101	HAI, fotemustine	Ocular	15	36	29% 2-year survival
Siegel et al. [40]	30	HAI, fotemustine	Ocular, n = 18 Cutaneous, n = 12	22 12	9/30 PR 10/30 SD 11/30 PD	–
Ueda et al. [41]	1	HAI, dacarbazine, nimustine, vincristine, cisplatin	Ocular	9	–	–
Cantore et al. [42]	8	HAI, carboplatin	Ocular	15	38	–
Bedikian et al. [43]	201	Systemic (143) HAI (38) Chemoembolization (64) Embolization (2)	Ocular	7	1 PR, 7 MR, 27 SD, 108 PD 2 PR, 4 MR, 10 SD, 22 PD 1 CR, 15 PR, 10 MR, 6 SD, 12 PD 2 PD	–
Sato et al. [44]	13	Immunoembolization, GM-CSF	Ocular, n = 12 Cutaneous, n = 1	–	1 CR, 4 PR, 5 SD, 3 PD	–
Carrasco et al. [45]	2	TACE, cisplatin/polyvinyl sponge	Ocular	6, 19 (DFS)		–
Mavligit et al. [46]	30	TACE, cisplatin/polyvinyl sponge	Ocular	11	46	–
Agarwala et al. [47]	19	HAI +/– TACE	Ocular	8.5	16 (3 PR, 13 SD, 1 PD)	
Feun et al. [48]	3	TACE, cisplatin, thiotepa lipiodol	Ocular	3, 16 (DFS)	2 PR	–
Patel et al. [49]	30*	TACE, BCNU	Ocular	5.2	16.7 (1 CR, 4 PR, 13 SD, 6 PD)	
Alexander et al. [50]	4	IHP, melphalan + TNF	Ocular	–	1 CR, 2 PR, 1 MR	–
Libutti et al. [51]	8	IHP, melphalan + TNF	Ocular	–	Not specifically reported	–
Alexander et al. [52]	22	IHP, melphalan +/– TNF	Ocular	11	62 (from 21 patients)	
Noter et al. [53]	8	IHP, melphalan	Ocular	9.9	50	–
Ravikumar et al. [54]	2	HAI with hepatic vein isolation, fluorouracil, doxorubicin	Unspecified	–	Not specifically reported	–
Pingpank et al. [55]	13	HAI with hepatic vein isolation, melphalan	Ocular, n = 10 Cutaneous, n = 3	–	50 (ocular)	–

Abbreviations used: HAI, hepatic artery infusion; TACE, transarterial chemoembolization; IHP, isolated hepatic perfusion; CR, complete response; PR, partial response; MR, minor response; SD, stable disease; PD, progressive disease; DFS, disease-free survival.
*Twenty-four patients were evaluable in this study, see discussion. As indicated in this table, intention-to-treat included 30 patients.

Several investigators [41, 42, 43] have reported on hepatic arterial infusion therapy using chemotherapeutics agent other than fotemustine. Cantore et al. [42, 43] reported a series of patients with ocular melanoma metastatic to the liver who were treated with intra-arterial monotherapy using carboplatin 300 mg/m² delivered once every 2 weeks. The overall response was 38% and the median survival time was 15 months. The regimen was relatively well tolerated, with the principle toxicity being myelosuppression. Evidence-based conclusions are difficult to be drawn from this series, however, as the study included only eight patients. Intra-arterial chemotherapy with cisplatin, vinblastine, and dacarbazine has been attempted in individuals, but has never proved effective [43, 44].

In addition to cytotoxic chemotherapeutic agents, regional infusion of immunotherapeutic agents has also been investigated. Keilholz et al. [57, 45] reported a phase Ib trial of high-dose infusion of interleukin-2 into the splenic artery or intravenous infusion with subsequent transfer of lymphokine-activated killer (LAK) cells into the portal vein or the hepatic artery. Trafficking studies revealed homogeneous distribution of the LAK cells within the liver. The treatment was tolerated relatively well, with no liver-limiting toxicity. One partial and two complete responses were observed in nine patients with metastases from cutaneous melanoma, however, none of the six patients with ocular melanoma metastases responded. In a separate study, Sato et al. [44, 46] described a new immuno-embolization approach using granulocyte-macrophage colony-stimulating factor (GM-CSF). GM-CSF was used to stimulate antigen-presenting cells in the liver metastases. Thirteen patients with metastatic melanoma in the liver (12 with uveal melanoma and 1 with cutaneous melanoma). Among the 12 assessable patients, one patient had a complete response, while four had a partial response and five had stable disease. Based on these findings, the investigators have initiated a phase II clinical trial.

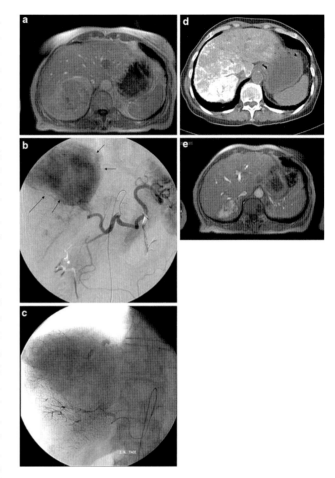

Fig. 16.1 (**a**) T1-weighted contrast-enhanced image of a moderately hypervascular uveal melanoma metastatic to the liver. (**b**) Angiogram displaying hypervascularity of the metastatic lesion. (**c**) Angiography of right hepatic artery. TACE was performed using mitomycin C and lipiodol, followed by microspheres for vascular occlusion. (**d**) CT scan showing hyperattenuated lesion due to retention of lipiodol. (**e**) MRI demonstrating 50% volume reduction of tumor following three cycles of TACE. Reprinted from: Vogl T, Eichler K, Zangos S, et al. Preliminary experience with transarterial chemoembolization (TACE) in liver metastases of uveal malignant melanoma: local tumor control and survival. J Cancer Res Clin Oncol. 2007; 133(3): 177–84. With kind permission of Springer Science and Business Media

Transarterial Hepatic Artery Chemoembolization

Transarterial chemoembolization (TACE) takes advantage of the fact that most macroscopic lesions derive the majority of their blood supply from the hepatic artery (see Fig. 16.1). In addition to delivering higher concentrations of cytotoxic agents, TACE also interrupts the blood supply. Disruption of the afferent blood supply not only induces ischemic necrosis of the tumor, but also is associated with longer retention times of the drug in the target lesion. As such, drug concentrations during chemoembolization can reach 10–25 times those obtained with intra-

arterial infusion alone. In addition, when cytotoxic chemotherapeutic agents are mixed with lipiodol—an iodized poppy-seed oil that destroys the capillary bed—tumor necrosis may be even more pronounced. No absolute contraindications to TACE exist. Good clinical judgment must be exercised, however, in selecting patients. In general, patients should have liver-only or liver-predominant disease and adequate hepatic reserve. Although in the past portal vein thrombosis was considered a contraindication to TACE, more recent reports have noted that TACE can be performed safely in patients with portal vein thrombosis using more selective catheterization techniques [45, 47, 48, 58].

Carrasco et al. [59, 49] published the first experience with chemoembolization for liver metastases of malignant melanoma. Two patients with metastatic melanoma to liver were treated with chemoembolization using cisplatin and polyvinyl sponge (PVS) and were noted to have tumor regression. Based on these preliminary findings, Mavligit et al. [46, 50] subsequently treated 30 patients with ocular melanoma metastatic to the liver with hepatic arterial chemoembolization using a similar admixture of cisplatin and PVS. The total response rate was noted to be 46%; tumor regression was complete in 1 patient and 13 patients had a partial (>50%) response. The median survival for the entire group was 11 months. Vogl et al. [51, 60] reported on 12 patients with liver metastases of uveal malignant melanoma treated with superselective TACE consisting of mitomycin C, lipiodol, and an injection of resorbable microspheres for vascular occlusion. The TACE was well tolerated. Three patients had a partial response (>50%), five patients had stable disease, and four patients had progressive disease. Mean survival following the embolization therapy was 19.5 months.

In a separate study, The University of Texas M.D. Anderson Cancer Centre [43, 44] reported that chemoembolization using cisplatin-based regimens demonstrated a markedly better response rate (36%) compared to systemic chemotherapy (1%) in patients with uveal melanoma metastatic to the liver. Chemoembolization was associated with a median response duration of 14.5 months. In contrast, a separate study by Agarwala et al. [52, 47] using a similar regimen of intrahepatic arterial infusion with cisplatin and chemoembolization with cisplatin and PVS failed to reproduce previous data. In this study, chemoembolization with cisplatin and PVS demonstrated an overall response rate of only 16%. In addition, many patients experienced dose-limiting toxicities related to renal, hepatic, and hematological effects. More recently, Feun et al. [48, 53] conducted a phase I trial of TACE using cisplatin, thiopeta, and lipiodol in 30 patients with both primary and metastatic liver tumors. Three patients with ocular melanoma were included in the study. Two of the three patients with ocular melanoma had partial responses in the liver metastases for 3 and 16 months. Similar to the study by Agarwala et al. [17, 52], toxicity in the Feun et al. [48, 53] study was noteworthy. Out of the 30 patients treated, there were 4 early deaths related to sepsis, respiratory failure, and myocardial infarction. Other toxicities included abdominal pain, elevation of serum creatinine, bilirubin, and transaminases, as well as ototoxicity and peripheral neuropathy. The authors concluded that, while chemoembolization of the liver with cisplatin, thiopeta, and lipiodol may affect a therapeutic response, it can also be associated with significant toxicity.

Patel et al. [49, 54] reported a new chemoembolization approach using 1,3-bis (2-chloro-ethyl)-1-nitrosourea (BCNU) dissolved in ethiodized oil followed by occlusive gelatin sponge particles. In this phase II trial of patients with uveal melanoma metastatic to the liver, 24 patients completed at least one treatment to all targeted liver metastases and were evaluable for hepatic response. Eighteen of these 24 patients experienced regression or stabilization of hepatic metastasis for at least 6 weeks (1 complete response; 4 partial responses; 13 stable disease). The overall response rate, including both complete and partial responders, was about 20%. The median overall survival was 21.9 months for patients with responsive disease compared with 8.7 months and 3.3 months for patients with stable disease and progressive disease, respectively. Seven patients had mild (grade 1 or 2) toxicity while eight patients experienced grade 3 or 4 toxicity. Specifically, the grade 3 or 4 toxicities included vascular thrombosis ($n=3$), partial splenic infarction ($n=1$), thrombocytopenia ($n=1$), acute renal failure ($n=1$), major liver dysfunction ($n=2$). Grade 3 or 4 side-effects were more likely to be seen in patients with more than 50% liver involvement with metastatic uveal lesions.

Isolated Hepatic Perfusion

Isolated hepatic perfusion (IHP) involves complete isolation of the liver from the systemic circulation, thereby permitting high-dose cytotoxic agents to be administered to the liver with minimal exposure to the systemic circulation [55, 61]. The operative procedure is rather extensive and involves complete mobilization of liver as well as the inferior vena cava. In order to fully isolate the liver, all the venous tributaries to the cava, phrenic veins, and right adrenal vein must be identified and ligated. Following dissection of the porta hepatis, the gastroduodenal artery is identified and used as the arterial cannulation site. After placing the patient on veno-venous bypass, the inferior vena cava is occluded with supra- and infra-hepatic clamps. A retrohepatic cannula is used to collect the venous effluent below the level of the hepatic veins. The cytotoxic agent of choice is then infused via the arterial catheter. Upon completion of treatment, the liver is flushed and the vessels decannulated.

Although still largely relegated to highly specialized centres, IHP therapy has been specifically advocated for the treatment of melanoma metastases isolated to the liver. The National Cancer Institute has reported several phase I and II trials using melphalan with and without tumor necrosis factor for patients with ocular melanoma metastatic to the liver [50, 51, 52, 56, 57, 58, 59, 62]. In one study [50, 57] that evaluated the efficacy and systemic and regional toxicities of hyperthermic IHP using melphalan and TNF, the investigators reported no operative mortality and one treatment-related mortality (3%) due to hepatic venoocclusive disease. In 33 assessable patients, the overall response rate was 75% (complete response, 1 patient [3%]; partial response, 26 patients [72%]). With a median potential follow-up of 15 months, the mean duration of response was 9 months (range, 2–30 months). In a separate study [52, 59], 22 patients with ocular melanoma metastatic to liver were treated with a 60-min hyperthermic IHP using melphalan alone (*n* = 11) or with TNF (*n* = 11). Via a laparotomy, IHP inflow was via the hepatic artery alone (*n* = 17) or hepatic artery and portal vein (*n* = 5) and outflow from an isolated segment of inferior vena cava. Most patients had advanced tumor burden with a mean percentage of hepatic replacement of 25% (range, 10–75%) and a median number of metastatic nodules of 25 (range, 5 to >50). There was one treatment-related mortality. The overall response rate in 21 patients was 62% including 2 radiographic complete responses (9.5%) and 11 partial responses (52%). The overall median duration of response was 9 months (range, 5–50) and was significantly longer in those treated with TNF than

without (14 months vs. 6 months, respectively). Overall median survival was 11 months.

The use of isolated hepatic perfusion with high-dose melphalan for the treatment of uveal melanoma metastases confined to the liver has also been reported in Europe [53, 60]. In this study, eight patients with uveal melanoma metastases confined to the liver underwent IHP with high-dose melphalan (200 mg) for 1 h. The tumor response rate (complete or partial remission) was 50%. The median time to progression was 6.7 months (range, 1.7–16.9 months). The overall median survival was 9.9 months (range, 4.7–34.6 months), with a 1-year survival of 50% and a 2-year survival of 37.5%. Three patients experienced grade 3 or 4 hepatotoxicity that was transient and resolved within 3 months.

More recently there has been an interest in trying to simplify IHP through the adoption of a percutaneous approach (see Fig. 16.2). Using this technique, the liver is perfused using a percutaneously place catheter placed in

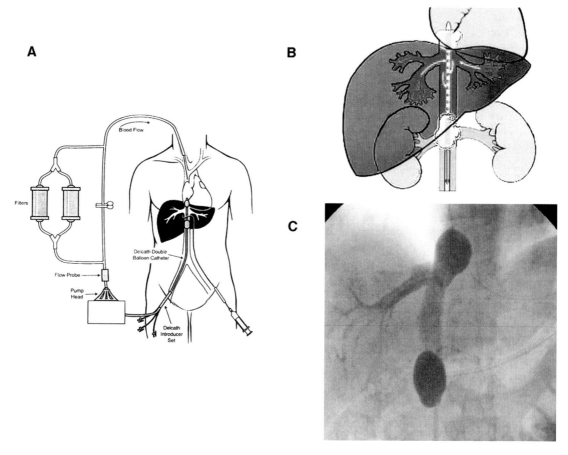

Fig. 16.2 (**a**) Diagram of percutaneous catheter-based approach to isolated hepatic perfusion. The cytotoxic drug of choice is administered via the hepatic artery through a percutaneous catheter while the hepatic venous effluent is collected via a caval balloon and sent through a filtration system. (**b**) Depiction of isolated retrohepatic vena cava showing how hepatic venous outflow is isolated by two inflating balloons. (**c**) Fluoroscopic image of the isolated retrohepatic IVC segment. Reprinted from: Pingpank JF, Libutti SK, Chang R, et al. Phase I study of hepatic arterial melphalan infusion and hepatic venous hemofiltration using percutaneously placed catheters in patients with unresectable hepatic malignancies. J Clin Oncol. 2005; 23(15): 3465–74. With permission from the American Society of Clinical Oncology

the proper hepatic artery. Hepatic venous effluent blood is isolated using a novel percutaneous double-balloon inferior vena cava catheter that then passes the blood through a detoxification filtration cartridge in the venovenous bypass circuit [54, 55, 61, 62]. The advantage of the percutaneous approach is that IHP can be achieved without a major operation and filtration of the hepatic venous effluent can reduce systemic exposure of cytotoxic chemotherapy by 80–90% compared with hepatic artery infusion alone [55, 62].

Several centres have reported their results using percutaneous catheter-based approaches to IHP therapy for unresectable malignancies metastatic to the liver, including metastatic melanoma [54,55, 61, 62]. Ravikumar et al. [54, 61] reported on 21 patients—two of whom had metastatic melanoma to the liver. Twelve patients received dose escalations of fluorouracil (5-FU) and nine received dose escalations of doxorubicin. The authors demonstrated that the percutaneous catheter system functioned efficiently throughout the proscribed dose ranges with no procedure associated mortality and reasonable toxicity. Significant tumor response was seen in two patients receiving doxorubicin. The investigators concluded that the double-balloon catheter technique was technically feasible and safe to isolate and detoxify hepatic venous blood during intra-asterial therapy of unresectable liver tumors. In a separate study, Pingpank and colleagues [55, 62] reported on 28 patients treated with hepatic arterial melphalan infusion and hepatic venous hemofiltration using percutaneously placed catheters. In this study, 13 patients had metastatic melanoma to the liver (ocular, $n = 10$; cutaneous, $n = 3$). Transient grade 3 or 4 hepatic and systemic toxicity was seen after 19% and 66% of treatments, respectively. An overall radiographic response rate of 30% was observed in treated patients. In the ten patients with ocular melanoma, a 50% overall response rate was observed, including two complete responses. The authors concluded that delivery of melphalan via a percutaneous system that employed hepatic venous hemofiltration was feasible, with limited, manageable toxicity and evidence of antitumor activity.

Surgical Resection

Most clinicians traditionally have discouraged resection of hepatic melanoma metastasis, noting that surgery is not warranted due to the dismal prognosis associated with stage IV disease. Other investigators have suggested that resection may only be appropriate in patients with an ocular primary, due to the worse clinical course of patients with cutaneous melanoma [6, 37]. Although the

role of hepatic resection for melanoma metastasis still remains somewhat poorly defined, there have been several studies reporting on resection of hepatic metastasis from melanoma. Unfortunately, most studies reporting on hepatic metastasis from melanoma have either been case reports [63, 64, 65, 66] or small case series (see Table 16.2) [30, 67, 68, 69, 70, 71, 72, 73, 74].

Aoyama et al. [69] reported a case series that included 12 patients who underwent surgical resection of metastatic ocular melanoma—nine of whom had liver metastases. In looking at the entire cohort of 12 patients, the median recurrence-free and overall survival after complete resection were 19 months and 27 months, respectively.

In a collective review of the melanoma experience from the John Wayne Cancer Institute and the Sydney Melanoma Unit, Rose et al. [8] identified 1,750 patients with hepatic metastases. Of these patients, 34 (2%) underwent exploration with intent to resect the metastases. Ultimately, 24 underwent hepatic resection and 10 underwent exploration but not resection. Eighteen patients underwent complete surgical resection, while the remaining six underwent palliative or debulking procedures with incomplete resection. The median disease-free and overall survival in the 24 patients who underwent surgical resection were 12 months and 28 months, respectively. Patients who had liver-only disease, and those who had undergone a hepatic resection with complete micro- and macroscopically negative margins (e.g., R0) had a significantly better disease-free and overall survival. Specifically, patients who had the presence of extrahepatic disease at the time of liver resection had a median overall survival of 15 months compared with 37 months for patients with liver-only metastasis. Similarly, patients who had a positive surgical margin following hepatic resection had a median survival of 13 months compared with 37 months for patients who had an R0 resection. Rivoire and colleagues [72, 75] confirmed the importance of an R0 resection in their study of 28 patients with uveal melanoma liver metastasis. In this study, in which 14 patients had an R0 liver resection and 14 patients had R2 surgery, R0 status was a strong predictor of a better prognosis following hepatic resection (see Fig. 16.3).

More recently the John Wayne Cancer Institute has published their updated experience on hepatic resection of metastases from intraocular melanoma[73]. The authors identified 112 patients with metastatic melanoma from an intraocular site that were enrolled in various treatment protocols; 78 patients had metastatic melanoma to the liver. Overall, 24 patients underwent resection of the metastatic lesions while other patients were treated with non-surgical therapy. At a median follow-up of 11 months, the overall median survival was 11 months

Table 16.2 Results of select studies investigating hepatic resection of metastatic melanoma to the liver

Author	Number of patients	Primary tumor site	Median survival (months)	Five-year survival (%)
Rose et al. [8]	34	Not specified	10	20
Pawlik et al. [30]	40	Ocular, $n = 16$	29.4	20.5
		Cutaneous, $n = 24$	23.6	0
Duh et al. [63]	1	Ocular	Resection of multiple lesions	Died 5 years after liver involvement diagnosed, 15 months after resection
Mondragon-Sanchez et al. [64]	1	Cutaneous	3 resections	NED at 2 years
Gunduz et al. [65]	1	Ocular	2 resections	NED at 2 years
Vauthey et al. [66]	1	Cutaneous	–	Alive at 60 months
Papachristou and Fortner [67]	3	Ocular	16	–
Stoelben et al. [68]	2	Not specified	1 alive at 3 years, 1 alive at 12 years	–
Aoyama et al. [69]	9	All ocular	>27 months	53.3
Fournier et al. [70]	2	Ocular	1 alive at 1 year, 1 survived 3 years	–
Herman et al. [72]	10	Ocular, $n = 5$	22	–
		Cutaneous, $n = 5$		
Hsueh et al. [73]	24	Ocular	11	7
Crook et al. [74]	5	Not specified	2 died from disease at 4, 7 months	3 alive, disease-free at 76, 92, 147 months

Fig. 16.3 Survival of patients with hepatic metastasis from primary uveal melanoma. R0 hepatic resection is associated with the best overall survival. In fact, there was no difference in survival between patients who underwent an R2 resection and those who received only best supportive care. Reprinted from Rivoire M, Kodjikian L, Baldo S, et al. Treatment of liver metastases from uveal melanoma. Ann Surg Oncol. 2005; 12(6): 422–8. With kind permission of Springer Science and Business Media

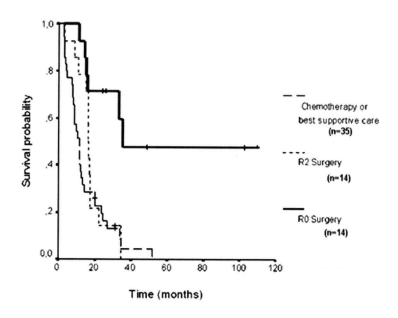

and the 5-year survival was 7%. On univariate analysis, liver metastasis was associated with a worse prognosis compared to other metastatic sites, although on multivariate analysis, site of metastasis did not remain significant. The median survival and the 5-year survival rates were 38 months and 39%, respectively, for surgical patients, versus 9 months and 0%, respectively, for non-surgical patients. The investigators concluded that

resection may prolong survival in certain select patients with metastases from ocular primary melanoma.

A large ($n = 40$) multicentre analysis of patients with either metastatic cutaneous or ocular melanoma has been reported [30]. In this study, the investigators specifically compared patients with ocular versus cutaneous melanoma who underwent hepatic metastasectomy with a curative intent. The primary tumor was ocular in

16 patients and cutaneous in 24. The median disease-free interval from the time of primary tumor treatment to hepatic metastasis was the same for both groups (ocular, 62.9 months; cutaneous, 63.1 months; $p = 0.94$). Most patients underwent either an extended hepatic resection (37.5%) or hemihepatectomy (22.5%). Twenty-six patients (65%) received perioperative systemic therapy. Thirty (75.0%) of 40 patients developed tumor recurrence. The median time to recurrence after hepatic resection was 8.3 months (ocular, 8.8 months; cutaneous, 4.7 months; $p = 0.3$). Patients with primary ocular melanoma were more likely to experience recurrence within the liver (53.3% vs. 17.4%; $p = 0.02$), whereas patients with a cutaneous primary tumor more often developed extrahepatic involvement. Although patients with metastatic cutaneous melanoma had a slightly shorter median overall survival (23.6 months), their 2-year and 5-year survival rates were significantly shorter. Of note, the 5-year survival rate for patients with a primary ocular melanoma was 20.5%, whereas there were no 5-year survivors for patients with cutaneous melanoma (see Fig. 16.4). The authors concluded that patterns of recurrence and prognosis after resection of hepatic melanoma metastasis differ depending on whether the primary melanoma is ocular or cutaneous.

Selection of appropriate patients for hepatic resection of metastatic melanoma must be individualized and include an extensive evaluation of the extent of disease.

Based on currently available data, there are several factors that can help determine the most appropriate candidates for hepatic resection of metastatic melanoma to the liver. Specifically, liver resection for metastatic melanoma should be considered only when the patient may be rendered disease-free by the procedure. That is, an R0

resection should be feasible. Patients with extrahepatic disease should not be categorically excluded from consideration, as several studies suggest that metastasectomy in selected patients may provide a survival benefit if both the intra and extrahepatic disease can be completely removed [74, 75, 76 ,77]. However, it must be kept in mind that patients with an increased tumor burden (multiple lesions, size > 5 cm, multiple sites of disease) may potentially derive relatively less benefit from surgical resection. Metastatic ocular and cutaneous melanomas also have important clinical differences that should be considered at the time of treatment. Although the majority of patients recur, resection of metastatic melanoma to the liver may be associated with improved survival in selected patients. Currently, patients with limited metastatic disease who can be rendered surgically free of disease should be considered for potential hepatic resection. Resection, however, should be performed as part of a multidisciplinary approach possibly in conjunction with systemic or locoregional therapy.

Conclusion

The management of patients with metastatic melanoma to the liver is complex and requires a multimodality approach. Because melanoma responds poorly to systemic treatment, resection remains the only chance at cure. However, the potential benefit of hepatic resection for melanoma metastases has not been established by any large series or prospective trials. Although data are limited, patients with ocular melanoma seem to benefit more from liver-directed therapy compared with patients who have metastatic cutaneous melanoma. These data are

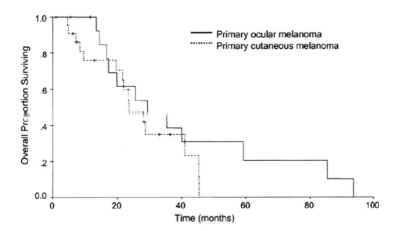

Fig. 16.4 In one study by Pawlik et al. [30], patients with a primary ocular melanoma had a slightly longer median survival (29.4 months) compared with patients with a primary cutaneous melanoma (23.6 months). While the 5-year survival rate for patients with a primary ocular melanoma was 20.5%, there were no 5-year survivors for patients with a cutaneous primary tumor ($p = 0.03$). Reprinted from Pawlik TM, Zorzi D, Abdalla EK, et al. Hepatic resection for metastatic melanoma: distinct patterns of recurrence and prognosis for ocular versus cutaneous disease. Ann Surg Oncol. 2006; 13(5): 712–20. With kind permission of Springer Science and Business Media

difficult to interpret, though, because the experience with resection of cutaneous melanoma metastatic to the liver is limited. In general, hepatic resection should be considered for patients with limited liver-only disease that is amenable to an R0 resection. Based on the aggregate data, resection can be performed safely, and in this select group of patients, appears to be associated with improved survival. Patients with limited tumor burden (few metastatic lesions, no extrahepatic disease, low LDH, etc.) may benefit the most from hepatic resection. For those patients with more extensive hepatic disease, locoregional therapies, including hepatic arterial infusion, TACE, or IHP, should be considered. Regardless of whether hepatic resection or other liver-directed therapies are used to treat liver-predominant disease, the incorporation of more effective systemic chemotherapeutic agents will be critical in the future as most patients ultimately recur at an extrahepatic site.

References

1. Jemal A, Tiwari RC, Murray T, et al. Cancer statistics, 2004. CA Cancer J Clin. 2004; 54(1): 8–29.
2. Singh AD, Topham A. Incidence of uveal melanoma in the United States: 1973–1997. Ophthalmology 2003; 110(5): 956–61.
3. Reintgen DS, Cox C, Slingluff CL Jr, Seigler HF. Recurrent malignant melanoma: the identification of prognostic factors to predict survival. Ann Plast Surg. 1992; 28(1): 45–9.
4. Soong SJ, Harrison RA, McCarthy WH, et al. Factors affecting survival following local, regional, or distant recurrence from localized melanoma. J Surg Oncol. 1998; 67(4): 228–33.
5. Becker JC, Terheyden P, Kampgen E, et al. Treatment of disseminated ocular melanoma with sequential fotemustine, interferon alpha, and interleukin 2. Br J Cancer. 2002; 87(8): 840–5.
6. Leiter U, Meier F, Schittek B, Garbe C. The natural course of cutaneous melanoma. J Surg Oncol. 2004; 86(4): 172–8.
7. Cohn-Cedermark G, Mansson-Brahme E, Rutqvist LE, et al. Metastatic patterns, clinical outcome, and malignant phenotype in malignant cutaneous melanoma. Acta Oncol. 1999; 38(5): 549–57.
8. Rose DM, Essner R, Hughes TM, et al. Surgical resection for metastatic melanoma to the liver: the John Wayne Cancer Institute and Sydney Melanoma Unit experience. Arch Surg. 2001; 136(8): 950–5.
9. Branum GD, Epstein RE, Leight GS, Seigler HF. The role of resection in the management of melanoma metastatic to the adrenal gland. Surgery. 1991;109(2): 127–31.
10. Mosimann F, Fontolliet C, Genton A, et al. Resection of metastases to the alimentary tract from malignant melanoma. Int Surg. 1982; 67(3): 257–60.
11. de Wilt JH, McCarthy WH, Thompson JF. Surgical treatment of splenic metastases in patients with melanoma. J Am Coll Surg. 2003; 197(1): 38–43.
12. Lejeune FJ, Lienard D, Sales F, Badr-el-Din H. Surgical management of distant melanoma metastases. Semin Surg Oncol. 1992; 8(6): 381–91.
13. Wong JH, Euhus DM, Morton DL. Surgical resection for metastatic melanoma to the lung. Arch Surg. 1988; 123(9): 1091–5.
14. Augsberger JJ, Damato BE, Bornfeld N. Uveal melanoma. In: Yanoff M, Duker JS, Augsberger JJ, eds. Ophthalmology. St. Louis: Mosby; 2004.
15. Patel JK, Didolkar MS, Pickren JW, Moore RH. Metastatic pattern of malignant melanoma. A study of 216 autopsy cases. Am J Surg. 1978; 135(6): 807–10.
16. Rajpal S, Moore R, Karakousis CP. Survival in metastatic ocular melanoma. Cancer. 1983; 52(2): 334–6.
17. Seregard S, Kock E. Prognostic indicators following enucleation for posterior uveal melanoma. A multivariate analysis of long-term survival with minimized loss to follow-up. Acta Ophthalmol Scand. 1995; 73(4): 340–4.
18. Conway RM, Chua WC, Qureshi C, Billson FA. Primary iris melanoma: diagnostic features and outcome of conservative surgical treatment. Br J Ophthalmol. 2001; 85(7): 848–54.
19. Singh AD, Shields CL, Shields JA. Prognostic factors in uveal melanoma. Melanoma Res. 2001; 11(3): 255–63.
20. Bedikian AY, Kantarjian H, Young SE, Bodey GP. Prognosis in metastatic choroidal melanoma. South Med J. 1981; 74(5): 574–7.
21. Albert DM, Niffenegger AS, Willson JK. Treatment of metastatic uveal melanoma: review and recommendations. Surv Ophthalmol. 1992; 36(6): 429–38.
22. Gragoudas ES, Egan KM, Seddon JM, et al. Survival of patients with metastases from uveal melanoma. Ophthalmology. 1991; 98(3): 383–9; discussion 390.
23. Einhorn LH, Burgess MA, Gottlieb JA. Metastatic patterns of choroidal melanoma. Cancer. 1974; 34(4): 1001–4.
24. Shields JA, Augsburger JJ, Donoso LA, et al. Hepatic metastasis and orbital recurrence of uveal melanoma after 42 years. Am J Ophthalmol. 1985; 100(5): 666–8.
25. Sato T, Babazono A, Shields JA, et al. Time to systemic metastases in patients with posterior uveal melanoma. Cancer Invest. 1997; 15(2): 98–105.
26. Diener-West M, Reynolds SM, Agugliaro DJ, et al. Development of metastatic disease after enrollment in the COMS trials for treatment of choroidal melanoma: Collaborative Ocular Melanoma Study Group Report No. 26. Arch Ophthalmol. 2005; 123(12): 1639–43.
27. Ries LG, Harkins D, Krapcho M, et al. SEER Cancer Statistics Review 1975–2003. National Cancer Institute; http://seer.cancer.gov/csr/1975_2003/ posted 2006.
28. Leong SP, Cady B, Jablons DM, et al. Clinical patterns of metastasis. Cancer Metastasis Rev. 2006; 25(2): 221–32.
29. Albert DM, Ryan LM, Borden EC. Metastatic ocular and cutaneous melanoma: a comparison of patient characteristics and prognosis. Arch Ophthalmol. 1996; 114(1): 107–8.
30. Pawlik TM, Zorzi D, Abdalla EK, et al. Hepatic resection for metastatic melanoma: distinct patterns of recurrence and prognosis for ocular versus cutaneous disease. Ann Surg Oncol. 2006; 13(5): 712–20.
31. Del Prete SA, Maurer LH, O'Donnell J, et al. Combination chemotherapy with cisplatin, carmustine, dacarbazine, and tamoxifen in metastatic melanoma. Cancer Treat Rep. 1984; 68(11): 1403–5.
32. Chapman PB, Einhorn LH, Meyers ML, et al. Phase III multicenter randomized trial of the Dartmouth regimen versus dacarbazine in patients with metastatic melanoma. J Clin Oncol. 1999; 17(9): 2745–51.
33. O'Day SJ, Kim CJ, Reintgen DS. Metastatic melanoma: chemotherapy to biochemotherapy. Cancer Control. 2002; 9(1): 31–8.
34. Nathan FE, Sato T, Hart E, et al. Response to combination chemotherapy of liver metastases from choroidal melanoma compared with cutaneous melanoma. Amer Soc Clin Oncol. 1994; 13: 396.

35. Pyrhonen S. The treatment of metastatic uveal melanoma. Eur J Cancer. 1998; 34(Suppl 3): S27–30.
36. Nathan FE, Berd D, Sato T, et al. BOLD + interferon in the treatment of metastatic uveal melanoma: first report of active systemic therapy. J Exp Clin Cancer Res. 1997; 16(2): 201–8.
37. Feldman ED, Pingpank JF, Alexander HR, Jr. Regional treatment options for patients with ocular melanoma metastatic to the liver. Ann Surg Oncol. 2004; 11(3): 290–7.
38. Leyvraz S, Spataro V, Bauer J, et al. Treatment of ocular melanoma metastatic to the liver by hepatic arterial chemotherapy. J Clin Oncol. 1997; 15(7): 2589–95.
39. Peters S, Voelter V, Zografos L, et al. Intra-arterial hepatic fotemustine for the treatment of liver metastases from uveal melanoma: experience in 101 patients. Ann Oncol. 2006; 17(4): 578–83.
40. Siegel R, Hauschild A, Kettelhack C, et al. Hepatic arterial Fotemustine chemotherapy in patients with liver metastases from cutaneous melanoma is as effective as in ocular melanoma. Eur J Surg Oncol. 2007; 33(5): 627–32.
41. Ueda H, Hamagami H, Tanaka H, et al. Combination hepatic arterial infusion therapy is effective for ocular melanoma metastasis to the liver. Oncol Rep. 2005; 14(6): 1543–6.
42. Cantore M, Fiorentini G, Aitini E, et al. Intra-arterial hepatic carboplatin-based chemotherapy for ocular melanoma metastatic to the liver. Report of a phase II study. Tumor. 1994; 80(1): 37–9.
43. Bedikian AY, Legha SS, Mavligit G, et al. Treatment of uveal melanoma metastatic to the liver: a review of the M. D. Anderson Cancer Center experience and prognostic factors. Cancer. 1995; 76(9): 1665–70.
44. Sato T, Terai M, Huandong Y. Systemic immune response after immunoembolization of liver metastasis with granulocyte-macrophage colony stimulating factor (GM-CSF). Proc Am Assoc Cancer Res. 2002; 43: 914.
45. Carrasco CH, Wallace S, Charnsangavej C, et al. Treatment of hepatic metastases in ocular melanoma. Embolization of the hepatic artery with polyvinyl sponge and cisplatin. JAMA. 1986; 255(22): 3152–4
46. Mavligit GM, Charnsangavej C, Carrasco CH, et al. Regression of ocular melanoma metastatic to the liver after hepatic arterial chemoembolization with cisplatin and polyvinyl sponge. JAMA. 1988; 260(7): 974–6.44.
47. Agarwala SS, Panikkar R, Kirkwood JM. Phase I/II randomized trial of intrahepatic arterial infusion chemotherapy with cisplatin and chemoembolization with cisplatin and polyvinyl sponge in patients with ocular melanoma metastatic to the liver. Melanoma Res. 2004; 14(3): 217–22.
48. Feun LG, Reddy KR, Scagnelli T, et al. A phase I study of chemoembolization with cisplatin, thiotepa, and lipiodol for primary and metastatic liver cancer. Am J Clin Oncol. 1999; 22(4): 375–80.
49. Patel K, Sullivan K, Berd D, et al. Chemoembolization of the hepatic artery with BCNU for metastatic uveal melanoma: results of a phase II study. Melanoma Res. 2005; 15(4) 297–304.
50. Alexander HR Jr, Bartlett DL, Libutti SK, et al. Isolated hepatic perfusion with tumor necrosis factor and melphalan for unresectable cancers confined to the liver. J Clin Oncol. 1998;16(4):1479–89.
51. Libutti SK, Barlett DL, Fraker DL, Alexander HR. Technique and results of hyperthermic isolated hepatic perfusion with tumor necrosis factor and melphalan for the treatment of unresectable hepatic malignancies. J Am Coll Surg. 2000; 191(5): 519–30.
52. Alexander HR, Libutti SK, Bartlett DL, et al. A phase I-II study of isolated hepatic perfusion using melphalan with or without tumor necrosis factor for patients with ocular melanoma metastatic to liver. Clin Cancer Res. 2000; 6(8): 3062–70.
53. Noter SL, Rothbarth J, Pijl ME, et al. Isolated hepatic perfusion with high-dose melphalan for the treatment of uveal melanoma metastases confined to the liver. Melanoma Res. 2004; 14(1): 67–72.
54. Ravikumar TS, Pizzorno G, Bodden W, et al. Percutaneous hepatic vein isolation and high-dose hepatic arterial infusion chemotherapy for unresectable liver tumors. J Clin Oncol. 1994; 12(12): 2723–36.
55. Pingpank JF, Libutti SK, Chang R, et al. Phase I study of hepatic arterial melphalan infusion and hepatic venous hemofiltration using percutaneously placed catheters in patients with unresectable hepatic malignancies. J Clin Oncol. 2005; 23(15): 3465–74.
56. Fety R, Lucas C, Solere P, et al. Hepatic intra-arterial infusion of fotemustine: pharmacokinetics. Cancer Chemother Pharmacol. 1992; 31(2): 118–22.
57. Keilholz U, Scheibenbogen C, Brado M, et al. Regional adoptive immunotherapy with interleukin-2 and lymphokine-activated killer (LAK) cells for liver metastases. Eur J Cancer. 1994; 30A(1): 103–5.
58. Pentecost MJ, Daniels JR, Teitelbaum GP, Stanley P. Hepatic chemoembolization: safety with portal vein thrombosis. J Vasc Interv Radiol. 1993; 4(3): 347–51.
59. Ramsey DE, Kernagis LY, Soulen MC, Geschwind JF. Chemoembolization of hepatocellular carcinoma. J Vasc Interv Radiol. 2002; 13(9 Pt 2): S211–21.
60. Vogl T, Eichler K, Zangos S, et al. Preliminary experience with transarterial chemoembolization (TACE) in liver metastases of uveal malignant melanoma: local tumor control and survival. J Cancer Res Clin Oncol. 2007; 133(3): 177–84.
61. Grover A, Alexander HR Jr. The past decade of experience with isolated hepatic perfusion. Oncologist. 2004; 9(6): 653–64.
62. Alexander HR Jr, Bartlett DL, Libutti SK. Isolated hepatic perfusion: a potentially effective treatment for patients with metastatic or primary cancers confined to the liver. Cancer J Sci Am. 1998; 4(1): 2–11.
63. Duh EJ, Schachat AP, Albert DM, Patel SM. Long-term survival in a patient with uveal melanoma and liver metastasis. Arch Ophthalmol. 2004; 122(2): 285–7.
64. Mondragon-Sanchez R, Barrera-Franco JL, Cordoba-Gutierrez H, Meneses-Garcia A. Repeat hepatic resection for recurrent metastatic melanoma. Hepatogastroenterology. 1999; 46(25): 459–61.
65. Gunduz K, Shields JA, Shields CL, et al. Surgical removal of solitary hepatic metastasis from choroidal melanoma. Am J Ophthalmol. 1998; 125(3): 407–9.
66. Vauthey JN, Winter MW, Blumgart LH. Solitary metastasis from cutaneous melanoma to the liver: resection by extended left hepatectomy (trisegmentectomy) with clearance of tumor from the portal vein. HPB Surg. 1994; 8(1): 53–6.
67. Papachristou DN, Fortner JJ. Surgical treatment of metastatic melanoma confined to the liver. Int Surg. 1983; 68(2): 145–8.
68. Stoelben E, Sturm J, Schmoll J, et al. [Resection of solitary liver metastases of malignant melanoma]. Chirurg. 1995; 66(1): 40–3; discussion 43–4.
69. Aoyama T, Mastrangelo MJ, Berd D, et al. Protracted survival after resection of metastatic uveal melanoma. Cancer. 2000; 89(7): 1561–8.
70. Fournier GA, Albert DM, Arrigg CA, et al. Resection of solitary metastasis. Approach to palliative treatment of hepatic involvement with choroidal melanoma. Arch Ophthalmol. 1984; 102(1): 80–2.
71. Harrison LE, Brennan MF, Newman E, et al. Hepatic resection for noncolorectal, nonneuroendocrine metastases: a fifteen-year experience with ninety-six patients. Surgery. 1997; 121(6): 625–32.

72. Herman P, Machado MA, Montagnini AL, et al. Selected patients with metastatic melanoma may benefit from liver resection. World J Surg. 2007; 31(1): 171–4.

73. Hsueh EC, Essner R, Foshag LJ, et al. Prolonged survival after complete resection of metastases from intraocular melanoma. Cancer. 2004; 100(1): 122–9.

74. Crook TB, Jones OM, John TG, Rees M. Hepatic resection for malignant melanoma. Eur J Surg Oncol. 2006; 32(3): 315–7.

75. Rivoire M, Kodjikian L, Baldo S, et al. Treatment of liver metastases from uveal melanoma. Ann Surg Oncol. 2005; 12(6): 422–8.

76. Gutman H, Hess KR, Kokotsakis JA, et al. Surgery for abdominal metastases of cutaneous melanoma. World J Surg. 2001; 25(6): 750–8.

77. Essner R, Lee JH, Wanek LA, et al. Contemporary surgical treatment of advanced-stage melanoma. Arch Surg. 2004; 139(9): 961–6; discussion 966–7.

Thomas A. Aloia

Introduction

Over the past 30 years the face of liver surgery has been transformed by the management of colorectal liver metastases. Uniquely, this is a malignancy where surgical cure of stage IV disease is not only possible, but is now common [1, 2, 3]. In addition, selected patients with large volume or ill-located colorectal liver metastases who respond to systemic chemotherapy can also achieve a survival benefit from hepatectomy [4].

The technical advances achieved through experience with colorectal liver metastasis surgery have encouraged hepatobiliary surgical oncologists to apply this treatment modality to patients with liver metastases from other primary sites. Included in the largest recent review of the surgical treatment for non-colorectal, non-endocrine liver metastases, commissioned by the French Surgical Association (L'Association Française de Chirurgie), were 460 patients operated for breast cancer liver metastases. The second largest group in this dataset was non-colorectal gastrointestinal liver metastases, accounting for 230 of the 1,452 total patients studied (16%) [5].

These 230 cases were collected over a 20-year period (1984–2004), emphasizing how infrequently these metastases are amenable to hepatic resection. The differential incidence of liver resection for non-colorectal versus colorectal liver metastases can be accounted for by several factors. First, colorectal cancer is more common than other gastrointestinal primary tumors. The most recent US cancer epidemiology data indicate that the only non-colorectal gastrointestinal cancer among the top ten cancers in incidence for US men and women is pancreatic cancer, which ranks #10 for US males [6]. Second, in contrast to colorectal cancer, most other gastrointestinal malignancies are diagnosed when they have already reached an advanced

stage. Of the 12 cancer types reported on by Jemal et al., esophageal, gastric, and pancreas cancers are the only primary cancer sites that more commonly present with metastatic (stage IV) disease than localized (stages I–II) disease [6]. Third, non-colorectal gastrointestinal tumors tend to be refractory to systemic chemotherapy. For example, despite decades of dedicated research, chemotherapy response rates and survivals for patients with pancreatic cancer continue to be dismal [7, 8]. Together these factors strongly contribute to the finding that non-colorectal gastrointestinal malignancies are associated with the highest all-stage mortality rates of any malignancy, rivaled only by those of lung and bronchus cancers [6].

Based on the portal venous and lymphatic drainage of the gut, some non-colorectal gastrointestinal malignancies metastasize to the liver via similar mechanisms and pathways as do colorectal cancers. However, there is much more variability in the metastatic pathways for most non-colorectal gastrointestinal malignancies. Lymphatic drainage to upper para-aortic and thoracic nodes is common in esophageal, gastric, and duodenopancreatic cancers. As well, systemic dissemination is more common for these tumor sites.

Given the variable mechanisms for metastases, the three most common presentations for non-colorectal gastrointestinal liver metastases are as follows:

Synchronous discovery on staging radiology at the time of diagnosis of the primary tumor

- Synchronous discovery of radiographically occult liver metastases at the time of surgical staging or primary tumor resection
- Metachronous discovery during follow-up from primary tumor treatment

Few single institutions have significant experience with liver metastases from non-colorectal gastrointestinal sites. Most of the outcome data available for these tumors are included in the reports of global liver metastases' surveys

T.A. Aloia (✉)
Assistant Professor of Surgery, Department of Surgery, Weill-Cornell Medical College, The Methodist Hospital, Houston, TX, USA

Table 17.1 Relative contribution of each gastrointestinal primary tumor site to five large series reporting on the surgical treatment of non-colorectal liver metastases

| Primary site | Reference | | | | |
	Reddy [11]	*Ercolani* [9]	*Weitz* [12]	*Elias* [10]	*Adam* [5]
Esophagus/GEJ	1	3	0	0	45
Gastric	1	10	3	11	64
Duodenum/SB	0	2	1	0	13
Bile ducts	1	0	2	7	43
Pancreas	0	3	5	0	40
Total	82	83	141	147	1452

Abbreviations: GEJ, gastroesophageal junction; SB, small bowel.

from major centres and from multi-institutional registry studies. Four recent large single-institution series are available for analysis of outcomes following resection in patients with non-colorectal liver metastases [9, 10, 11, 12]. In total, these four series account for 453 cases. However, the proportion of cases contributed by non-endocrine gastrointestinal primary sites to each of these series is small, ranging from only 4% of cases [11] to 22% of cases [9] (Table 17.1, Fig. 17.1). In some cases, these series offer specific prognostic information regarding individual tumor types; however, most only report the prognostic factors for the larger group of non-colorectal liver metastases.

Of note, for a discussion of carcinoid and other endocrine metastases that frequently arise in digestive organs the reader is referred to Chapter 13. Likewise, the reader is referred to Chapter 14 for the discussion of liver metastases from gastrointestinal stromal tumors (GIST).

Esophageal and Gastroesophageal Junction Cancer

Background and Epidemiology

Over the past several decades there has been an epidemiologic shift in the spectrum of disease for patients with esophageal and gastroesophageal junction cancers. Distal esophageal and gastroesophageal junction adenocarcinomas are now far more common than the previously prevalent upper esophageal squamous cell cancers [13]. Both for the proximity of distal esophageal lesions to the portal lymphatic pathways and the propensity for adenocarcinoma to thrive in the hepatic parenchyma, these tumors are frequently associated with liver metastases [14].

As with most of the non-colorectal gastrointestinal primary liver metastases, those from esophageal and gastroesophageal junction cancers are rarely solitary or isolated, and therefore, are seldom considered resectable. Although there are more reports of complete radiographic response to chemoradiotherapy than successful hepatic resections, in select patients with chemosensitive tumors, hepatic resection has been used as a treatment option, usually in combination with hepatic arterial chemotherapy.

Presentation and Diagnosis

As many as 35% of patients with esophageal and gastroesophageal junction cancers will have synchronous liver metastases at the time of diagnosis [14]. When synchronous metastases are present, the liver involvement may be radiographically apparent or occult; frequently discovered at the time of staging laparoscopy or definitive

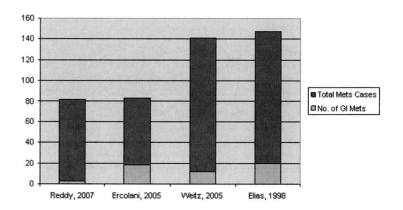

Fig. 17.1 Four recent international reports documenting outcomes for patients with non-colorectal liver metastases treated with hepatic resection and the relative contribution of gastrointestinal primary tumor metastases to each series

surgical resection. Usually this finding contraindicates esophagectomy for cure and relegates the patient to palliative procedures.

A second group of patients with esophageal carcinoma will develop metachronous liver disease following treatment of their primary lesion. In these cases, hepatic metastases tend to be multiple and be associated with extrahepatic disease, again contraindicating hepatic resection. Only occasionally, hepatic metastases will be solitary or limited to one liver section, allowing treating physicians to contemplate resection as part of a multimodality treatment strategy.

Typical of other adenocarcinoma metastases, those from esophageal and gastroesophageal junction cancers tend to be lobulated hypoattenuating lesions on cross-sectional imaging that are readily distinguishable from benign and malignant primary liver tumors (Fig. 17.2).

Role of Surgery

Prior to 2006, less than 20 cases of hepatic resection for esophageal and gastroesophageal cancer liver metastases had been reported [9, 15, 16]. Most of these were single case reports and none of these contained analyses of prognostic factors. In 2006, Adam et al. reported on a multi-institutional experience of 20 patients with resected liver metastases from esophageal cancer [5]. This

experience included patients with both esophageal squamous cell and adenocarcinoma metastases. Only 32% of patients were alive for more than 3 years following resection. Likewise, resection of gastroesophageal junction cancer liver metastases in 25 patients was associated in this series with a 5-year survival of only 12% [5]. These survivals were among the poorest in their global analysis of 1,452 resections for non-colorectal, non-endocrine liver metastases from multiple sites. The nature of this study and the low numbers of patients did not allow for an analysis of prognostic factors.

The only favorable reports of outcome following hepatic resection for esophageal cancer liver metastases come from Japanese surgical units in the form of case reports. Typically, patients with intermediate-term survivals have solitary liver metastases that are responsive to chemotherapy, usually given via both systemic and hepatic arterial routes. For example, Yamamoto and colleagues reported in 2001 on a patient with a solitary esophageal cancer liver metastasis treated with resection and postresection hepatic arterial chemotherapy with cisplatinum and 5-fluorouracil [15]. The patient was alive 15 months after surgery, although with recurrent disease.

These limited data suggest that, in the vast majority of cases, resection of esophageal and gastroesophageal junction cancer metastases provides little survival benefit. Only selected cases with durable responses to chemotherapy should be considered for hepatic resection.

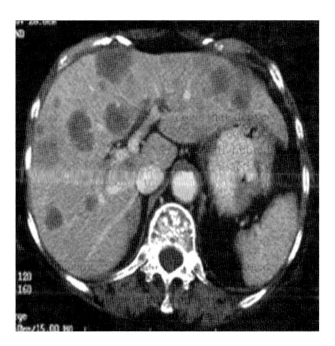

Fig. 17.2 Computed tomography image of multiple bilateral liver metastases in a patient with esophageal cancer

Role of Adjuvant Therapies

Hepatic metastases may be responsive to both chemotherapy and radiation therapy. Chemotherapy is delivered systemically, and may also be given via hepatic arterial infusion. Regimens typically include 5-fluorouracil, platinum derivatives, and/or taxanes.

Recent Novel Approaches

Based on the literature, the only novel surgical approach to patients with esophageal cancer liver metastases is a theoretical multimodality construct in patients with technically resectable hepatic disease. Good-performance status patients with technically resectable synchronous liver metastases could be submitted to a protocol that begins with systemic chemotherapy with or without primary tumor-directed radiotherapy. Patients with responsive disease at the primary site and stable or responding hepatic disease would undergo esophagectomy and placement of a hepatic arterial chemotherapy pump. Those who remained resectable following intra-arterial hepatic chemotherapy could be submitted to subsequent hepatic resection. A similar construct for selected patients with limited metachronous liver disease, involving systemic and hepatic arterial chemotherapy followed by resection, can also be envisioned.

Gastric Cancer

Background and Epidemiology

Since 1930, when gastric cancer was a leading cause of mortality for men and women in the United States, the incidence of death from gastric cancer has sharply declined [6]. The vast majority of gastric malignancies are adenocarcinomas, with gastrointestinal stromal tumors (GIST) and lymphomas representing less common histologies. Currently, the incidence of gastric adenocarcinoma is less than 5 per 100,000, ranking below both pancreatic cancer and hepatocellular carcinoma in prevalence in the United States [6]. Although likely related to differing etiologic factors, gastric cancer is also a predominant malignant histology in other parts of the world; most notably in Japan. Owing to the rich lymphatic drainage of the stomach, nodal metastases are the most common site of extragastric spread. The liver is the most common organ site of gastric cancer metastases [14], however, the majority of patients with liver involvement also have other sites of extrahepatic distant disease. In addition to lymphatic or hematologic seeding of the liver, direct extension from the lesser curve of the stomach to the left liver is also a common presentation.

Presentation and Diagnosis

Primary disease in the stomach usually begins with insidious symptoms of epigastric discomfort and weight loss, progressing in advanced stages to pain, subacute or acute bleeding, and less commonly, obstructive symptoms. Liver involvement, and the frequently associated peritoneal involvement, may be detected on physical exam and/or on cross-sectional imaging with approximately 75% accuracy. Endoscopic ultrasound may help to define direct extension to the left liver as well as lymph node involvement. Otherwise, synchronous liver metastases are usually detected during staging laparoscopy or during exploration for definitive treatment.

Role of Surgery

Palliative hepatic resection for gastric cancer metastases is rarely justified. Hepatic resection with curative intent is possible in highly selected patients. A review of the literature finds documentation of such resections in over 350 patients, however, only 3 Western series comment on more than 10 patients [10, 17, 18]. The limited prognostic information from these series focuses on the disease-free interval from treatment of the primary tumor to development of isolated liver metastases. Patients with synchronous liver metastases, even when they are resectable and represent the only overt metastatic disease, have a relatively poor prognosis, compared to patients resected for metachronous liver metastases [17].

In contrast to the Western experience, multiple single-institution experiences from Japan have recently been published on the treatment of patients with gastric cancer liver metastases [19, 20, 21, 22, 23]. Together these 5 reports comment on 122 treated patients, with 5-year survival rates ranging from 18% to 38% and recurrence rates between 75% and 84%. In general, patients received systemic therapy prehepatectomy, posthepatectomy, or in both settings. The favorable prognostic factors identified within these studies included metachronous presentation, tumor number, tumor size, and a negative surgical margin.

Included in the recent French review from Adam et al. are 64 cases of hepatic resection for gastric cancer metastases [5]. The 5-year and median survivals in these patients were 27% and 15 months, respectively. At each time point in follow-up half of alive patients had recurred. Long-term survivors typically had low volume metachronous disease and an absence of extrahepatic metastases. Again, negative surgical margin was an important prognostic factor (Table 17.2).

Role of Adjuvant Therapies

The majority of gastric cancer patients with localized disease receive multimodality therapy with varying combinations of chemoradiotherapy and surgery. Active systemic regimens include 5-FU and platinum-containing compounds. For patients with metachronous liver metastases, systemic therapy is warranted prior to and following liver resection.

Table 17.2 Selected studies documenting survivals and prognostic factors for patients with gastric cancer liver metastases treated with hepatic resection

Author, year	N	Survivals	Favorable prognostic factors
Elias, 1998 [10]	12	3-yr: 35%	NR
Ambiru, 2001 [19]	40	2-yr: 27%	Metachronous
Saiura, 2002 [21]	10	3-yr: 30%	Lack of nodal metastases
Okano, 2002 [20]	19	3-yr: 34%	Solitary, metachronous, pseudocapsule
Shirabe, 2003 [22]	36	3-yr: 26%	Primary tumor without LVI, <3 LM
Sakamoto, 2003 [23]	22	3-yr: 38%	Solitary, size <5 cm
Adam, 2006 [5]	64	5-yr: 27%	Lack of extrahepatic metastases

Abbreviations: yr, year; NR, not reported; LVI, lymphovascular invasion; LM, liver metastases.

Recent Novel Approaches

For patients with gastric cancer, who frequently enter preoperative chemoradiotherapy protocols, there is a role for pre-treatment staging laparoscopy. The sensitivity of this procedure to diagnose intraperitoneal metastatic disease is 20–30% greater than that of CT scan and/or EUS [24]. One recent study involving 416 patients with radiographically resectable gastric and esophageal cancers found advanced disease in 84 patients (20.2%) [25]. Of these 84 cases, 13 were excluded from resectability due to small volume liver metastases and an additional 5 patients were excluded due to the combination of liver and peritoneal disease identified at staging laparoscopy. Of caution, however, was the finding that 15 of the 27 false negative staging laparoscopies were from patients with gastric cardia and gastroesophageal junction tumors. Based on these data, it appears that laparoscopy is an important adjunct in the staging and surgical treatment of patients with gastric cancers, but may have relatively less accuracy in patients with proximal gastric cancers.

Finally, there are reports of ablative technologies being applied to gastroesophageal liver metastases [26], but long-term survivals following this approach have not been described.

Duodenal and Small Bowel Cancer

Background and Epidemiology

Although small bowel malignancy is ten times more common than primary duodenal cancer, because the spectrum of histologies for small bowel cancer (adenocarcinoma, stromal tumors, lymphoma, and neuroendocrine tumors) is broader than for duodenal cancer (typically adenocarcinoma), the incidence of adenocarcinoma at either site is rare. In both duodenal and small bowel adenocarcinoma the predominant site of metastases is regional lymph nodes, followed by the liver [27]. Traditionally, liver metastases in these cases have been treated with medical therapy only, using regimens similar to those used to treat other more common gastrointestinal adenocarcinomas. Reports of resection of hepatic metastases from non-endocrine duodenal and small bowel primary tumors are exceedingly rare.

Presentation and Diagnosis

The typical presenting symptoms for patients with duodenal and small bowel tumors are abdominal pain and obstruction. When present, hepatic metastases from duodenal and small bowel primary tumors are usually multiple and bilateral [27]. The diagnosis of hepatic metastases in these patients is usually made incidentally. For patients with synchronous disease this may be at the time of staging or during emergent operations to relieve obstruction.

Particularly in patients with duodenal cancer, that typically would require a pancreaticoduodenectomy to treat the primary tumor, careful operative planning is required. If hepatic metastases are diagnosed preoperatively, the ability to avoid initial operative management (in lieu of systemic therapy) is based on the degree of obstruction and the history or risk for tumor related hemorrhage. In cases with symptomatic obstruction, palliative local radiation therapy and operative bypass are therapeutic options.

Role Of Surgery

There is one case report of a patient with metastatic duodenal adenocarcinoma treated with simultaneous pancreaticoduodenectomy and hepatic resection, with a long-term survival of more than 5 years [28]. With the exception of this case, the literature contains very little information regarding the surgical treatment of duodenal and small bowel liver metastases. The largest recent global non-colorectal liver metastases resection reports from Elias [10], Reddy [11], Wietz [12], and Ercolani [9] include only one case of metastases from duodenal cancer and only two cases from small bowel primary tumors.

The French Surgical Association review from Adam et al. reports on 12 cases of duodenal liver metastases and 28 cases of small bowel liver metastases; however, only 13 of these 40 total cases were adenocarcinomas (7 duodenal and 6 small bowel) [5]. In 11 of these 13 patients the metastases were solitary and in 7 of 13 cases the lesions were metachronous with a mean interval between treatment of the primary tumor and discovery of metastases of 3 years. The 5-year overall survival for these 13 patients was 30%, with 3 patients alive 5 years after first hepatectomy. Interestingly, all three of these patients experienced a treatment response to pre-hepatectomy chemotherapy. Compared to the favorable 5-year postliver resection survival of 49% for all patients with small bowel liver metastases (all histologies, $n = 28$), the subset with small bowel adenocarcinoma fared worse with a 5-year survival of 23%.

Role of Adjuvant Therapies

Based on these data it appears that the vast majority of cases of metastatic duodenal and small bowel adenocarcinoma have been treated with palliative therapies. The mainstay of this approach is systemic chemotherapy, with a role for local radiotherapy in cases of symptomatic unresectable duodenal tumors. Certainly, patients with metachronous liver metastases and no evidence of local recurrence should be treated with preoperative systemic therapy. The series from Adam et al. suggests that a response to pre-hepatectomy systemic therapy may predict a long-term benefit for patients who are subsequently resected [5].

Recent Novel Approaches

Given the rarity of this clinical scenario, novel surgical strategies are absent in the literature. Theoretically, radiofrequency ablation could be used to treat small metastases; however, radiofrequency ablation for this indication has not been described. With the development of multiple new effective systemic therapies, including anti-angiogenic drugs and other biologic agents, there is hope that more patients with metastatic disease from duodenal and small bowel adenocarcinoma could be converted from an unresectable situation to a resectable one with systemic therapy.

Biliary Cancers

Background And Epidemiology

Extrahepatic biliary malignancy, including gallbladder, extrahepatic bile duct, and ampullary cancers present some of the most difficult challenges to the hepatobiliary surgeon. With the exception of distal bile duct tumors, which may present early in development with biliary obstruction, most malignancies of the biliary tract are discovered at an advanced stage. The mechanisms for intrahepatic metastasis formation are multiple and likely to include lymphatic spread, portal translocation, and systemic dissemination. In the previous two mentioned scenarios, there is a higher possibility that disease may be localized in the liver with less extrahepatic spread. This fact, combined with the increased incidence of biliary tract malignancy relative to other gastrointestinal tumors, may explain the larger number of reports of liver resection for biliary cancer metastases compared to other primary gastrointestinal sites.

Presentation and Diagnosis

Extrahepatic biliary tract cancers typically present with local symptoms including right upper quadrant abdominal pain, jaundice, cholangitis, and manifestations of local extension to adjacent structures including the duodenum and colon. Cross-sectional imaging prior to endobiliary or percutaneous biliary procedures/stenting is advised [29, 30]. These studies can be supplemented by cholangiography, endoscopic ultrasound, and biopsy to complete the diagnostic and staging evaluation. Frequently, local invasion of adjacent structures and peritoneal metastases that are occult on radiographic staging are identified at laparoscopic staging. Laparoscopy also allows for intra-abdominal ultrasound examination which may detect liver metastases not previously imaged [31].

Patients with gallbladder cancer also typically present with advanced stage disease. Except for those who are incidentally found to have early stage disease at the time of cholecystectomy, the survival rate for patients with gallbladder cancer is dismal [32, 33, 34]. As well, patients with advanced stage gallbladder cancer and liver metastases frequently present with simultaneous invasion of other local structures, peritoneal dissemination, advanced age, and poor performance status. Occasionally, patients with presumed stage III disease, treated with major hepatectomy, radical cholecystectomy, and portal lymphadenectomy will have liver metastases discovered in the operative specimen. Otherwise, there are very few reports in the literature describing the surgical treatment of metastatic gallbladder cancer [35].

Role of Surgery

Combined, the reported number of liver resections for extrahepatic biliary cancer hepatic metastases is only 45 cases (gallbladder: 28, bile duct: 5, and ampullary: 12). For patients with metastatic gallbladder cancer, the three largest series (Elias, $n = 7$ [10], Morrow, $n = 8$ [36], Yamada, $n = 6$ [37]) report only one long-term survivor. Importantly, the majority of patients resected for gallbladder liver metastases had synchronous disease and underwent a simultaneous resection of the primary and metastatic disease. These complex resections were associated with an elevated operative mortality, as high as 33% [37].

Reported operative mortality rates and survivals following resection of Klatskin [38] and mid-bile duct cancer liver metastases were equivalent to those of gallbladder primaries [36, 37, 39]. In contrast, reports on liver-directed treatment of ampullary cancer more commonly focus on patients with metachronous disease. In addition, none of the reported hepatectomies for ampullary cancer liver metastases were associated with a perioperative death. Of the 12 reported cases of ampullary cancer metastasis resections, 3 patients are 3-year survivors [40, 41, 42] and 1 patient has achieved a 5-year survival following resection [40].

Of the 1,452 non-colorectal liver metastases patients reported on by Adam et al. in 2006, 43 cases (3%) were from patients with biliary tract primary cancers [5]. Again, the majority of gallbladder cancer cases involved synchronous disease and the majority of mid and lower bile duct cases were metachronous. The only perioperative mortality was reported in the gallbladder cancer group. For all sites of biliary cancer, the posthepatectomy recurrence rates were high. The 3-year survivals for gallbladder cancer were less than 30%. Only one patient in the mid-bile duct cancer group survived more than 2 years following hepatectomy. In contrast, patients undergoing resection for ampullary cancer liver metastases

experienced a 46% 5-year survival rate with a median survival of 38 months. The survivals in the ampullary cancer subset of bile duct primary tumors were among the longest recorded in this series.

Role of Adjuvant Therapies

Of the total reported cases of liver resection for bile duct cancer metastases less than 20% of patients received preoperative systemic or radiation therapy. Approximately 60% of patients are reported to have received postoperative adjuvant therapies. Systemic regimens include 5-FU, adriamycin, and/or platinum derivatives, although these tumors are typically chemoresistant.

Recent Novel Approaches

Two important technical advances have been developed to treat patients with extrahepatic biliary tract cancer. First is an emphasis on a surgical approach that minimizes potential displacement of tumor cells from the porta hepatis to the liver parenchyma. These "minimal-touch" techniques aim to assess resectability of hilar biliary tumors, dividing biliary and portal pedicles as far from the tumor as possible and include a thorough portal lymphadenectomy and neurectomy [43].

The second advance in the treatment of these patients is the use of preoperative portal vein embolization to induce a hypertrophy of the future liver remnant when the intended resection involves a large portion of the liver parenchyma [44]. More recently, the technique has been enhanced by the ability to extend the embolization to segment IV portal branches, focusing the hypertrophy in the left lateral bisegment in patients intended to have an extended right hepatectomy [45]. This technique has been widely used in colorectal liver metastases' resection cases, and also for patients with biliary tract cancers [46].

Pancreatic Cancer

Background and Epidemiology

Pancreatic adenocarcinoma is an aggressive malignancy that affects approximately 32,000 Americans per year [6]. It represents the tenth leading cause of cancer-related mortality in men [6]. The disease is most frequently discovered in advanced stages, with invasion of local neurovascular structures, nodal metastases, and distant metastases. Liver metastases are common, but usually observed in the setting of other peritoneal or distant disease. Occasionally, isolated intraparenchymal liver metastases are identified. Selected patients with apparently isolated liver disease following pancreatic resection that do not progress during systemic therapy have been submitted to liver resection.

Presentation and Diagnosis

Synchronous liver metastases, frequently in the form of capsular implants are generally identified during staging laparoscopy or open exploration, and are considered a contraindication to extirpative pancreatic surgery. These patients may undergo palliative bypass procedures and are then treated with systemic therapy. Rarely, patients with synchronous liver metastases have been treated with simultaneous pancreatic and liver resection [47].

In contrast, the clinical scenario that usually presents for liver resection consideration is that of metachronous disease presenting during or following completion of postoperative systemic treatment. These metastases may be suspected when the serum CA 19.9 level rises, and can be confirmed with cross-sectional imaging or positron-emission tomograms. Even when isolated metachronous liver metastases are identified, the disease is frequently considered systemic at this point. Based on this paradigm, these patients are recommended to undergo additional systemic therapies with careful restaging to detect extrahepatic disease. The subset of these patients who remain with isolated intrahepatic disease may be considered for liver resection.

Role of Surgery

In the four recent reviews of non-colorectal liver metastases resections a total of only eight cases of pancreatic metastases have been reported (Weitz, $n = 5$ [12]; Ercolani, $n = 3$ [9]; Elias, $n = 0$ [10]; Reddy, $n = 0$ [11]). Of the 15 patients with actual 5-year survival in Ercolani's study, none were operated for pancreatic cancer metastases; however, 2 of the 24 actual 5-year survivors in the Weitz study came from the group of 5 patients resected for pancreatic cancer metastases. In total, 38 cases have been reported between 1982 and 2005, with only 5 patients (13%) reported to survive beyond 5 years following resection of pancreatic cancer liver metastases.

The largest single-institution series of liver resection for hepatic pancreas cancer metastases comes from Takada et al. in 1997 [47]. This group reported on 11 patients treated with simultaneous pancreaticoduodenectomy and hepatectomy for synchronous metastases. Following this aggressive approach they observed a small, but clinically insignificant, survival advantage (median survivals: 4 vs. 6 months).

In the recent report from Adam and colleagues [5], a total of 40 liver resections for non-endocrine pancreatic cancer metastases are documented [5]. Half of these patients were diagnosed with synchronous hepatic metastases, and 18 underwent simultaneous pancreatic and hepatic resections. The median survival for these 40 patients was 20 months with three patients surviving beyond 5 years from resection.

Role of Adjuvant Therapies

Adjuvant therapies are an integral part of the treatment of pancreatic adenocarcinoma. Debate continues regarding the optimal treatment sequence, and multiple clinical trials are ongoing to determine the efficacy of novel systemic agents (i.e., gemcitabine) [48]. Based on the available data it is advisable to initiate the treatment of patients diagnosed with pancreatic cancer liver metastases with systemic therapy. This allows for a "test of time" to determine if treatment refractory disease will develop at other distant sites.

Recent Novel Approaches

Independent of treatment with novel systemic therapies, there has been little innovation in the treatment of liver metastases from pancreatic cancer. There are only isolated reports of ablative technologies being applied to pancreas metastases, with no long-term survivors reported. Likewise, intra-arterial hepatic chemotherapy appears to have little efficacy [49].

Conclusion

With the exception of a relative few long-term survivors, the history of hepatic resection for non-colorectal, non-endocrine gastrointestinal metastases is marked by early recurrences and poor overall survivals (Fig. 17.3). In particular, hepatic resection of liver metastases from

Fig. 17.3 Patient survivals
following hepatic resection of
non–colorectal non–endocrine
gastrointestinal cancer liver
metastases. Courtesy of
Professor René Adam

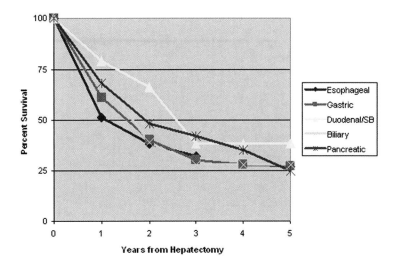

esophageal, gastric, biliary, and pancreatic cancers is
unlikely to prolong survival. In contrast, patients with
small bowel adenocarcinoma metastases may be more
likely to experience favorable outcomes. Based on the
similar mechanism of metastases (portal), organ type
(bowel), and histology (adenocarcinoma) as colorectal
cancer, it is not surprising that these two primary sites
share similar long-term prognoses following hepatic
metastatectomy.

Despite the generally poor postresection outcomes
observed in patients with non-colorectal gastrointestinal
liver metastases, these patients should continue to be
presented at multidisciplinary tumor boards that include
hepatobiliary surgical oncologists. Occasionally, a patient
with favorable tumor biology may be identified who will
benefit from liver directed therapy. Patients successfully
treated with liver resection are characterized as having
low-volume, systemic therapy-responsive tumors, which
are isolated and resectable with negative margins.

The treatment of solid tumors is an ever-changing environment. The success of multimodality treatment strategies
for the treatment of colorectal liver metastases has taught
us that as more effective systemic agents are developed, the
importance of hepatic resection of liver metastases will
increase. Hopefully, in the future a similar pattern of development will occur for patients with liver metastases from
other gastrointestinal primary malignancies.

References

1. Choti MA, Sitzmann JV, Tiburi MF, et al. Trends in long-term
   survival following liver resection for hepatic colorectal metastases. Ann Surg. 2002; 235(6): 759–66.
2. Fernandez FG, Drebin JA, Linehan DC, et al. Five-year survival after resection of hepatic metastases from colorectal cancer
   in patients screened by positron emission tomography with F-
   18 fluorodeoxyglucose (FDG-PET). Ann Surg. 2004; 240(3):
   438–47.
3. Pawlik TM, Scoggins CR, Zorzi D, et al. Effect of surgical
   margin status on survival and site of recurrence after hepatic
   resection for colorectal metastases. Ann Surg. 2005; 241(5):
   715–22, discussion 22–4.
4. Adam R, Delvart V, Pascal G, et al. Rescue surgery for unresectable colorectal liver metastases downstaged by chemotherapy: a model to predict long-term survival. Ann Surg. 2004;
   240(4): 644–57.
5. Adam R, Chiche L, Aloia T, et al. Hepatic resection for non-
   colorectal nonendocrine liver metastases: analysis of 1,452
   patients and development of a prognostic model. Ann Surg.
   2006; 244(4): 524–35.
6. Jemal A, Siegel R, Ward E, et al. Cancer statistics, 2007. CA
   Cancer J Clin. 2007; 57(1): 43–66.
7. Linder S, Bostrom L, Nilsson B. Pancreatic cancer in Sweden 1980–2000: a population-based study of hospitalized
   patients concerning time trends in curative surgery and
   other interventional therapies. J Gastrointest Surg. 2006;
   10(5): 672–8.
8. Jemal A, Clegg LX, Ward E, et al. Annual report to the nation
   on the status of cancer, 1975–2001, with a special feature
   regarding survival. Cancer. 2004; 101(1): 3–27.
9. Ercolani G, Grazi GL, Ravaioli M, et al. The role of liver
   resections for noncolorectal, nonneuroendocrine metastases:
   experience with 142 observed cases. Ann Surg Oncol. 2005;
   12(6): 459–66.
10. Elias D, de Albuquerque CA, Eggenspieler P, et al. Resection of
    liver metastases from a noncolorectal primary: indications and
    results based on 147 monocentric patients. J Am Coll Surg.
    1998; 187(5): 487–93.
11. Reddy SK, Barbas AS, Marroquin CE, et al. Resection of
    noncolorectal nonneuroendocrine liver metastases: a compara-
    tive analysis. J Am Coll Surg. 2007; 204(3): 372–82.
12. Weitz J, Blumgart LH, Fong Y, et al. Partial hepatectomy for
    metastases from noncolorectal, nonneuroendocrine carcinoma.
    Ann Surg. 2005; 241(2): 269–76.
13. Blot WJ, Devesa SS, Kneller RW, Fraumeni JF Jr. Rising
    incidence of adenocarcinoma of the esophagus and gastric
    cardia. JAMA. 1991; 265(10): 1287–9.
14. Quint LE, Hepburn LM, Francis IR, et al. Incidence and dis-
    tribution of distant metastases from newly diagnosed esopha-
    geal carcinoma. Cancer. 1995; 76(7): 1120–5.

15. Yamamoto T, Tachibana M, Kinugasa S, et al. Esophagectomy and hepatic arterial chemotherapy following hepatic resection for esophageal cancer with liver metastasis. J Gastroenterol. 2001; 346(8): 560–3.
16. Hanazaki K, Kuroda T, Wakabayashi M, et al. Hepatic metastasis from esophageal cancer treated by surgical resection and hepatic arterial infusion chemotherapy. Hepatogastroenterology. 1998; 45(19): 201–5.
17. Laurent C, Rullier E, Feyler A, et al. Resection of noncolorectal and nonneuroendocrine liver metastases: late metastases are the only chance of cure. World J Surg. 2001; 25(12): 1532–6.
18. Zibari GB, Riche A, Zizzi HC, et al. Surgical and nonsurgical management of primary and metastatic liver tumors. Am Surg. 1998; 64(3):211–20; discussion 20–1.
19. Ambiru S, Miyazaki M, Ito H, et al. Benefits and limits of hepatic resection for gastric metastases. Am J Surg. 2001; 181(3): 279–83.
20. Okano K, Maeba T, Ishimura K, et al. Hepatic resection for metastatic tumors from gastric cancer. Ann Surg. 2002; 235(1): 86–91.
21. Saiura A, Umekita N, Inoue S, et al. Clinicopathological features and outcome of hepatic resection for liver metastasis from gastric cancer. Hepatogastroenterology. 2002; 49(46): 1062–5.
22. Shirabe K, Shimada M, Matsumata T, et al. Analysis of the prognostic factors for liver metastasis of gastric cancer after hepatic resection: a multi-institutional study of the indications for resection. Hepatogastroenterology. 2003; 50(53): 1560–3.
23. Sakamoto Y, Ohyama S, Yamamoto J, et al. Surgical resection of liver metastases of gastric cancer: an analysis of a 17-year experience with 22 patients. Surgery. 2003; 133(5): 507–11.
24. Lowy AM, Mansfield PF, Leach SD, Ajani J. Laparoscopic staging for gastric cancer. Surgery. 1996; 119(6): 611–4.
25. de Graaf GW, Ayantunde AA, Parsons SL, et al. The role of staging laparoscopy in oesophagogastric cancers. Eur J Surg Oncol. 2007; 33(8): 988–92.
26. Wood TF, Rose DM, Chung M, et al. Radiofrequency ablation of 231 unresectable hepatic tumors: indications, limitations, and complications. Ann Surg Oncol. 2000; 7(8): 593–600.
27. Dabaja BS, Suki D, Pro B, et al. Adenocarcinoma of the small bowel: presentation, prognostic factors, and outcome of 217 patients.Cancer. 2004; 101(3): 518–26.
28. Bakaeen FG, Murr MM, Sarr MG, et al. What prognostic factors are important in duodenal adenocarcinoma? Arch Surg. 2000;135(6): 635–41; discussion 41–2.
29. Aloia TA, Charnsangavej C, Faria S, et al. High-resolution computed tomography accurately predicts resectability in hilar cholangiocarcinoma. Am J Surg. 2007; 193(6): 702–6.
30. Khan SA, Davidson BR, Goldin R, et al. Guidelines for the diagnosis and treatment of cholangiocarcinoma: consensus document. Gut. 2002; 51(Suppl 6): VI1–9.
31. Weber SM, DeMatteo RP, Fong Y, et al. Staging laparoscopy in patients with extrahepatic biliary carcinoma. Analysis of 100 patients. Ann Surg. 2002; 235(3): 392–9.
32. Jarnagin WR, Ruo L, Little SA, et al. Patterns of initial disease recurrence after resection of gallbladder carcinoma and hilar cholangiocarcinoma: implications for adjuvant therapeutic strategies. Cancer. 2003; 98(8): 1689–700.
33. Bartlett DL, Fong Y, Fortner JG, et al. Long-term results after resection for gallbladder cancer. Implications for staging and management. Ann Surg. 1996; 224(5): 639–46.
34. Perpetuo MD, Valdivieso M, Heilbrun LK, et al. Natural history study of gallbladder cancer: a review of 36 years experience at M. D. Anderson Hospital and Tumor Institute. Cancer. 1978; 42(1): 330–5.
35. Eriguchi N, Aoyagi S, Fukuda S, et al. A long-term survival patient with advanced gallbladder cancer massively metastasizing to the liver. Kurume Med J. 1999; 46(1): 83–6.
36. Morrow CE, Grage TB, Sutherland DE, Najarian JS. Hepatic resection for secondary neoplasms. Surgery. 1982; 92(4): 610–4.
37. Yamada H, Katoh H, Kondo S, et al. Hepatectomy for metastases from non-colorectal and non-neuroendocrine tumor. Anticancer Res. 2001; 21(6A): 4159–62.
38. Klatskin G. Adenocarcinoma of the hepatic duct at its bifurcation within the porta hepatis. An unusual tumor with distinctive clinical and pathological features. Am J Med. 1965; 38: 241–56.
39. Cobourn CS, Makowka L, Langer B, et al. Examination of patient selection and outcome for hepatic resection for metastatic disease. Surg Gynecol Obstet. 1987; 165(3): 239–46.
40. Berney T, Mentha G, Roth AD, Morel P. Results of surgical resection of liver metastases from non-colorectal primaries. Br J Surg. 1998; 85(10): 1423–7.
41. Le Treut YP, Sebag F, Hardwigsen J. [Surgery of liver metastases of non-colorectal origin]. Ann Chir. 1998; 52(1): 88–91.
42. Fujii K, Yamamoto J, Shimada K, et al. Resection of liver metastases after pancreatoduodenectomy: report of seven cases. Hepatogastroenterology. 1999; 46(28): 2429–33.
43. Nagino M, Kamiya J, Arai T, et al. "Anatomic" right hepatic trisectionectomy (extended right hepatectomy) with caudate lobectomy for hilar cholangiocarcinoma. Ann Surg. 2006; 243(1): 28–32.
44. Abdalla EK, Barnett CC, Doherty D, et al. Extended hepatectomy in patients with hepatobiliary malignancies with and without preoperative portal vein embolization. Arch Surg. 2002; 137(6): 675–80; discussion 80–1.
45. Madoff DC, Abdalla EK, Gupta S, et al. Transhepatic ipsilateral right portal vein embolization extended to segment IV: improving hypertrophy and resection outcomes with spherical particles and coils. J Vasc Interv Radiol. 2005; 16(2 Pt 1): 215–25.
46. Nagino M, Kamiya J, Nishio H, et al. Two hundred forty consecutive portal vein embolizations before extended hepatectomy for biliary cancer: surgical outcome and long-term follow-up. Ann Surg. 2006; 243(3): 364–72.
47. Takada T, Yasuda H, Amano H, et al. Simultaneous hepatic resection with pancreato-duodenectomy for metastatic pancreatic head carcinoma: does it improve survival? Hepatogastroenterology. 1997; 44(14): 567–73.
48. El Kamar FG, Grossbard ML, Kozuch PS. Metastatic pancreatic cancer: emerging strategies in Chemotherapy and palliative care. Oncologist. 2003; 8(1): 18–34.
49. Vogl TJ, Schwarz W, Eichler K, et al. Hepatic intraarterial chemotherapy with gemcitabine in patients with unresectable cholangiocarcinomas and liver metastases of pancreatic cancer: a clinical study on maximum tolerable dose and treatment efficacy. J Cancer Res Clin Oncol. 2006; 132(11): 745–55.

Index

A

Abdalla, E. K., 28, 39–47, 165
Ablation
    for breast cancer liver metastases, 152–153
    cryo-, 39–40
    for metastatic CRC treatment, 63–64
    5-FU-based, 64
    FUDR-based, 63
    HAI therapy and, 64
    irinotecan-based, 63–64
    PEI, 46
    radiofrequency (RFA)
        for breast cancer liver metastases, 152–153
        for CRC, 10–12, 40–45
        imaging and follow-up aspects, 10–12
    See also Hepatic artery infusion (HAI)
Acute phase proteins (APP), 112
Adam, R., 26, 32, 34, 69–80, 114, 150, 152, 170–176
Adjuvant therapies
    for non-colorectal gastrointestinal liver metastases
        biliary cancers, 175
        duodenal and small bowel cancer, 174
        esophageal and gastroesophageal junction cancers, 171–172
        gastric cancer, 172
        pancreatic cancer, 176
    HAI infusion of chemotherapy with/without systemic
        chemotherapy after resection, 83–84
    systemic chemotherapy after resection, 84–85
    See also Locoregional therapies; Neoadjuvant chemotherapy;
        Systemic treatment
Agarwala, S. S., 159, 161
Aging liver, *see* Elderly
Ahmad, S. A., 15–22
Alba, E., 1–12
Alberts, S. R., 71
Alexander, H. R., 159
Allen, P. J., 35
Allen-Mersh, T. G., 62
Aloia, T. A., 31, 43, 169–177
Ambiru, S., 173
Amersi, F. F., 42–43
Anatomic versus wedge resection, 31
Anaya, D. A., 39–48
Anderson, J. E., 106
Ando, N., 140
Anesthesia, 29–30
Angiography
    hepatic, 102–103

See also Radiation treatment
Anti-angiogenetic therapy
    VEGF antibody, 94–95
    VEGFR and multiple tyrosine kinase inhibitors, 95
    See also EGFR-targeted therapy
Anxiety
    hospital anxiety and depression scale (HADS), 123
    See also Depression; Health-related quality of
        life (HRQoL)
Aoyama, T., 163–164
Apoptosis, 20
Arena, E., 150
Audisio, R.A., 111
Auerbach's plexus, 137
Avastin, 21
    See also Bevacizumab

B

Bak gene, 20
Baldo, S., 164
Basement membrane (BM), 18
Bax gene, 20
Bcl-2 expression, 20
Bcl-X_L expression, 20
Becker, J. C., 157
Bedikian, A. Y., 159
Bendelow, J., 129–133
Benoist, S., 32
Berman, R. S., 15–22
β (beta)-catenin, 16–17
Bevacizumab, 22
    as anti-angiogenetic therapy for CRC, 94–95
    effect on VEGF, 54
    FOLFOX plus, 54
    for metastatic CRC treatment, 54–55
    locoregional, 65
    neoadjuvant chemotherapy and, 87
    resectability improvement aspects, 71
    surgical resection and, 34
    See also Cetuximab; Panitumumab
Bilateral CLM, 26
Bilchik, A. J., 59–66
Biliary cancer
    adjuvant therapies, 175
    background and epidemiology, 174
    presentation and diagnosis, 174–175
    recent novel approaches, 175

Biliary cancer (*cont.*)
    surgery, 175
    See also Duodenal and small bowel cancer; Esophageal and
            gastroesophageal junction cancer; Gastric cancer;
            Pancreatic cancer
Biopsy, 140
Bipat, S., 4
Blanchard, R. J. W., 106
Blanke, C., 137–146
Blazer III, Dan G., 39–48
Body surface area (BSA) method, 101
Bose, D., 155–166
Brachytherapy, 99, 106
    See also Radiation treatment
Breast cancer liver metastases, 149–153
    liver ablation, 152–153
    liver resection, 151–152
    patient selection aspects, 150–151
    radiation treatment, 105
    See also Colorectal liver metastases (CLM); Non-colorectal
            gastrointestinal liver metastases
Brief Edinburgh Depression Scale (BEDS), 124
Brunicardi, F. C., 42
Byrd, D., 137–146
Byrne, C., 117–127

C
Calcified liver metastases, 3
Cantore, M., 159–160
Capecitabine, 52–53
Carcinoembryonic antigen (CEA)
    determination, 10
    level, 77
Carcinoid syndrome
    detecting metastatic, 129
    quality of life and, 133
    treatment
        chemoembolisation, 131
        resection, 130–131
        somatostatin analogues, 131–132
        systemic therapies, 133
        targeted nuclear treatments for, 132–133
Carino, N. de Liguori, 111–115
Carlini, M., 150
Carrasco, C. H., 159, 161
Central venous pressure (CVP), 29
Cervantes, A., 71
Cetuximab, 21–22
    dose for EGFR, 34
    effect on EGFR, 55
    EGFR-targeted therapy, 92
    for metastatic colorectal cancer treatment, 55
    in pretreated patients with metastatic colorectal cancer, 91
    resectability improvement aspects, 71
    surgical resection and, 34
    See also Bevacizumab; Panitumumab
Chang, A. E., 62
Chang, R., 162
Chemoembolization
    for carcinoid syndrome treatment, 131
    hepatic arterial (HACE), 145–146
    transarterial (TACE), 160–161
Chemotherapy
    adjuvant, 83–85
    associated steatohepatitis (CASH), 86–87

cytotoxic, 141
FOLFIRI-based, 32
FOLFOX-based, 32
for initially irresectable disease, 32
for initially resectable disease, 32
for unresectable liver metastases, 70–72
induced liver injury, 32–33
irinotecan-based, 32–33
locoregional, 59–65
neoadjuvant, 57, 85–87, 143
oxaliplatin-based, 32–33
resectability improvement aspects, 70–72
c-kit mutations, 138
Coagulation
    ILP, 46
    MCT, 45
Cohen, A. M., 64
Coldwell, D. M., 99–107
Colorectal cancer (CRC)
    calcified metastases, 3
    diagnosis and staging, 1
    follow-up of patients after surgical resection of, 10
    imaging, *see* Radiological imaging
    non-operable, 51–57
    treatment
        locoregional chemotherapy, 59–66
        systemic, *see* Systemic treatment
Colorectal liver metastases (CLM), 15, 25
    anti-angiogenetic therapy
        VEGF antibody, 94–95
        VEGFR and multiple tyrosine kinase inhibitors, 95
    apoptosis and, 20
    cell–cell and cell–matrix interactions, alteration of, 15–18
    destructive therapies for, 39–47
    EGFR-targeted therapy, 91–94
        in pretreated patients, 91–92
        in untreated patients, 92
    epithelial to mesenchymal transition (EMT), 15–18
    formation, 15
    growth factors
        EGF, 19
        VEGF, 19–20
    in elderly, 111–115
    invasion and metastasis, 18
    migration and motility, 18
    patients selection for hepatic resection
        patients' general medical fitness, 25
        tumor resectability and anticipated extent of resection
            assessment, 25–26
    QOL and, *see* Health-related quality of life (HRQoL)
    radiation treatment aspects of, 104
    Src in, 18
    surgery for, 25
    See also Resection
    treatment
        anti-VEGF therapy, 20–21
        EGF inhibitors, 21–22
    See also Adjuvant therapies; Breast cancer liver metastases;
            Non-colorectal gastrointestinal liver metastases
Contrast agents
    ferumoxides, 5
    gadolinium, 5–6
    SPIO, 5
Couinaud's segments, 7, 31
CPT-11 for metastatic CRC, 62
Crook, T. B., 164

Cryoablation, 39–40
Cryoshock effects, 40
Cryotherapy, 73
CT scan, *see under* Radiological imaging
Cummings, L. C., 114
Cunningham, D., 21, 62
Curley, S. A., 42
Cutaneous melanoma, 156–157
    See also Ocular melanoma
Cytotoxic chemotherapy, 141

D

Dacarbazine, 157
de Haas, R. J., 69–80
de la Camera J., 71
DeMatteo, R., 140
Depression
    Edinburgh depression scale (EDS), 123–124
    hospital anxiety and depression scale (HADS), 123
    screening for, 123
    symptom in palliative care, 122–123
    See also Health-related quality of life (HRQoL)
Depression, 122–124
    See also Anxiety
Destructive therapies
    cryoablation, 39–40
    HIFU, 46–47
    ILP, 46
    MCT, 45–46
    PEI, 46
    radiation therapy, 47
    RFA, 40–45
    See also Local treatment; Systemic treatment
Distress
    psychological, 121–122
    See also Anxiety; Depression
Dose delivery
    radiation treatment and, 102
Dromain, C., 11
Duh, E. J., 164
Duodenal and small bowel cancer
    adjuvant therapies, 174
    background and epidemiology, 173
    presentation and diagnosis, 173
    recent novel approaches, 174
    surgery, 173–174
    See also Biliary cancer; Esophageal and gastroesophageal
        junction cancer; Gastric cancer; Pancreatic cancer

E

E-cadherin expression, 15–18
Edinburgh depression scale (EDS), 123–124
Efficace, F., 124
EGF (epidermal growth factor)
    CRC metastases and, 19
    inhibitors for CRC treatment, 21–22
    See also VEGF (vascular endothelial growth factor)
EGFR (epidermal growth factor receptor)
    cetuximab
        dose for, 34
        effect on, 55
    panitumumab and, 55
    tumor angiogenesis and, 19
EGFR-targeted therapy

EGFR antibodies
    in pretreated patients with metastatic CRC, 91–92
    in untreated patients, 92
    toxicity, 92
    preclinical markers for efficacy, 92
    tyrosine kinase inhibitors, 92–94
    See also Anti-angiogenetic therapy
Eichler, K., 160
Elderly
    CLM treatment in
        comorbidity, 112–113
        epidemiology of aging and CRC in Western world,
            111–112
        outcome, 113–115
        physiological changes in aging liver, 112
        resection techniques, 113
    See also Systemic treatment
Elias, D., 27, 44, 150, 170, 173–176
Emmanouilides, C., 71
Empiric method calculation, 101
    See also Radiation treatment
Endoscopic ultrasound (EUS), 140
Epithelial to mesenchymal transition (EMT), 15–18
Ercolani, G., 170, 174, 176
Erlotinib, 93
Esophageal and gastroesophageal junction cancer
    adjuvant therapies, 171
    background and epidemiology, 170
    presentation and diagnosis, 170–171
    recent novel approaches, 171–172
    role of surgery, 171
    See also Biliary cancer; Duodenal and small bowel cancer;
        Gastric cancer; Pancreatic cancer
Esophageal GISTs, 139
Ethanol injection, *see* Percutaneous ethanol injection (PEI)
Ettore, 112
European Organisation for Research and Treatment of Cancer
        (EORTC)
    EORTC QLQ-C30 Questionnaire, 119, 121, 125
    neoadjuvant chemotherapy and, 86
    See also health-related quality of life (HRQoL)
External-beam radiation therapy (EBRT), 47
Extracellular matrix (ECM), 18
Extrahepatic disease
    presence
        FDG-PET–CT, 9–10
        PET–CT, 9–10
    surgical resection aspects, 27
    See also Liver metastases
Extreme liver resections
    resectability improvement aspects, 74
    See also Liver resection

F

FDG PET, 4, 102
    extrahepatic disease presence, 9–10
    FDG-PET–CT, 9–11
    for CLM, 25–26
    See also Radiological imaging
Ferumoxides MRI, 5
Feun, L. G., 159, 161
Flt-1 upregulation, 20
18-Fluorodeoxyglucos (FDG), *see* FDG PET
Focal lesions, sub-centimeter, 6
Focal steatosis, 6

FOLFIRI, 53
    based chemotherapy, 32
    EGFR-targeted therapy, 92
    for unresectable liver metastases
        two-stage hepatectomy and PVE (case report), 76–77
        two-stage hepatectomy, PVE, and RFA (case report), 80
    See also 5-FU (5-Fluorouracil); FUDR (Floxuridine)
FOLFOX, 21
    based chemotherapy, 32
    EGFR-targeted therapy, 92
    FOLFOX4, 32, 53, 62
    FOLFOX6, 53
    for unresectable liver metastases
        hepatic resection combined with local treatment (case report), 75
        two-stage hepatectomy and PVE (case report), 76–77
        two-stage hepatectomy, PVE, and RFA (case report), 77, 79–80
    in pretreated patients with metastatic colorectal cancer, 91
    neoadjuvant chemotherapy and, 86–87
    plus bevacizumab, 54
Follow-up, *see* Recurrent metastatic disease follow-up
Folprecht, G., 71, 91–95
Fong, Y., 27, 114
Fortner, J. J., 164
Fotemustine, 158, 160
Fournier, G. A., 164
Freeny, P. C., 10
5-FU (5-Fluorouracil), 51, 91
    based ablative techniques, 64
    based HAI, 62–63
        primary therapy for metastatic CRC, 62
        secondary therapy for metastatic CRC, 62
    for metastatic colorectal cancer treatment, 51–52
    5-FU/leucovorin, 21–22, 32, 51–54, 56–57, 59, 70, 84–86, 104, 107, 120
    FUDR plus systemic 5-FU, 63
    See also FOLFIRI; FOLFOX
FUDR (Floxuridine), 57
    based HAI, 61–63
        adjuvant therapy postresection aspects, 63
        primary therapy for metastatic CRC, 62
        secondary therapy for metastatic CRC, 62–63
    based ablative techniques, 63
    plus systemic 5-FU, 63
Functional Assessment of Cancer Therapy-General (FACT-G) questionnaire, 119, 121
Future liver remnant (FLR)
    measurement, 28
    standardized (sFLR), 28
    See also Portal vein embolization (PVE)

G
Gadolinium MRI, 5–6
Gastric cancer
    adjuvant therapies, 172
    background and epidemiology, 172
    presentation and diagnosis, 172
    recent novel approaches, 173
    surgery, 172
    See also Biliary cancer; Duodenal and small bowel cancer; Esophageal and gastroesophageal junction cancer; Gastrointestinal stromal tumors (GISTs); Pancreatic cancer
Gastric tumors, 139

Gastroduodenal artery (GDA) insertion site, 60
Gastroesophageal junction cancers, *see* Esophageal and gastroesophageal junction cancer
Gastrointestinal liver metastases, *see* Non-colorectal gastrointestinal liver metastases
Gastrointestinal stromal tumors (GISTs), 137
    clinical disease, 139
    diagnosis
        biopsy, 140
        endoscopic ultrasound (EUS), 140
        imaging, 139–140
    epidemiology, 138–139
    light microscopy and immunohistochemistry, 137–138
    molecular pathology, 138
    organ specific studies, 139
    pathology, 137
    treatment
        cytotoxic chemotherapy, 141
        drug resistance mechanisms, 144
        hepatic arterial chemoembolization, 145–146
        imatinib, 141–144
        masitinib, 145
        nilotinib, 145
        sunitinib malate, 144
        surgery, 140–141
        surgery plus imatinib, 143
    See also Duodenal and small bowel cancer; Esophageal and gastroesophageal junction cancer; Gastric cancer
Gefitinib, 93
Giacchetti, S., 71
Giantonio, B. J., 21, 62
Glisson's capsule, 31
Gray, B. N., 107
Grothey, A., 56
Gunduz, K., 164

H
Hamady, Z. Z., 26
Health-related quality of life (HRQoL), 117–127
    anxiety aspects, 122
    defined, 118
    depression aspects, 122–124
    EORTC QLQ-LMC21 questionnaire, 119
    FACT Hep questionnaire, 119
    liver metastases and palliative care
        advanced stages of liver metastases, 125–126
        caregivers and palliative care in liver metastases, 126–127
    measurements
        EORTC QLQ-C30 questionnaire, 119
        FACT-G questionnaire, 119
        modular approach, 118–119
        Spitzer QLI, 118
    methodological issues
        baseline data and missing data, 120
        data analysis and interpretation, 120
        implications for advanced CRC clinical trials, 119
        lack of a priori hypothesis about possible QoL changes before trial's commencement, 120
        rationale for specific measure selection, 120
        reporting results, 120–121
        timing, 120
    psychological distress and, 121–122
    social functioning and, 124–125
    spiritual aspects, 124
    See also Palliative care

Heaney, J. P., 74
Hemangioma, 6
Hepatectomy
    laparoscopic, 31–32
    repeat, 29
    two-stage
        for unresectable liver metastases, 73, 75–80
        surgical resection and, 28–29
Hepatic arterial chemoembolization (HACE)
    GISTs treatment, 145–146
    See also Transarterial chemoembolization (TACE)
Hepatic artery infusion (HAI)
    chemotherapy with/without systemic chemotherapy after
        resection, 83–84
    for carcinoid syndrome treatment and, 131
    for melanoma, 158–160
    for metastatic CRC treatment, 59–64
        ablative techniques, 63–64
        adjuvant therapy postresection, 63
        FOLFOX-4-based, 62
        5-FU/LV-based, 62–63
        FUDR-based, 61–63
        placement technique, 60–61
        primary therapy, 62
        randomized clinical trials, 61–63
        secondary therapy, 62–63
    localized treatment strategy, 56–57
    See also Ablation; Isolated hepatic perfusion (IHP);
        Neoadjuvant chemotherapy; Systemic treatment;
        Transarterial chemoembolization (TACE)
Hepatic metastases, see Liver metastases
Hepatotoxicity, chemotherapy-associated, 86–87
Herman, P., 164
HGF (hepatocyte growth factor), 18
    See also EGF (epidermal growth factor)
High-intensity focused ultrasound (HIFU)
    CLM and, 46–47
Hilar lymph node involvement, 7
Ho, W. M., 71
Hoff, P. M., 51–57
Hohn, D. C., 62
Hospital anxiety and depression scale (HADS), 123
Hsueh, E. C., 164
Huang, Y., 64
Hurwitz, H. I., 21

I
Imaging, see Radiological imaging
Imatinib
    escalating doses and GISTs, 143
    GIST treatment, 141–145
        assessing response to imatinib, 144
        escalating doses of imatinib, results from, 143
        for locally advanced and metastatic GIST, 142
        mutational assessment and imatinib use, 142–143
        neoadjuvant imatinib, 143
        surgery plus imatinib, 143
    See also Sunitinib malate
Inferior vena cava (IVC), 74
Intensity modulated radiation therapy (IMRT), 104
Interstitial laser photocoagulation (ILP), 46
Intraoperative ultrasound (IOUS), 31
Invasion, 18
Irinotecan
    based ablative techniques, 63–64

based chemotherapy, 32–33
    for metastatic colorectal cancer treatment, 53
    irinotecan/5-FU/leucovorin (IFL), 21, 53
    IROX, 53
    See also FOLFIRI; FOLFOX
Isolated hepatic perfusion (IHP)
    for melanoma, 161–163
    See also Hepatic artery infusion (HAI); Transarterial
        chemoembolization (TACE)

J
Jaundice, 125
Jemal, A., 169
Jones, L., 129–133

K
Kabbinavar, F., 21
Keilholz, U., 160
Kemeny, N., 62–64
Kennedy, A. S., 99–107
Kesmodel, S. B., 94
Kim, Y. S., 105
KIT protein, 138, 142, 137
Klatskin, G., 175
Kobayashi, K., 145
Kodjikian, L., 164
Kokudo, N., 26
Kondo, S., 150
Koniaris, L. G., 47
Kopetz, S., 51–57
k-ras mutant tumors, 92

L
Laparoscopy
    GISTs treatment, 141
    laparoscopic hepatectomy, 31–32
Large bowel GISTs, 139
Laser-induced interstitial thermotherapy (LITT), 99
    See also Radiation treatment
Lencioni, R., 42–43
Leucovorin, 21
Leyvraz, S., 158–159
Libutti, S. K., 159, 162
Light microscopy, 137
Liver disease
    chemotherapy-induced, 32–33
    radiation-induced (RILD), 47, 103
Liver metastases
    diagnosis and staging, 1
    imaging, see Radiological imaging
    surgery, see Resection
    unresectable
        definition, 69–70
        oncosurgical strategies, 69–80
        preoperative chemotherapy for, 70–72
        resectability improvement aspects, 72–74
        treatment, 74–80
        unresectability, 69–70
    See also Breast cancer liver metastases; Colorectal liver
        metastases (CLM); Non-colorectal gastrointestinal liver
        metastases
Livraghi, T., 42–43, 153
Lloyd-Williams, M., 117–127

Local treatment
    destructive treatments
        cryotherapy, 73
        resectability improvement aspects, 73
        RFA, 73
    hepatic resection combined with local treatment (case report), 75
    for non-operable liver metastasis
        HAI, 56–57
        neoadjuvant chemotherapy, 57
    See also Systemic treatment
Locoregional therapies
    for melanoma
        HAI, 158–160
        IHP, 161–163
        TACE, 160–161
    historical perspective, 61
    placement technique, 59–61
    randomized clinical trials
        ablative techniques, 63–64
        adjuvant therapy, 63
        agents via HAI, 64–65
        primary therapy, 61–62
        secondary therapy, 62–63
    resectability improvement aspects, 73
    RFA, 73
    See also Ablation; Systemic treatment; Unresectable liver
        metastases
Lorenz, M., 62–63
Lugli, A., 17
Lymph node involvement, hilar, 7

M
Macro-aggregated albumin (MAA), 101, 103
    See also Radiation treatment
Maguire, P., 122
Maksan, S. M., 150
Makuuchi, M., 72
Martin, J. K., 62
Martínez, L., 1–12
Masi, G., 71
Masitinib, 145
Matrix metalloproteinases (MMPs), 18
Matsuo, M., 5
Mavligit, G., 159, 161
Mazzaferro, V., 42
Mazzoni, G., 114–115
MDACC criteria, 144
Melanoma, 155
    locoregional therapies for
        HAI, 158–160
        IHP, 161–163
        TACE, 160–161
    primary tumor site
        cutaneous, 156
        ocular, 155–156
    stage IV, 155
    surgical resection for, 163–165
    systemic chemotherapy, 157–158
    therapeutic options, 157–158
Menon, K. V., 113
Mentha, G., 35
Meta-iodobenzylguanidine (MIBG), 129, 132–133
Microsphere implantation, 106
    See also Radiation treatment
Microwave coagulation therapy (MCT), 45–46

Miettinen, M, 139, 141
Migration, cell, 18
Mondragon-Sanchez, R., 164
Monoclonal antibodies
    bevacizumab, 54–55
    cetuximab, 55
    panitumumab, 55–56
Morrow, C. E., 175
MRI, see under Radiological imaging
Muller, H. H., 62
Müller, J. H., 105
Multimodality therapy
    biologic agents, 34
    chemotherapy-induced liver injury, 32–33
    surgical resection and, 32–34
    systemic chemotherapy for
        initially irresectable disease, 32
        initially resectable disease, 32
Multinodular CLM, 26

N
Nathan, F. E., 157
Nausea, 125–126
Neoadjuvant chemotherapy
    drawbacks
        chemotherapy-associated hepatotoxicity, 86–87
        complete response before surgery, 86
    for resectable liver metastases
        rationale for neoadjuvant chemotherapy, 85–86
        results of neoadjuvant chemotherapy, 87–88
        therapy including targeted agents, 88
    See also Adjuvant therapies; Hepatic artery infusion (HAI)
Neoadjuvant imatinib, 143
Neuroendocrine tumor metastases, 105
Nickl, N., 140
Nilotinib, 145
Nilsson, B., 139
Non-colorectal gastrointestinal liver metastases, 169–176
    biliary cancers, 174–175
    duodenal and small bowel cancer, 173–174
    esophageal and gastroesophageal junction cancers, 170–172
    gastric cancer, 172–173
    pancreatic cancer, 175–176
    See also Breast cancer liver metastases; Colorectal liver
        metastases (CLM)
Non-operable colorectal cancer, 51–57
    See also Systemic treatment
Nordlinger, B., 83–88
Noter, S. L., 159
Nuclear medicine studies, 103
    See also Radiation treatment

O
Ocular melanoma, 155–156
    systemic chemotherapy for, 157
    See also Cutaneous melanoma
Okano, K., 173
Okaro, A. C., 150
Oncosurgical strategies, 69
    See also Unresectable liver metastases
Oshowo, A., 43–44
Oxaliplatin
    based chemotherapy, 32–33
    for metastatic colorectal cancer treatment, 53

locoregional, 65
surgical resection and, 34
See also FOLFOX

P
Palliative care
    anxiety symptom in, 122
    caregivers and palliative care in liver metastases, 126–127
    depression symptom in, 122–124
    liver metastases advanced stages and
        confusion and terminal phase, 126
        jaundice, 125
        nausea, 125–126
        pain, 125
        poor appetite, 126
        pruritus, 126
    psychological distress and, 121–122
    See also Health-related quality of life (HRQoL)
Pancreatic cancer
    adjuvant therapies, 176
    background and epidemiology, 175–176
    novel approaches, 176
    presentation and diagnosis, 176
    surgery, 176
    See also Biliary cancer; Duodenal and small bowel cancer;
            Esophageal and gastroesophageal junction cancer;
            Gastric cancer
Panitumumab
    effect on EGFR, 55
    for metastatic CRC treatment, 55–56
    in pretreated patients with metastatic CRC, 92
    See also Bevacizumab; Cetuximab
Papachristou, D. N., 164
Parenchymal transection methods, 30
Parker, C., 19
Patel, K., 159, 161
Pawlik, T. M., 27, 155–166
PDGFR (platelet derived growth factor receptor), 138
    mutations, 142
    See also Gastrointestinal stromal tumors (GISTs)
Peeters, M., 71
Penna, C., 83–89
Percutaneous ethanol injection (PEI), 46
    PET, *see under* Radiological imaging
Peters, S., 159
Photocoagulation, interstitial laser (ILP), 46
Pingpank, J. F., 159, 162–163
Pocard, M., 150–151
Pompili, M., 42
Portal vein embolization (PVE), 28
    for unresectable liver metastases (case report)
        two-stage hepatectomy, 75–77
        two-stage hepatectomy, PVE, and RFA, 77–80
    resectability improvement aspects, 72, 73
    surgical resection and, 28
    See also Future liver remnant (FLR); Two-stage hepatectomy
Portier, G., 85
Poston, G. J., 111–115, 129–133
Pozzo, C., 71
Pruritus, 126
Psychological distress measurement, 121–122
    See also Anxiety; Depression
Pulmonary metastases
    surgical resection, 26–27
    See also Liver metastases

Q
Quality of life (QoL), *see* Health-related quality of life
            (HRQoL)
Quenet, F., 71
Questionnaires
    EORTC QLQ-C30. *See also* health-related quality of life
            (HRQoL), 119
    EORTC QLQ-LMC21, 119
    FACT Hep, 119
    FACT-G. *See also* health-related quality of life
            (HRQoL), 119
    module specific to CLM patients, 119
    See also Health-related quality of life (HRQoL)

R
Raab, R., 150
Radiation treatment
    breast cancer metastases, 105
    colorectal cancer metastases, 47, 104–105
    dose delivery aspects, 102
    empiric method, 101
    external-beam (EBRT), 47
    LITT, 99
    liver metastases, 99–107
    hepatic angiography, 102–103
    imaging studies, 102
    IMRT, 104
    laboratory studies, 102
    microsphere implantation, 106
    neuroendocrine tumor metastases, 105
    nuclear medicine studies, 103
    patient selection aspects, 103–104
    planning, 100–101
    radioactive material for, 100
    radioactivity formula
        activity required, 101
        dose, 101
    selective internal (SIRT), 47, 107
    toxicity aspects, 103
    See also Brachytherapy; Radiofrequency ablation (RFA);
            Systemic treatment
Radiation induced liver disease (RILD), 47, 101
    toxicity aspects, 103
Radiofrequency ablation (RFA), 99
    breast cancer liver metastases, 152–153
    CLM and, 45
    for CLM, 40–44
    imaging and follow-up after, 10–12
    resectability improvement aspects, 73
    resection and, 43–45
    two-stage hepatectomy, PVE, and RFA for unresectable liver
            metastases (case report), 77–80
    See also Hepatic artery infusion (HAI); Portal vein embolization
            (PVE); Two-stage hepatectomy
Radiological imaging, 1
    CT scan
        for carcinoid syndrome detection, 129
        for CLM, 25–26
        GISTs, 140
        helical (HCT), 3–4, 6, 9
        multidetector (MDCT), 4–6
        PET–CT, 9–10
        radiation treatment and, 102
    detection modalities, 3
    differential diagnosis

Radiological imaging (*cont.*)
    focal steatosis, 6
    hemangioma, 6
    sub-centimeter focal lesions, 6
   FDG PET, 4, 9–11, 25–26, 102
   follow-up for recurrent metastatic disease
    follow-up of patients after surgical resection of CRC hepatic
      metastases, 10
    imaging and follow-up after RFA, 10–12
   GISTs, 139–140
   liver metastases from colorectal cancer, 1–3
   MRI, 4–6, 26
    ferumoxides contrast agent, 5
    for carcinoid syndrome detection, 129
    gadolinium contrast agent, 5–6
    SPIO contrast agent, 5
    T1-weighted, 5
    T2-weighted, 5
   PET, 102
    for carcinoid syndrome detection, 129
    GISTs, 140
    PET–CT, 9–11, 129
   radiologic–pathologic correlation, 2–3
   staging in potentially resectable patients
    extrahepatic disease presence, 9
    FDG-PET–CT, 9–10
    liver volumetry, 9
    possible hilar lymph node involvement, 7
    possible liver metastases evaluation, 7
    vascular invasion assessment, 8
   ultrasound
    endoscopic (EUS), 140
    for carcinoid syndrome detection, 129
    high-intensity focused (HIFU), 46–47
    intraoperative (IOUS), 31
    liver metastases, 4
Ravikumar, T. S., 40, 159, 163
RECIST (response evaluation criteria in solid tumors) criteria, 102
   assessing GISTs response to imatinib, 144
   See also Radiation treatment
Recurrent metastatic disease follow-up
   after radiofrequency ablation, 10–12
   of patients after surgical resection of CRC hepatic metastases, 10
Reddy, S. K., 170, 174, 176
Repeat hepatectomy, 29
Resectability
   definitely unresectable, 70
   easily resectable, 70
   marginally resectable, 70
   See also Resection
Resectability improvement
   downstaging with preoperative chemotherapy
    chemotherapy combined with biological agents, 71
    conversion to resectability, 70
    risks related to preoperative chemotherapy, 71–72
   techniques
    cryotherapy, 73
    extreme liver resections, 74
    local destructive treatments, 73
    PVE, 72–73
    RFA, 73
    two-stage hepatectomy, 73
Resectable liver metastases
   neoadjuvant chemotherapy for, 86
    rationale for neoadjuvant chemotherapy, 85–86
    results of neoadjuvant chemotherapy, 87–88

    therapy including targeted agents, 88
   See also Unresectable liver metastases
Resection
   adjuvant therapy postresection, 63
   breast cancer liver metastases, 151–152
   CLM respectability and anticipated extent of resection
    assessment, 26
   CRC in elderly and, 113
   cryoablation and, 39–40
   for carcinoid syndrome treatment, 130–131
   for CLM
    anatomic versus wedge resection considerations, 31
    anesthesia considerations, 29–30
    biologic agents, 34
    chemotherapy-induced liver injury, 32–33
    extrahepatic disease sites, 27
    FLR measurement, 28
    hepatic and pulmonary metastases, 26–27
    IOUS considerations, 31
    laparoscopic hepatectomy considerations, 31–32
    multimodality therapy aspects, 32
    multinodular and/or bilateral disease, 26
    operative considerations, 29–32
    parenchymal transection method considerations, 30
    patients selection aspects, 25–26
    prognostic factors, 27
    PVE and, 28
    repeat hepatectomy strategy, 29
    respectability definition, 26
    size > 5 cm, 26
    surgical margin, 26
    synchronous CLM management, 35
    systemic chemotherapy for initially irresectable disease, 32
    systemic chemotherapy for initially resectable disease, 32
    two-stage hepatectomy strategy, 28–29
   for melanoma, 163–165
   HAI chemotherapy after resection of hepatic metastases, 83–84
   MCT and, 45–46
   patients selection for hepatic resection, 25
   RFA and, 43–45
   systemic chemotherapy after resection of hepatic metastases,
    84–85
   unresectability definition, 70
   See also Locoregional therapies; Systemic treatment
Ribero, D., 25–35
Rivoire, M., 163–164
Rose, D. M., 163–164
Rossier, P. H., 105
Rougier, P., 62
Rubbia-Brandt, L., 27
Ruiz, S., 1–12

S
Saiura, A., 173
Sakamoto, Y., 150–151, 173
Saline-linked cautery (SLC), 30
Saltz, L. B., 21
Santoro, E., 150
Sargent, D. J., 56
Sarlomo-Rikala, M., 137
Sato, T., 156, 159–160
Scappaticci, F. A., 94
Schwartz, L. H., 42
Seifert, J. K., 150
Selective internal radiation therapy (SIRT), 47, 107

Selzner, M., 150
Shah, A. N., 15–22
Shibata, T,, 45
Shin Chun, Yun, 25–35
Shirabe, K., 173
Siegel, R., 158–159
Sielaff, T. D., 42
Small bowel cancer, 173
    small bowel GISTs, 139
    See also under Duodenal and small bowel cancer
Social functioning, 124
    See also Health-related quality of life (HRQoL)
Solbiati, L., 42–43
Somatostatin analogues, 131–132
Spaderna, S., 15
SPECT imaging, 102–103
    See also Radiation treatment
Spitzer Quality of Life Index (QLI), 118
Src, 18
Staging, 1
    extrahepatic disease presence, 9, 10
    liver volumetry, 9
    possible hilar lymph node involvement, 7
    possible liver metastases evaluation, 7
    vascular invasion assessment, 8
Standardized FLR volume (sFLR), 28
Steatohepatitis, chemotherapy-associated (CASH), 86–87
stem cell factor (SCF), 138
    See also Gastrointestinal stromal tumors (GISTs)
Stoelben, E., 164
Stromal tumors, *see* Gastrointestinal stromal tumors (GISTs)
Sub-centimeter focal lesions, 6
Sunitinib malate
    GISTs treatment, 144
    See also Imatinib
Superparamagnetic iron oxide (SPIO) MRI, 5
Surgery
    breast cancer liver metastases
      liver ablation, 152–153
      liver resection, 151–152
    CLM treatment in elderly, 111–115
    GISTs treatment, 140–141, 143
      laparoscopy, 141
      risk of recurrence, 141
    non-colorectal gastrointestinal liver metastases
      biliary cancers, 175
      duodenal and small bowel cancer, 173–174
      esophageal and gastroesophageal junction cancers, 171
      gastric cancer, 172
      pancreatic cancer, 176
    hepatic cryosurgery, 39
    See also Resection
Synchronous CLM management, 169
    surgical resection and, 35
    See also Non-colorectal gastrointestinal liver metastases
Systemic treatment
    chemotherapeutic agents
      5-FU, 51–52
      capecitabine, 52–53
      irinotecan, 53
      oxaliplatin, 53
    chemotherapy
      after resection of hepatic metastases, 83–85
      for duodenal and small bowel cancer, 174
      for esophageal and gastroesophageal junction cancers, 171
      for initially irresectable disease, 32

      for initially resectable disease, 32
      for melanoma, 157–158
    for biliary cancers, 175
    for carcinoid syndrome treatment, 133
    for pancreatic cancer, 176
    HAI chemotherapy with/without systemic chemotherapy after resection of hepatic metastases, 83–84
    monoclonal antibodies
      bevacizumab, 54–55
      cetuximab, 55
      panitumumab, 55–56
    recommendations for, 56
    See also Local treatment; Locoregional therapies

T
Takada, T., 176
Targeted treatment
    for carcinoid syndrome treatment, 132–133
    neoadjuvant therapies including targeted agents, 88
    See also EGFR-targeted therapy
Telian, S. H., 59–66
Thelen, A., 150–151
Total estimated liver volume (TELV), 28
Total vascular exclusion (TVE), 74
    See also Resection
Toxicity
    EGFR antibodies, 92
    radiation treatment and, 103
Transarterial chemoembolization (TACE)
    for melanoma, 160, 161
    See also Hepatic arterial chemoembolization (HACE); Hepatic artery infusion (HAI); Isolated hepatic perfusion (IHP)
Transection methods
    parenchymal, 30
    See also Resection
Tryggvason, G., 139
Two-stage hepatectomy
    for unresectable liver metastases
      PVE and two-stage hepatectomy (case report), 75–77
      resectability improvement aspects, 73
      two-stage hepatectomy, PVE, and RFA (case report), 77–80
    surgical resection and, 28–29
    See also Portal vein embolization (PVE); Radiofrequency ablation (RFA)
Tyrosine kinase inhibitors
    EGFR, 92–94
    VEGFR and multiple, 95

U
Ueda, H., 150
Ultrasound, *see under* Radiological imaging
Unresectable liver metastases
    definition, 69–70
      definitely unresectable, 70
      easily resectable, 70
      marginally resectable, 70
    oncosurgical strategies, 69–80
    preoperative chemotherapy for, 70–72
    resectability improvement aspects
      cryotherapy, 73
      extreme liver resections, 74
      PVE, 72–73
      RFA, 73
      two-stage hepatectomy, 73

Unresectable liver metastases (*cont.*)
   treatment (case reports)
      hepatic resection combined with local treatment, 75
      two-stage hepatectomy and PVE, 75–77
      two-stage hepatectomy, PVE, and RFA, 77, 79–80
   treatment strategies, 74
   unresectability, 69–70

V
Valls, C., 1–12
van Leeuwen, B. L., 111–115
van Oosterom, A. T., 142
Vascular invasion assessment, 8
   See also Staging
Vauthey J.-N., 25–38,164
VEGF (vascular endothelial growth factor)
   anti-angiogenetic therapy for CRC, 94–95
   anti-VEGF therapy for CRC treatment, 20–21
   bevacizumab effect on, 34, 54
   CRC metastases and, 19–20
   See also EGF (epidermal growth factor)
Vlastos, G., 149–153
Vogl, T. J., 46, 160–161
Volumetry
   liver, 9
   See also Staging

W
Wagman, L. D., 63
Warren, R. S., 20
Wedge resection
   versus anatomic resection, 31
   See also Resection
Weitz, J., 170, 174, 176
Wicherts, D. A., 69–80
Wong, S. C., 17
Wray, C. J., 15–22
Wright, B. E., 59–66

Y
Yamada, H., 175
Yoshimoto, M., 150
Yttrium-90, 100, 106
   See also Radiation treatment

Z
Zacharias, T., 114
Zangos, S., 160
Zieren, H. U., 113
Zorzi, D., 33, 149–153, 165

Printed in the United States of America